Parenteral and Enteral Nutrition

A PRACTICAL GUIDE

'A slender and restricted diet is always dangerous in chronic diseases, and also in acute diseases . . .'

Hippocrates,
Aphorisms, *c.* 400 BC

Parenteral and Enteral Nutrition
A PRACTICAL GUIDE

G. D. Phillips MB BS BSc (Med) FFARACS
Director of Intensive Care,
Flinders Medical Centre;
Associate Professor,
Department of Anaesthesia and Intensive Care,
The Flinders University of South Australia

C. L. Odgers BPharm FSHP
Department of Pharmacy,
Flinders Medical Centre;
Lecturer, School of Medicine,
The Flinders University of South Australia;
Honorary Associate,
South Australian Institute of Technology

THIRD EDITION

CHURCHILL LIVINGSTONE
EDINBURGH LONDON MELBOURNE AND NEW YORK 1986

CHURCHILL LIVINGSTONE
Medical Division of Longman Group Limited

Distributed in the United States of America by
Churchill Livingstone Inc., 1560 Broadway, New York,
N.Y. 10036, and by associated companies, branches and
representatives throughout the world.

First published 1980
Second edition 1982
Third edition 1986

ISBN 0 443 03294 7

British Library Cataloguing in Publication Data
Phillips, G. D.
  Parental and enteral nutrition: a practical guide.—3rd ed.
  1. Tube feeding   2. Parental feeding
  I. Title   II. Odgers, C. L.
  615.8'54   RM225

Library of Congress Cataloging in Publication Data
Phillips, G. D.
  Parenteral and enteral nutrition.

  Includes bibliographies and index.
  1. Parenteral feeding.   2. Enteral feeding.
3. Nutrition.   I. Odgers, C. L.   II. Title.
[DNLM: 1. Enteral Feeding.   2. Nutrition.
3. Parenteral Feeding. WB 410 P558p]
RM224.P48 1986   615.8'55   85-29931

Printed in Great Britain by Bell and Bain Ltd., Glasgow

Preface to the Third Edition

The success of the first and second editions of this book, published privately, has led to the third, completely revised edition, published by Churchill Livingstone.

The format of the book is unaltered, but it has been updated, and made more complete by the addition of further material on enteral nutrition, and by the addition of a new chapter, on the requirements of the hypermetabolic patient. New material has been added in several areas, such as parenteral and enteral nutrition during pregnancy, and in anorexia nervosa.

Considerable effort has been expended on relating parenteral and enteral nutrition to relevant practical issues, such as fluid, electrolyte and acid−base balance, and the medical condition of the patient. A large number of tables and figures has been included to allow rapid checking of useful points. As far as possible, reference to a broad spectrum of enteral and parenteral nutrition products from the USA, UK, Europe and Australasia has been made in the text.

G. D. Phillips
Adelaide, 1986
C. L. Odgers

Preface to the Second Edition

The Preface to the First Edition remains valid, but it is necessary to add our thanks to reviewers of the First Edition, and to those people who gave us constructive criticism, which has resulted in a completely revised, improved book. Omissions from the First Edition were chapters on the physiological and biochemical bases of nutrition, the metabolic effects of starvation, sepsis and trauma, and provision of a sample regimen, which have now been added. More information on nutrition substrates has been included, and the chapter on enteral nutrition considerably expanded. Areas of particular interest to the authors, and areas where rapid developments have occurred have been elaborated on, resulting in some chapters being larger than others. References up to February 1982 have been included, and the book has been typeset by word processor to allow rapid publication. As a result of the international acceptance of the First Edition, more information on internationally marketed products has been added. Although this edition is much larger than the first, the practical chapters remain concise, and the longer ones reflect an increase in the theory on which clinical nutrition is based.

We would like to acknowledge the assistance given by ADIS Press Australasia Pty. Ltd., Auckland, New Zealand, and Alan R. Liss, Inc., New York, in allowing us to use substantial amounts of our previously published material.

G. G. Phillips
C. L. Odgers

Adelaide, 1982

Preface to the First Edition

In 1977 some notes on 'Parenteral Nutrition and Gastric Tube Feeding' were printed for the use of our staff. The demand for them was so great that we decided to expand the text and add references. This is the result.

We would like to acknowledge the encouragement of our Department Heads, Professor M. J. Cousins and Mr M. L. Abbott, and the assistance of our colleagues.

We also acknowledge the work of Mr Alan Bentley, Department of Medical Illustration and Media, who designed the cover and prepared the illustrations, and the assistance of Mrs Marion Wallace, who typeset the manuscript, and Mrs Sue Johannsen who provided secretarial support.

This book is dedicated to patients who need nutrition.

G. D. Phillips

C. L. Odgers

Adelaide, 1980

Contents

List of Tables and Figures

Figures

Introduction

Over the last 10 years the literature on parenteral nutrition has proliferated. Hundreds of articles are published each year on the topic, together with one or two books and the proceedings of several meetings. Some of this information is the result of research into new aspects, and some is reiteration of old principles. Much of it relates to products available only in the country of origin, and much of it is difficult to interpret.

Gastric (and other) tube feeding (although a much older technique) has been taken for granted, and probably has been executed with less care than parenteral feeding. In recent years, however, with the availability of an increasing range of enteral feeds and improved delivery systems, more attention has been focused on tube feeding. The literature on this form of nutrition is now increasing.

The aims of this monograph are:
1. to present the principles of parenteral and enteral nutrition;
2. to elaborate on technical details;
3. to outline recent advances.

The book is intended as a practical guide for students and for nursing, medical, dietetic and pharmacy staff who are placed in the position of managing patients receiving parenteral and enteral nutrition. Key references have been selected so that readers may follow up areas of special interest.

1

Background and perspective

In the last four to five decades, new knowledge has shed light on what was described at the beginning of this century as the darkly yawning chasm of intermediary metabolism with its 'vast number of unresolved enigmas'. Amino acids required for growth, including those that are termed 'essential' according to the definition of Dr W C Rose, and their amounts, have been identified; certain fatty acids have been recognised as necessary dietary constituents; vitamins have been identified and synthesised; knowledge has accumulated regarding the enzymatic activities of specific proteins, and the roles of certain vitamins in the reactions these enzymes catalyse; and various trace metals have been recognised as necessary dietary constituents.

In spite of these advances, the application of this accumulated knowledge, together with the numerous technological advances that have occurred concurrently, to the nutritional well-being of hospitalised patients, is often neglected. It is assumed by many workers that patients receive adequate nutrition, or that inadequate nutrition is an essential part of illness. How often does the doctor or nurse know what intake a patient actually has, even if they have some idea of what is being presented to the patient? How often does one find a patient on intravenous glucose and saline for long periods with an energy intake of 1670 kJ (400 kcal) per day and no minerals other than sodium, chloride and potassium, and half the necessary vitamins? How often does one see semi-conscious patients having fluids poured down their throats?

Although the first descriptions of the definitive and remarkably successful use of parenteral preparations in meeting total human nutritional requirements were published approximately 20 years ago, parenteral nutrition had its beginning decades before (Table 1.1). In 1911, Kausch administered the first intravenous injection of glucose (5% and 10%) into man for nutritional purposes. Later, attempts were made to increase the peripherally infused calorie load. However, these were complicated by the development of phlebitis and thrombosis. It was not until the technique of catheterising the subclavian vein via the infraclavicular route, first described by Aubaniac in 1952, was adopted by Dudrick et al in 1968, that hypertonic glucose solutions could be infused without these complications.

Table 1.1   Some milestones in parenteral nutrition

Achievement	Worker	Year
Blood circulation and access		
Description of blood circulation	William Harvey	1616
Infusions given via catheter in superior vena cava	Bernard Zimmerman	1945
Subclavian catheterisation via infraclavicular route	Robert Aubaniac	1952
Development of teflon-silastic catheter for long-term use (the artificial gut)	Belding H. Scribner	1970
IV glucose as energy source		
Post-operative nutritional management of patients	W Kausch	1911
Relationship of infusion rate to renal threshold	R T Woodyatt	1915
Optimal calorie: nitrogen ratio defined	Francis Moore	1959
IV protein hydrolysates and amino acids		
Positive nitrogen balance in animals following infusion of protein hydrolysate	V Henriques/A C Andersen	1913
Oral amino acid metabolism and requirements defined	William C Rose	1934
Protein hydrolysates infused into man	Robert Elman	1937
Crystalline D- and L-amino acids infused into man	A T Shohl/K D Blackfan	1940
Synthetic manufacture of L-amino acids on industrial scale	Japanese Scientists	1950s
IV fat emulsions		
Infusion in dogs accompanied by decreased RQ, increased heat production	J R Murlin/ J A Riche	1915
Formulation and investigation in man	S Yamakawa	1920
Fat emulsions injected into babies	L Emmett Holt	1935
Development of safe metabolisable soybean oil emulsion	Arvid Wretlind	1961
Clinical application of TPN		
Growth, development, positive nitrogen balance achieved in man	Stanley J Dudrick	1968
Development of systems for long-term TPN maintenance at home	Belding H Scribner K N Jeejeebhoy	1970/ 1971

The first successful intravenous feeding of an experimental animal occurred in 1913. Henriques & Andersen demonstrated that the intravenous administration of protein hydrolysates, prepared from the enzymatic digest of goat muscle, together with glucose and salt, could be used to maintain normal weight and achieve positive nitrogen balance in a goat. Protein hydrolysates were first infused into man in 1937 by Robert Elman. In 1940 Shohl & Blackfan infused a complete mixture of dextro and laevo-forms of crystalline amino acids in infants, and this solution was found to be as effective in maintaining nitrogen balance as a commercially prepared protein hydrolysate solution. More recently, solutions of pure crystalline laevo-forms of essential and non-essential amino acids, combined according to the recommendations of Rose, have become available, and these have been shown to be more efficiently utilised in protein synthesis than the racemic solutions. Another advantage of these synthetic amino acids is that formulation of mixtures of amino acids for specific purposes, e.g. for renal failure or hepatic failure is made possible.

Early this century Murlin & Riche reported that non-emulsified fat given intravenously or subcutaneously to animals did not serve as a useful nutrient source, but that appropriate fat emulsions could be utilised. These initial studies were followed by a series of systematic investigations conducted in animals and humans by Yamakawa and his colleagues in the 1920s, using emulsions of castor oil. These Japanese workers also investigated methods for preparing fat emulsions. They found that, with the addition of a sufficient quantity of egg lecithin to act as an emulsifying agent, it was possible to make emulsions that would withstand heat sterilisation. They also found that by homogenisation it was possible to produce an emulsion with a particle size of less than 2 μ in diameter — small enough to pass through the lung capillaries.

In the intervening years to 1960, a number of fat emulsions were prepared using different fats such as sesame oil, cottonseed oil, cod liver oil, human body fat, coconut oil, peanut oil, lard oil, safflower oil, soybean oil and synthetic oils. Also, a very large number of natural and synthetic emulsifiers were investigated because the clinical use of intravenous fat emulsions was being hampered by the development of severe adverse reactions. It was not until Wretlind developed an emulsion from soybean oil and egg phospholipid that parenteral therapy with fat emulsions became a safe and acceptable component of parenteral nutrition.

By the early 1960s the major problems surrounding the safe infusion of adequate amounts of energy substrates and nitrogen had been overcome. In the last two decades, work towards the elucidation of man's specific nutritional requirements via the intravenous route, including vitamins and trace elements, during stress, following surgery, trauma, sepsis and thermal burns, and in paediatric and adult long-term nutrition has been gaining momentum. In extreme situations, total parenteral nutrition (TPN) has become a form of life support.

The practice of enteral nutrition (EN), has undergone equally dramatic improvements with respect to tubes and formulations. Using enteral nutrition, it is possible to meet the nutritional requirements of surgical and medical patients by tube feeding suitably formulated diets, provided access can be gained to the gastrointestinal tract, and there is present at least a segment of small bowel with mucosa capable of processing and absorbing nutrients. In many situations it is not exploited enough.

Enteral nutrition therapy may be administered by mouth, nasoenteric

Table 1.2   Some milestones in enteral nutrition

Achievement	Worker	Year
Naso-enteric tube nutrition		
Description of use of tube to deliver liquids into oesophagus	Capivacceus	1598
Use of hollow, flexible eel skin tube passed into stomach	John Hunter	1790
Use of India rubber tubing ($\frac{1}{8}$" bore) attached to suspended bottle	Clement Dukes	1876
Tube feeding of infants by gavage using a rubber catheter	L Emmett Holt	1894
Technique for feeding into duodenum	Max Einhorn	1910
Use of a nasogastric jejunal method for postoperative feeding	A Stengel/I Ravdin	1939
Requirements for a jejunal feed defined	W O Abbott	1939
Successful long-term nasogastric tube feeding in hospital and at home, using a 2.5 mm polyvinyl chloride catheter	M D Pareira	1954
Tube enterostomy nutrition		
First successful gastrostomy	Verneuil	1876
Jejunostomy first performed	Surmay	1879
Serosal tunnel technique	Witzel	1891
Use of concentric pursestring sutures around gastrostomy tube	Stamm	1894
First permanent gastrostomy	DePage	1901
and modifications	Janeway	1913
Use of jejunostomy for immediate postoperative nutrition	A F R Andresen	1918
Description of cervical oesophagostomy	C T Klopp	1951
Introduction of technique for needle catheter jejunostomy	H A McDonald	1954
Description of cervical pharyngostomy	D A Shumrick	1967
Use of anastomotic stapler	G Moss	1972
Introduction of duodenostomy tube feeding technique	J Alexander-Williams	1976

tube or tube enterostomy. Important developments in the evolution of the two latter techniques are summarised in Table 1.2.

Enteral nutrition by nasoenteric tube has been used since ancient times. It was reported to have been reintroduced in the latter half of the eighteenth century by Hunter to treat a patient with 'paralysis of the muscles of glutition'. Nasogastric tube feedings, although more commonly used, were poorly accepted because of patient intolerance and inadequate liquid diet preparations. Tube gastrostomy or jejunostomy became the methods of choice when long-term enteral nutrition was required.

The first successful human gastrostomy was performed by Verneuil in 1876, and the first permanent gastrostomy was described by Depage in 1901. Leakage of gastric contents was a common and serious complication of the initial gastrostomies. Several modifications of gastrostomy techniques have been reported over the years, including the use of the gastrointestinal anastomotic stapler. Gastrostomy has the advantage of permitting early decompression and drainage of the stomach after surgery, and then subsequent feeding.

One of the earliest feeding jejunostomies was constructed in 1885 by Gould for palliation of a patient with carcinoma of the stomach. Further innovations were reported in the first half of the twentieth century and in 1954 McDonald proposed the technique of needle catheter jejunostomy. The incidence of fistulae and intestinal obstruction has been reduced with this technique. Jejunostomy is used when prolonged enteral nutrition is anticipated.

In recent years, with the renewed interest in enteral nutrition, the range of formulae available has expanded considerably and includes blenderised, partially hydrolysed and elemental (defined formulae) diets. Diet selection should be based on the functional ability of the gastrointestinal tract to digest and absorb the required nutrients. Their administration has been facilitated by the development of fine bore nasoenteric tubes and infusion pumps and delivery systems designed specifically for enteral use. In 1976, Dobbie & Hoffmeister reintroduced the principles of continuous feeding through a small calibre tube placed nasogastrically through the pylorous into the small bowel.

Complications of enteral nutrition are fewer than with parenteral nutrition, monitoring is less exacting, and the cost may be as little as 10% of that of parenteral nutrition. However, there are situations in which inadequate nutritional intake for a short period is preferable to complicated attempts to feed.

In assessing the nutritional requirements of each patient, the following questions should be asked each day: what nutrition has this patient had in the last 24 hours?; does he need more nutrition?; can he eat, or is enteral feeding required?; is the gut unavailable and parenteral nutrition required?.

Because the scientific basis and technical details of parenteral nutrition have been explored to a far greater extent than enteral nutrition, this guide has been written around the former. The principles are applicable, in many cases, to enteral feeding, and specific aspects of the latter are presented in Chapter 27.

REFERENCES AND FURTHER READING

Dudrick S J, Wilmore D W, Vars H M, Rhoads J E Long-term total parenteral nutrition with growth, development, and positive nitrogen balance. Surgery 1968; 64: 134–142

Heymsfield S B, Bethel R A, Ansley J D, Nixon D W, Rudman D Enteral hyperalimentation: an alternative to central venous hyperalimentation. Ann Int Med 1979; 90: 63–71

Levenson S M, Smith Hopkins B, Waldron M, Canham J E, Seifter E Early history of parenteral nutrition. Fed Proc 1984; 43: 1391–1406

Randall H T Enteral nutrition: tube feeding in acute and chronic illness. JPEN 1984; 8: 113–136

Rombeau J L, Barot L R Enteral nutritional therapy. Surg Clin N Am 1981; 61: 605–620
Rose W C II: The sequence of events leading to the establishment of the amino acid needs
    of man. Am J Pub Health 1968; 58: 2020–2027
Schuberth O, Wretlind A Intravenous infusion of fat emulsions, phosphatides and
    emulsifying agents. Clinical and experimental studies. Acta Chir Scand 1961; 278
    (Suppl): 1–21
Shils M E Historical aspects of minerals and vitamins in parenteral nutrition. Fed Proc
    1984; 43: 1412–1416
Torosian M H, Rombeau J L Feeding by tube enterostomy. Surg Gynecol Obstet 1980;
    150: 918–927

2

Logistic considerations

Today, nutritional support has become accepted as a 'standard of care' for many disease states and circumstances (Ch 3), even though a critical evaluation of the scientific literature, as undertaken by Koretz in 1984, may lead one to question the validity of its application in certain situations. Nevertheless, the denial of nutritional support may raise questions as to the quality of care, particularly when the patient's condition worsens through increasing nutritonal deficits.

Thus, the physician, whether he is attending a patient in a small (private) acute care hospital, or a large university-affiliated acute care teaching centre, should be able to provide an acceptable level of nutritional care to ensure that malnutrition is recognised and safely and effectively treated. These minimum standards of nutritional care are summarised in Table 2.1 and include patient assessment, development of a therapeutic plan, implementation of this plan, patient monitoring and appropriate termination of therapy.

The degree of organisation of the actual provision of nutritional support will vary greatly between the small acute care hospital and the large teaching centre. Often, because of limited resources and/or limited patient numbers, the primary physician in the smaller hospital assumes the responsibility for providing and coordinating nutritional support — the 'ad hoc' approach. In contrast, many large hospitals have developed nutritional support teams to ensure that a planned approach to nutritional support is provided. An alternate approach adopted by some other hospitals is to appoint a nutritional committee to guide and monitor the provision of nutritional support — the supported approach.

THE AD-HOC APPROACH

A common method in many smaller hospitals with limited facilities and resources, is for the parenteral nutrition to be ordered each morning by a member of the team responsible for the patient. A multi-bottle system is used, with glucose in the main drip, amino acids (with or without carbohydrate) in a second side drip, lipid in another, albumin in another, and

7

Table 2.1 Minimum standards for nutrition support for hospitalised patients (adapted from the American Society for Parenteral and Enteral Nutrition — Standards for Nutrition Support, 1984)

Assess patient's
nutritional status
indications/contraindications for nutritional support
specific nutrient requirements

Develop therapeutic plan for patient
determine objectives for nutritional intervention
select appropriate access route
prescribe formulation appropriate to disease process and assessment

Implement therapeutic plan
establish access, document
commence routine care of access device, site
prepare prescribed formulation safely, accurately
administer formulation according to prescribed plan, patient's tolerance

Monitor patient for
therapeutic effects
adverse effects
clinical changes

Terminate therapy when patient
tolerates adequate nutrient requirement by gastrointestinal tract
complications take precedence over nutritional support
no longer benefits from nutritional support

possibly a crystalloid solution in another. Additives such as sodium and potassium, calcium and magnesium salts or phosphate, and vitamins are added to the glucose solution or the amino acids by the nursing staff in the ward. Modifications to the electrolyte content of the glucose are made when the daily electrolytes have been reported. This system is flexible and can be used in most hospital settings. However, the risks of bacterial and particulate contamination, incompatibilities, and prescription and calculation errors are potentially greater than when there is a planned approach to the provision of nutrition with the pharmacist assuming responsibility for pre-mixing solutions. Today, with the increasing availability of commercially prepared pre-mixed solutions, there is little justification for use of this multiple bottle system with ward-level additives.

The smaller hospital may or may not have developed written policies and procedures for catheter insertion and care, solution preparation and patient monitoring and assessment. In their absence, the physician assumes responsibility for providing appropriate guidelines to other members of the team responsible for caring for the patient.

THE SUPPORTED APPROACH

A number of hospitals, recognising the complexity and cost of parenteral nutrition, have established multidisciplinary nutritional support advisory committees to oversee the use of parenteral nutrition by specialty groups and primary physicians. Membership of such committees generally includes representatives of various medical and surgical specialties, as well as nursing, pharmacy and dietetics. Their responsibilities include the development of protocols for the procedures involved in the delivery of safe and effective nutritional support. In addition, the committee should ensure that in-service educational programmes are offered to staff so that they are familiar with the various protocols and guidelines.

Periodically, the committee should review and evaluate the quality and appropriateness of the nutritional support being provided in the hospital to document the need for revising protocols and procedures, expanding services and providing educational programmes to meet designated needs.

THE PLANNED APPROACH

A team approach to nutritional support has been adopted most successfully in some of the larger acute care centres. In this idealised system, the parenteral nutrition team co-ordinates the management of patients' feeding throughout the hospital. The team usually includes a physician, a pharmacist, a registered nurse and sometimes a dietitian. The minimum responsibilities of these team members are listed in Table 2.2.

Table 2.2   Organisation of nutrition support team

Personnel	Some minimum responsibilities
Physician	oversees activities of team
	responsible for development and implementation of protocols, procedures
	monitors metabolic and nutritional requirements of patients
	performs invasive procedures
	prescribes nutrition formulations
	periodically coordinates review of activities of team
	conducts in-service training programmes
Nurse	assists during invasive procedures
	adheres to procedures for catheter and site care and maintenance
	monitors solution administration
	interprets physician's orders for monitoring patient
	liaises between patient and other team members
	participates in in-service training/patient training programmes
Pharmacist	screens orders for physicochemical incompatibilities
	formulates and prepares nutrition solutions
	provides quality control programme for solution preparation
	monitors patient for drug-nutrient interactions
	participates in in-service training/patient training programmes
Dietitian	assists with nutritional assessment
	participates in design of enteral nutrition prescriptions
	responsible for preparation and delivery of enteral feeds
	monitors patient's response
	evaluates enteral formulae and feeding systems
	participates in in-service training/patient training programmes

Intravenous lines are inserted by a few authorised physicians and care of the system is entrusted to specially trained registered nurses. Results of laboratory investigations are assessed, together with the patient's clinical status, in the morning, and prescriptions for the next 24 hours' feeds written. In the pharmacy, feeding solutions are prepared under sterile conditions and sent to the ward. This approach reduces the risk of infection, particulate contamination, incompatibilities, and prescription and calculation errors. In addition, the team assumes responsibility for ensuring that the established protocols and guidelines are adhered to.

There is clearly a place for different systems for providing nutritional assessment and support under different circumstances. Patients in smaller hospitals can be fed intravenously safely using an ad-hoc approach, provided due care is taken. In major hospitals there are advantages to a planned approach, including:

— establishment of uniform criteria for institution and termination of parenteral nutrition
— establishment of uniform regimens
— maintenance of records
— education of medical and nursing staff in correct procedures
— establishment of a data base for clinical research projects.

As a result, an efficient, economic system can be established with proper auditing of complications and improved patient care.

In 1980, Nehme reported the results of a 2 year prospective study of two groups of patients, one managed exclusively by a nutrition support team and the other managed by a variety of physicians. From a comparison of the complication rates of the two groups, he concluded that the team approach to parenteral nutrition, when there was strict adherence to an established protocol, resulted in both a diminished risk and rate of complications. Other workers also have reported superior performance and improved patient care after forming a team which can accumulate experience more rapidly than an individual, provide a wider background of knowledge, offer formal training and create the opportunity to undertake research and participate in controlled trials.

REFERENCES AND FURTHER READING

Blackburn G L, Bothe A Jnr, Lahey M A Organization and administration of a nutrition support service. Surg Clin N Am 1981; 61: 709–719
Committee on Standards of Professional Practice, American Society for Parenteral and Enteral Nutrition. Standards for nutrition support. Hospitalized patients. American Society for Parenteral and Enteral Nutrition, Washington DC, 1984
Dalton M J, Schepers G, Gee J P, Alberts C C, Eckhauser F E, Kirking D M Consultative total parenteral nutrition teams: the effect on the incidence of total parenteral nutrition-related complications. JPEN 1984; 8: 146–152

Gilster S D The impact of a team approach on catheter-related infections. Nutr Supp Serv 1985; 5(4): 22–34

Koretz R L What supports nutritional support? Digest Dis Sci 1984; 29: 577–588

Kudsk K A, Thompson M, Tranbaugh R F, Sheldon G F Medical audit as an educational tool to improve intravenous nutritional support. J Med Education 1982; 57: 336–338

Nehme A E Nutritional support of the hospitalized patient: the team concept. JAMA 1980; 243: 1906–1908

Sanderson I, Deitel M Intravenous hyperalimentation without sepsis. Surg Gynecol Obstet 1973; 136: 577–585

Seltzer M H, Slocum B A, Cataldi-Betcher E L, Seltzer D L, Goldberger D J Specialized nutrition support: patterns of care. JPEN 1984; 8: 506–510

3

Indications and contraindications

There are many hotly debated topics in the field of parenteral and enteral nutrition, and one of these is the indications for such therapy. Traditionally, the question of who to feed was answered by listing disease states, which is analogous to listing the various disease states in which artificial ventilation might be used. Just as artificial ventilation is indicated for therapeutic respiratory failure (as in anaesthesia), or for respiratory failure due to disease, so are parenteral and enteral nutrition indicated for therapeutic nutritional failure (as in abdominal surgery or chemotherapy for malignant disease) or nutritional failure due to disease.

The indications for TPN may be absolute (as in total small bowel resection) or relative (as in a gastric fistula). Just as in respiratory failure, there are several ways of approaching nutritional failure. In many situations, enteral nutrition may be just as effective as TPN, but safer and cheaper.

Total parenteral nutrition has been employed in many disease states, but a commonly used rule of thumb is to consider it in any patient unable to receive nutrition by any other route for more than 3 or 4 days. In some situations, for example extensive small bowel resection, it should, of course, be started as soon as but not before fluid, electrolyte and acid-base abnormalities have been corrected.

A broad list of common indications for TPN is given in Table 3.1. The most pressing of these are:

— enterocutaneous fistulae
— pre-operative preparation of cachetic patients
— post-operative feeding of patients fed pre-operatively, or who cannot be fed via the gastrointestinal tract within 3 or 4 days
— inflammatory bowel disease
— as an adjunct to various forms of cancer therapy.

While these indications would be generally accepted, Goodgame has critically reviewed the indications for TPN using improvement of the outcome of illness in terms of reduction of mortality, morbidity and length of hospital stay, and comparison of TPN with other methods of nutrition as yardsticks. He concluded that while TPN is of proven value in several

Table 3.1 Common indications for parenteral nutrition

Pre-operatively
  Malnourished patients > 10–15% weight loss

Post-operatively
  Surgical complication, e.g. fistulae, prolonged ileus, peritoneal sepsis

Gastrointestinal diseases
  Inflammatory bowel diseases (Crohn's, ulcerative colitis), fistulae, pancreatitis

Conditions where inadequate oral intake
  Chronic vomiting, short bowel syndrome, anorexia nervosa

Post-trauma
  Hypermetabolic states, e.g. multiple injuries, severe burns

Unconsciousness, coma
  Tube feeding contraindicated

Depressed immune responses
  Cancer-associated malnutrition

Organ failure
  Renal or hepatic insufficiency

Paediatric conditions
  Prematurity, congenital malformations, necrotising enterocolitis

---

infant disease categories, it has been shown conclusively to be of value in adults with short bowel syndrome, inflammatory bowel disease and acute renal failure, but not other conditions. After considering claims that TPN decreases gastrointestinal secretions, corrects protein depletion, decreases mortality and increases spontaneous closure rates of gastrointestinal fistulae, he could find no evidence to support the claim that TPN was more efficacious than other methods of nutritional support. Likewise, there was no evidence that TPN per se altered the course of pancreatitis, liver failure, cancer or post-traumatic catabolism. A broad list of common indications for EN is given in Table 3.2.

Identification of which patients need TPN or EN usually can be made by a consideration of nutritional history, physical examination and simple

Table 3.2 Some indications for enteral nutrition

Neurological or psychiatric disorders
  Coma, severe depression, brainstem lesions

Oropharyngeal or oesophageal disorders
  Neoplasms, trauma, or fractures of the head and neck

Gastrointestinal disorders
  Gastrointestinal fistulae, short bowel syndrome, chronic pancreatic insufficiency

Post-trauma
  Head injuries, burns

Organ failure
  Renal or liver failure

---

laboratory tests such as serum albumin concentration. Existing or proposed drug, surgical or other therapy also influences the decision to feed. There are many increasingly sophisticated tests of nutritional status, but most of them only support clinical impression.

The value of nutritional assessment is being criticised increasingly. Review articles and editorials in the 'Journal of Parenteral and Enteral Nutrition' during 1982, 1983 and 1984 have highlighted some of the problems. Most studies of delayed cutaneous hypersensitivity skin testing were found to be poorly controlled and inconclusive. There is a wide range of 'normal' values, and no clear definition of what is a malnourished patient. Most clinical studies are carried out on small groups of patients of different ages, at different stages in different disease processes on different forms of therapy. Use of such measurements as skinfold thickness and arm muscle circumference has been criticised. Body chemistry is altered by many factors other than nutritional state.

There are many variations on the theme of the composition of parenteral and enteral nutrition solutions, so the question of what is indicated is often as difficult (or as easy) as who should receive it. The old concept of 'more is better' is disproven. Some 6300 mJ (1500 kcal) per day is more than enough to provide basal energy requirements in the well patient. More than that is of no value in the critically ill, septic or traumatised patient, since it cannot be utilised. High calorie/protein input is only of value in the recovering, mobile patient.

The duration of TPN which is of value is equally contentious. Feeding for a few days is of little value. Attempts to 'improve' a cachectic patient for surgery by forced feeding may only result in iatrogenic hypokalaemia and hypophosphataemia. Once commenced, feeding should continue until adequate enteral or normal nutrition is resumed.

Factors which influence decision-making in relation to enteral and parenteral nutrition are listed in Figure 3.1.

Despite these comments, it is important to bear in mind that many established forms of medical therapy have achieved general acceptance without being subjected to prospective double-blind trials. It is entirely logical to attempt to maintain patients in as good a nutritional state as possible during illness.

There are no absolute contraindications to parenteral nutrition except perhaps a functioning gastrointestinal tract. The volume and composition of feeds will require variation in different disease states, particularly in the presence of cardiac, renal or liver failure. It is most important to remember that it is very often the most complex patient who has the the greatest need for nutritional support, but it is these very patients who require the most careful assessment and often gradual introduction of TPN, particularly in relation to fluid volume, glucose content and content of ingredients known to be consumed rapidly in the depleted patient — potassium, phosphate, magnesium, zinc, folic acid.

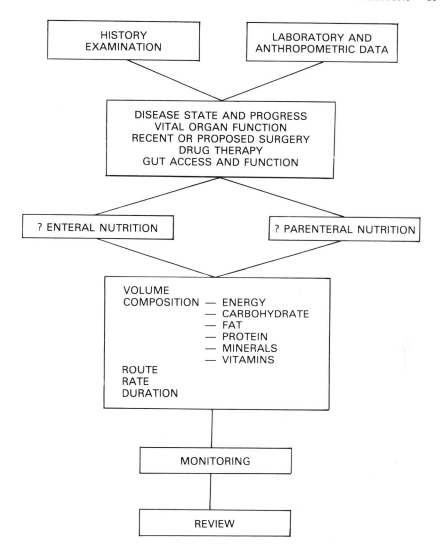

Fig. 3.1 Enteral and parenteral nutrition — factors influencing decisions.

Before TPN is commenced, and when it is periodically reviewed, consideration should be given to the following factors:

1. Is the gastrointestinal tract available by any route, including nasogastric tube, gastrostomy or jejunostomy?
2. Has a goal been set? Parenteral nutrition is inappropriate if it prolongs death rather than helps towards recovery.
3. Careless parenteral nutrition may be worse than no nutrition.

REFERENCES AND FURTHER READING

Goodgame J T Jnr A critical assessment of the indications for total parenteral nutrition. Surg Gynecol Obstet 1980; 151:433–441

Kirby D F, Craig R M The value of intensive nutritional support in pancreatitis. JPEN 1985; 9: 353–357

McLaren D S, Meguid M M Nutritional assessment at the crossroads. JPEN 1983; 7: 575–579

Muggia-Sullam M, Fischer J E Current concepts of indications for preoperative parenteral nutrition. In: Biebuyck J F Nutritional Aspects of Anaesthesia. Clin Anaesthesiol 1983; 1: 579–598

4

Venous access

Although peripheral veins may be used for administration of TPN solutions, particularly if they are not excessively hyperosmolar, a central venous catheter is regarded as essential for total parenteral nutrition in adults because of the irritation caused to peripheral veins by the hypertonic solutions used. The subclavian route generally is chosen because the catheter is easy to secure and it is comfortable for the patient. Contraindications to insertion are local infection and a bleeding disorder. Central venous catheters may be inserted via the jugular, median cubital or femoral veins, but these routes are associated with a higher complication rate than the subclavian route. This chapter describes the procedure we have adopted, although we accept it has infinite variations.

PATIENT PREPARATION

After explaining the proposed procedure to the patient, he lies flat on the bed with no pillow, and is tilted head down to minimise the risk of air embolism during insertion. The arms are positioned straight by the sides, and a rolled towel can be placed beneath the middle of the back, between the scapulae, to allow the shoulder to fall posteriorly, if necessary. The skin of the shoulder, chest and neck is shaved, if necessary, and prepared with aqueous povidone iodine (Betadine®) 1% solution, and the area draped. The operator, gowned, masked and gloved, infiltrates skin and subcutaneous tissues below a point just medial to the mid-point of the clavicle, and continues into the tissues between the clavicle and first rib and across towards the midline, using 5–8 ml of 1% lignocaine.

CATHETER INSERTION

A fine, 6.3 cm (2.5″)–7.6 cm (3″) short bevel needle is inserted, with a 10 ml syringe attached, through the anaesthetised skin, and advanced in a cephalad direction until it has passed between clavicle and first rib. It is then redirected towards the suprasternal notch and advanced horizontally until blood can be withdrawn from the subclavian vein. The syringe is

17

detached, and a flexible tip guidewire inserted into the vein via the needle. The needle is then withdrawn, and a 20 cm (8″) catheter inserted over the wire, and then the wire is withdrawn. If there is any risk of air embolism, for example in a dehydrated or shocked patient, or one who is hyperventilating, the patient is asked to hold his breath while the risk exists, or the gloved thumb is placed over the hub of the catheter. The drip tubing is attached to the hub via a Luer lock fitting, and the catheter is flushed. The catheter is sutured to the skin and a sterile transparent dressing is applied to cover the wound and the drip tubing-catheter hub connection. A loop of drip tubing is taped to the patient to avoid traction on the catheter (Fig. 4.1). The drip is now turned fully on, fluid flow is checked and the bag of fluid lowered below the patient. A flashback of blood indicates that the catheter is in the vein.

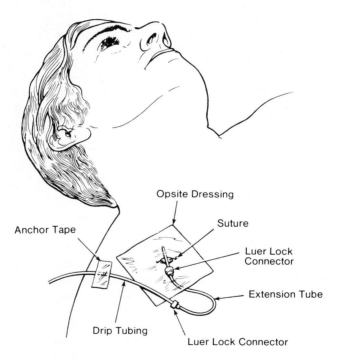

Fig. 4.1 Subclavian catheter dressing.

A chest X-ray is taken to confirm the presence of the catheter tip in the superior vena cava and to exclude a pneumothorax (Fig. 4.2).

Use of a 20 cm (8″) catheter locates the tip of the catheter in the superior vena cava in most patients, especially if the right subclavian vein is used. A 30 cm (12″) catheter is useful in the obese, but the catheter tip may enter the right ventricle, causing arrhythmias (Fig. 4.3)

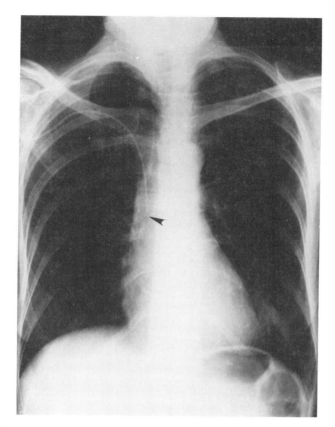

Fig. 4.2 X-ray showing position of catheter tip and absence of pneumothorax.

Recently, we have altered our protocol to include a short Luer lock connector between the drip set and the subclavian catheter hub. This is kept sterile by the assistant who connects it to the drip tubing and flushes it. When the syringe is disconnected the Luer lock connection is made with the catheter hub. Part of the connection tube is included in the occlusive dressing. The extension tube is then secured, and subsequent essential manipulations are performed between between the drip set and the extension tube, thus avoiding disturbance of the original dressing. There are many variations on this theme. It is now accepted by most workers that catheter-through-needle units should not be used because of the risk of catheter embolism. Investigations proceed as to the best catheter material, and polyurethane is regarded by many as superior even to silicone elastomer. A great variety of prepacked kits is available, and prices have become competitive. The more common use of straight and curved flexible tip guidewires has made venous access easier and safer than probing with wide-bore needles.

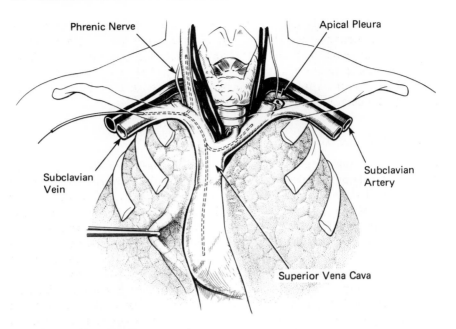

Fig. 4.3 Some possible catheter positions.

OTHER TECHNIQUES

Other techniques of central venous catheterisation used include the supra-clavicular subclavian and internal jugular veins. The former suffers from problems of a higher incidence of pneumothorax than the infraclavicular approach, potential damage to the thoracic duct on the left side, and more difficult immobilisation and dressing. The latter has a lower incidence of vascular and pleural damage, but is more difficult to dress and maintain. The external jugular vein may be used, but insertion is sometimes difficult, even with a flexible J-tipped guidewire.

Implantable catheters such as the Port-a-Cath® have been used as an alternative to the subcutaneously tunnelled catheters for long-term nu-trition. This device is buried subcutaneously and consists of a small stainless steel chamber sealed at the top by a rubber disc, and a thin silicone catheter which is inserted into a central vein. TPN can be infused via a needle inserted percutaneously through the rubber diaphragm of the portal. At the end of infusion, portal and catheter are heparinised and the needle removed.

While surgical implantation of the Broviac or Hickman catheter is commonly used when long-term access is required, percutaneous tunnelling techniques have been employed for intermediate term use. It is debatable whether or not this approach is of any value in reducing the incidence of catheter infection. In some centres, all the techniques used for venous access for haemodialysis have been employed for long-term TPN. In infants, it is common to infuse solutions containing up to 12.5% glucose via peripheral veins, with frequent change of infusion site. Fine bore silastic or polyurethane catheters, inserted via a peripheral vein, also have been used. Many of the subclavian catheters available have been reviewed by Burri & Ahenefeld (1978) (Appendix 1).

CATHETER CARE

Catheter care regimens vary enormously. We have evolved a system in which the original sterile dressing is not changed unless it becomes dirty or lifts, or if there is evidence of haemorrhage or infection at the catheter entry site. When this occurs, the dressing is changed using a sterile procedure in the same manner as on insertion of the catheter, and the drip tubing is also changed. The issue of catheter site dressings has been examined in some detail over the past few years. A recent review of use of sterile transparent polyurethane dressing for the catheter site found that, using a specific dressing technique, the average time interval between dressing changes was 4.3–5.3 days depending on catheter material, and that the incidence of catheter induced sepsis was 1%. Regular application of topical antibiotic or antifungal ointment to the catheter entry site is debated. Blood is not sampled from the line. Side drips and drug injections into the feeding line are avoided if possible. In the critically ill patient, this counsel of perfection cannot always be followed. If at any time the line is broken, the patient is placed head down to avoid air embolism.

COMPLICATIONS

Complications relating to the catheter itself are listed in Table 4.1. Catheter complications are minimised if the insertion is carried out by an expert, and if patient care is performed by staff familiar with the procedure. A chest X-ray must always be taken and seen following catheter insertion, to exclude complications, and to note the position of the catheter. In several large series, the major technical complication rate has been less than 1%. However, the rare complication of perforation of the heart has a mortality of 85%.

Catheter material is a dilemma, since soft floppy catheters are more difficult to insert, while the firmer catheters are more likely to perforate the vessel. Catheter embolism cannot occur if catheter-through-needle sets are not used. Air embolism is extremely rare if the head-down position is used during insertion, if the catheter is not left open to air and if Luer lock connections are used. Delayed vessel perforation due to pressure has been reported days after insertion, resulting in pneumothorax, haemothorax, hydrothorax, and mediastinitis. The two major, unpredictable complications are venous thrombosis and sepsis.

Table 4.1   Some catheter complications

Damage to adjacent structures by needle
  pleura, resulting in pneumothorax
  thoracic duct, resulting in chylothorax
  adjacent artery, resulting in haemomediastinum
  adjacent nerves

Perforation by catheter tip
  vena cava, resulting in haemomediastinum
  right atrium, resulting in haemopericardium
  pleura, resulting in hydrothorax

Embolism
  air
  catheter

Thrombosis
  subclavian
  vena caval

Cardiac arrhythmias

Sepsis
  local
  wound (if tunnelled)
  systemic
  endocarditis

Malposition of catheter

Venous thrombosis

Subclavian vein thrombosis was first reported as a complication of indwelling subclavian catheters in 1971 by McDonough & Altemeier. In another prospective study, 6 of 22 patients were shown to have central vein thrombosis by contrast venography, but only 1 patient had clinical evidence of thrombosis. If thrombosis occurs in this situation, usually it is recommended that the catheter be removed, and the patient systemically heparinised. If there is any question of infection, antibiotics should be given. Recently, a technique of dispersing the thrombus using either urokinase or streptokinase injected into the catheter has been described. Central vein thrombosis is not necessarily a bar to subsequent central venous cannulation. Many factors may contribute to thrombosis, including infection, catheter material, underlying disease affecting blood coagulation and infusion of irritating solutions. Silastic, polyurethane and other catheters have been introduced to prevent the problem of thrombosis, but none of these has been universally successful.

In a comparison between long silicone elastomer and polyurethane catheters inserted via the cubital fossa, the incidence of clinical thrombophlebitis was some seven times greater with the silicone catheters. However, there was no significant difference between the catheters with regard to the number and size of radiologic thrombi in peripheral or central veins, catheter occlusion rate, and platelet adhesion to the inner side of catheter tips on withdrawal. The value of the addition of low dose heparin to TPN solutions to decrease venous thrombosis is debated.

Sepsis

Sepsis is an ever-present threat to the patient on parenteral nutrition. While thrombophlebitis is a common problem with peripherally inserted cannulae or catheters, septicaemia often is the presentation of infection involving a central catheter.

Right sided endocarditis has been reported recently as a complication of central venous catheterisation.

Sepsis can be prevented only by meticulous attention to detail in several areas (Table 4.2). As far as sepsis is concerned, an issue which has been debated increasingly is the question of diagnosis of catheter related sepsis. Catheters may become infected either because of infection at the catheter insertion site or of the catheter hub-dripset connection, or because of infection of the catheter thrombus by circulating organisms. The former is the more important. Semi-quantitative culture of the catheter exit site has predictive value in identifying patients at risk of developing catheter sepsis. Semi-quantitative culture of the transcutaneous catheter segments has greater predictive value than culture of catheter tips. There appears to be best correlation between catheter hub infection and catheter sepsis.

Table 4.2 Measures advocated to decrease catheter sepsis

Aseptic insertion
Minimal line breaching
Aseptic handling of fluid pathway
Strict dressing protocol
Observation for site sepsis
Observation for systemic sepsis
? Tunnelling of catheter
? Heparin for thrombosis prophylaxis

If septicaemia is suspected in a previously well patient, the catheter should be removed immediately, and only reintroduced after blood cultures have been taken and the catheter cultured. In catheter associated sepsis, removal of the catheter is often enough to solve the problem, without administration of antibiotics. The patient clearly requires close observation and antibiotics may be required if the patient does not improve following catheter removal. In a patient who has an obvious cause for septicaemia, for example, intra-abdominal sepsis, there may be no indication to remove a central venous catheter just because of fever and leucocytosis.

Subcutaneous tunnelling of catheters has been recommended as a method of reducing sepsis. In one study using this technique, the incidence of staphylococcus epidermidis infections increased, while those due to other organisms decreased. Reinfection of replaced catheters has led to delay of recatheterisation for 24–48 hours after removal of the infected catheter. In another prospective study, subcutaneous tunnelling was not shown to influence the rate of sepsis. In the management of catheter sepsis, it has been proposed that removal and reinsertion of a new catheter over a guidewire is a safe and effective measure. This method requires further evaluation before it can be recommended.

CATHETER REMOVAL

It has been our routine to culture the catheter tip on removal, a practice of doubtful value (see above). The patient should be supine while the catheter is removed and a dressing applied. After 24 hours the dressing should be removed.

REFERENCES AND FURTHER READING

Baumgartner T G, Sitren H S, Hall J, Lottenberg R The stability of urokinase in parenteral nutrition solutions. Nutr Supp Serv 1985; 5(1): 41–43

Bozzetti F, Scarpa D, Terno G, Scotti A, Ammatuna M, Bonalumi M G, Ceglia E Subclavian vein thrombosis due to indwelling catheters: a prospective study on 52 patients. JPEN 1983; 7: 560–562

Burri C, Ahnefeld F W The caval catheter. Springer-Verlag, Berlin, 1978

Dunbar R D Radiologic appearance of compromised thoracic catheters, tubes, and wires. Radiol Clin N Am 1984; 22: 699–722

Linares J, Sitges-Serra A, Garau J, Perez J L, Martin R Pathogenesis of catheter sepsis: a prospective study with quantitative and semiquantitative cultures of catheter hub and segments. J Clin Microbiol 1985; 21: 357–360

Linder L–E, Curelaru I, Gustavsson B, Hansson H–A, Stenqvist O, Wojciechowski J Material thrombogenicity in central venous catheterization: a comparison between soft, antebrachial catheters of silicone elastomer and polyurethane. JPEN 1984; 8: 399–406

Meguid M M, Eldar S, Wahba A The delivery of nutritional support. A potpourri of new devices and methods. Cancer 1985; 55: 279–289

Moyer M A, Edwards L D, Farley L Comparative culture methods on 101 intravenous catheters; routine, semiquantitative, and blood cultures. Arch Intern Med 1983; 143: 66–69

Parsa M H, Ferrer J M, Habif D V Safe central venous nutrition. Guidelines for prevention and management of complications. Charles C Thomas, Springfield, 1974

Pettigrow R A, Lang S D R, Haydock D A, Parry B R, Bremner D A, Hill G L Catheter-related sepsis in patients on intravenous nutrition: a prospective study of quantitative catheter cultures and guidewire changes for suspected sepsis. Br J Surg 1985; 72: 52–55

Raaf J H Results from use of 826 vascular access devices in cancer patients. Cancer 1985; 55: 1312–1321

Rosen M, Latto I P, Ng W S Handbook of percutaneous central venous catheterisation. W B Saunders, London, 1981

Ryan J A Jnr, Abel R M, Abbott W M, Hopkins C C, Chesney TMcC, Colley R, Phillips K, Fischer J E Catheter complications in total parenteral nutrition: a prospective study of 200 consecutive patients. New Engl J Med 1974; 290: 757–761

Vazquez R M, Jarrard M M Care of the central venous catheterization site: the use of a transparent polyurethane film. JPEN 1984; 8: 181–186

Wilson S E, Stabile B E, Williams R A, Owens M L Current status of vascular access techniques. Surg Clin N Am 1982; 62: 531–551

5

Physiological and biochemical bases of nutrition

An understanding of the normal metabolic requirements of man, and the integration of metabolism between organs, is essential to permit estimation of the patient's daily metabolic requirements and administration of adequate nutritional therapy. In this chapter it is intended to provide an overview of these requirements and processes in the healthy young adult, so that the reader is able to understand better the account of the alterations in these metabolic processes, and hence nutritional requirements, in the presence of starvation, sepsis, trauma or organ failure, as presented in Chapter 6.

THE FEEDING STATE

When man eats, the first requirement is to provide fuel for intermediary metabolism. The second requirement is to expand glycogen reserves in liver and muscle and also to replace protein broken down in various tissues, particularly muscle, since the last meal. The third requirement is to convert excess energy ingested as carbohydrate, protein or fat into triglycerides and to store these in adipose tissue.

Attainment of these requirements is facilitated through the changes that feeding induces in the plasma concentrations of the hormones insulin and glucagon. The insulin concentration increases in response to feeding, thus accelerating the deposition of glycogen in the liver and, to a lesser extent, in muscle. Carbohydrate becomes the main energy source in these tissues.

THE FASTING STATE

During the fasting state, these requirements are reversed. The plasma insulin concentration falls progressively, while the glucagon concentration rises with fasting. As a consequence of the decreasing insulin concentration, less glycogen is deposited in liver and muscle, while lipase in adipose tissue is activated, causing release of large amounts of free fatty acids and glycerol. The increased concentration of glucagon enhances hepatic uptake of these free fatty acids and their subsequent conversion to ketone bodies. At the same time, the conversion of hepatic glycogen stores to glucose is accelerated. Consequently, free fatty acids and ketone bodies replace glucose as the major fuel available to muscle, with ketone bodies becoming the preferred energy substrate as fasting progresses. Meanwhile, the muscle fibres, as a result of inadequate oxygenation or stimulation by adrenaline, release increasing quantities of lactate, which is converted in the liver to glucose and used by the muscle to replenish glycogen stores (the Cori cycle). Thus, during fasting, the body draws selectively on its extensive supply of energy stored in adipose tissue and spares the breakdown of proteins, particularly those associated with nervous tissues, the heart and liver. Proteins involved in muscle contractility and enzyme systems also are spared.

At maturity, these anabolic and catabolic phases of metabolism normally are balanced so that weight is maintained constant. This fine balance however, may be disrupted easily by starvation, severe illness, trauma or sepsis and nutritional intervention, enteral or parenteral, may be indicated.

INTERMEDIARY METABOLISM

When food is ingested the absorptive process begins through the action of intraluminal and brush border enzymes which break down complex carbohydrates, lipids and proteins to their constituent sugars, fatty acids and amino acids. Parenteral administration of carbohydrate, protein and fat delivers the basic nutrients directly into the bloodstream, thus bypassing intestinal absorption and the portal venous system. The substrates glucose, amino acids and fatty acids then are available to the normal intermediary metabolic pathways via which they are oxidised to provide energy necessary to maintain body temperature and to maintain intracellular adenosine triphosphate (ATP) concentrations so that cellular, tissue and organ function may be maintained.

CARBOHYDRATE METABOLISM

The primary function of carbohydrates in the body is to provide a source of energy. Most of the reactions coupled to ATP synthesis are involved in the metabolism of carbohydrates.

Dietary carbohydrate constitutes approximately 40–45% of the total dietary intake. It consists mainly of the polysaccharides amylose and amylopectin, with small amounts of free glucose and fructose. The polysaccharides are degraded in the gut to the monosaccharides glucose, fructose and lactose, which are absorbed mainly in the proximal small bowel by an active transport process. Fructose and galactose are converted rapidly by the liver to glucose, the major carbohydrate of human metabolism. Most of this glucose enters the blood circulation to be taken up by body cells and metabolised for energy.

Virtually all human tissues catabolise carbohydrate (glucose) via the

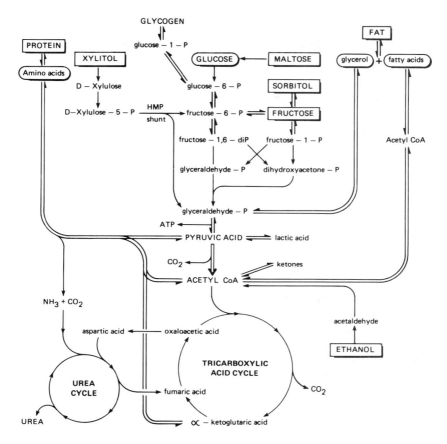

Fig. 5.1 Intermediary metabolism. (Adapted from Phillips & Odgers, 1982, with permission of ADIS Press Australasia Pty Ltd)

Embden-Meyerhoff (glycolytic) pathway, leading to pyruvic acid or lactic acid (Fig. 5.1). The formation of pyruvic acid is dependent on an adequate oxygen supply to the cell (*aerobic glycolysis*). If the oxygen supply is inadequate, lactic acid is formed (*anaerobic glycolysis*). The overall reaction of glycolysis yielding pyruvate results in a net gain of 2 moles of nicotinamide adenine dinucleotide (NADH) and 2 moles of ATP per mole of glucose. Anaerobic glycolysis to lactate yields only 2 moles of ATP.

The second portion of glucose degradation involves the conversion of pyruvic acid to carbon dioxide and water via the tricarboxylic acid cycle (TCA cycle, Krebs cycle) (Fig. 5.2). These reactions occur in the presence of oxygen, and also result in the synthesis of ATP. The total yield of ATP is 36 or 38 moles per mole of glucose oxidised to carbon dioxide and water.

Glucose also can be stored in liver and muscle cells in the form of the glucose polysaccharide glycogen (*glycogenesis*). Glucose is converted to

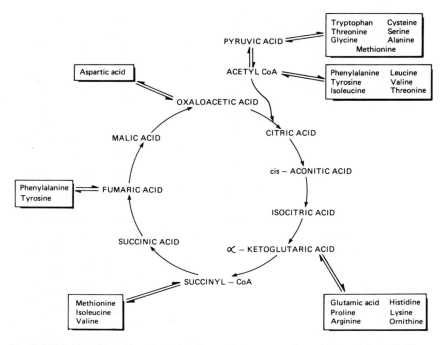

Fig. 5.2 Tricarboxylic acid cycle and amino acid interconversions. (Adapted from Phillips & Odgers, 1982, with permission of ADIS Press Australasia Pty Ltd)

glucose-6-phosphate and then can be converted to glycogen or proceed via the Embden-Meyerhoff pathway to pyruvic acid. The process of glycogenesis is coupled to the influx of potassium ions into the cell. Glycogen provides a means of storing glucose molecules in the cell, and acts as a source for glucose-6-phosphate when glucose supply to the cell is inadequate.

The liver stores only enough glycogen to supply the body with glucose for 12–24 hours. To meet the body's demands for glucose during prolonged fasting, the liver, kidneys and intestinal endothelium can form glucose from glycerol (derived from triglyceride hydrolysis) and from the alpha-keto acids pyruvate and oxaloacetate (derived from amino acid catabolism). Formation of glucose in this manner is termed *gluconeogenesis*.

An amino acid that can be converted to glucose via gluconeogenesis is termed *glucogenic* or *glycogenic* (see Table 9.4). To undergo gluconeogenesis, an amino acid must be broken down to pyruvic acid, 3-phosphoglyceric acid or an intermediate in the tricarboxylic acid cycle. Alanine is the major gluconeogenic precursor in the liver and glutamine is an important precursor in the renal cortex. Sufficient dietary carbohydrate results in protein sparing, because amino acid breakdown for gluconeogenesis is reduced.

In adipose tissue glucose is utilised for de novo synthesis of long chain fatty acids which are esterified with glycerol (derived from glucose) to form triglycerides (*lipogenesis*). The liver also synthesises a significant amount of triglycerides which are transported to adipose tissue by very low density lipoprotein molecules to be stored as fat.

Organs that actively synthesise fatty acids and steroids, such as the liver, adipose tissue, lactating mammary gland and adrenal cortex, channel a significant proportion of their glucose into the hexose monophosphate (HMP) shunt (Fig. 5.3). Products of this pathway include pentose sugars and nicotinamide adenine dinucleotide phosphate (reduced form) (NADPH). Other reactions rearrange triose, pentose, hexose and heptulose sugars. This shunt can oxidise glucose-6-phosphate completely to carbon dioxide and water.

Glucose does not penetrate readily through cell membranes of most human tissues and insulin must be present to facilitate its entry. Insulin also promotes amino acid uptake by cells and stimulates protein synthesis, thereby reducing the amino acid pool available for gluconeogenesis. In addition, insulin promotes *glycogenesis*, enhancing the capacity of the liver to retain glucose as glycogen. Insulin is the only hormone that acts to lower serum glucose concentrations as well as to promote glucose storage.

Growth hormone antagonises insulin activity and acts as a glucose-mobilising hormone, raising the serum glucose concentration. The glucocorticoids promote hyperglycaemia by stimulating gluconeogenesis. They promote protein and amino acid breakdown and also stimulate the liver to

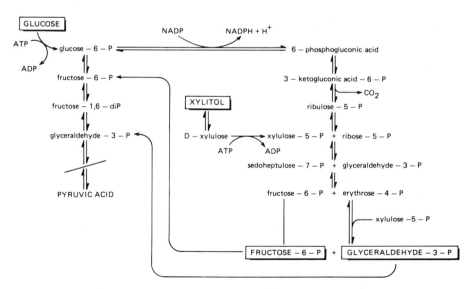

Fig. 5.3 Hexose monophosphate (HMP) shunt (including the metabolic pathway of xylitol). (Adapted from Phillips & Odgers, 1982, with permissions of ADIS Press Australasia Pty Ltd)

produce more gluconeogenic enzymes. Adrenaline and glucagon also are glucose-mobilising hormones, stimulating *glycogenolysis* via cyclic adenosine monophosphate (c-AMP) in the liver and kidneys, as well as by inhibiting glycogenesis.

The increase in serum glucose concentration after administration of carbohydrate triggers insulin release from the pancreas while inhibiting the glucose-mobilising enzymes. During fasting, little or no insulin is detectable in the serum and glucagon and adrenaline maintain the serum glucose concentration via glycogenolysis for only 6–24 hours. After the hepatic stores are depleted, glucagon and the glucocorticoids assume the dominant role in stimulating hepatic glucose production via gluconeogenesis.

PROTEIN METABOLISM

Proteins are the chief organic components of cellular structure and metabolism. Their metabolism is, essentially, the metabolism of amino acids:

— to provide the building blocks for protein metabolism in all tissues
— to provide precursors for the synthesis of numerous small nitrogenous molecules
— to be deaminated when in excess, to provide nitrogen for urea formation.

Regulation of their metabolism requires the interaction of many tissues, particularly intestinal mucosa, liver, muscle and kidney.

On ingestion, protein is broken down first by proteolytic enzymes and then by pancreatic proteases to free amino acids, which are absorbed by the mucosal cells of the small intestine, and peptides, which are absorbed and hydrolysed in the mucosal cells to free amino acids. Glutamic acid and aspartic acid are transaminated in the gut wall to the corresponding keto acids. Oxaloacetic acid and alanine also are produced. The amino acids are conveyed to the liver where oxidation of the essential amino acids, excluding the branched chain amino acids (BCAA) leucine, isoleucine and valine, to urea occurs (Fig. 5.4). Alanine is processed in the liver to provide carbon for gluconeogenesis and nitrogen for urea formation. In addition, a proportion of these amino acids is used for the synthesis of plasma proteins and a further proportion is retained temporarily as liver protein.

The branched chain amino acids undergo minimal degradation in the liver, but undergo transamination in the peripheral tissues such as kidney, brain and muscle. It has been estimated that the proportion of branched chain amino acids needed for re-synthesis of muscle protein is approximately 20% of the dietary protein intake. The non-essential amino acids enter a number of different metabolic pathways and their oxidation occurs at many tissue sites.

The metabolism of amino acids in the liver is modulated in accordance with body needs and the plasma amino acid concentration is normally

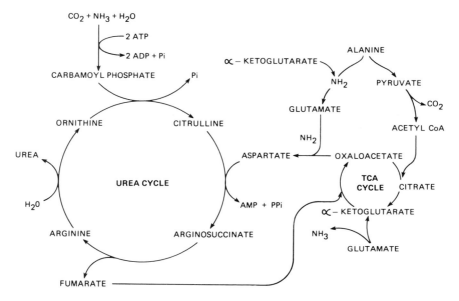

Fig. 5.4 The urea cycle and its interrelationships with tricarboxylic acid cycle. (Adapted from Phillips & Odgers, 1982, with per·ission of ADIS Press Australasia Pty Ltd)

0.3–0.4 mmol/l. However, the liver does not completely eliminate a rise in the plasma amino acid concentration when excess of an essential amino is consumed.

Dietary carbohydrate, administered orally or parenterally, also affects the plasma amino acid concentration by facilitating the deposition of amino acids in muscle through an insulin-dependent mechanism. This response to carbohydrate is maximal for the branched chain amino acids. Thus alterations in the plasma free amino acid pattern caused by the administration of amino acids and carbohydrate can affect significantly the availability of amino acids to the peripheral tissues. The plasma amino acid concentration also is regulated by glucocorticoids and growth hormone.

The plasma amino acid concentration is supplemented further by breakdown of tissue proteins, in particular, skeletal muscle protein (*proteolysis*). Alanine and glutamine each account for approximately 30–40% of the amino acids released from muscles of fasting subjects. A proportion (c. 50%) of the glutamine then is converted in the small intestine to alanine, which, together with the alanine coming directly from muscle and tissues, becomes the substrate in the liver for gluconeogenesis (the *glucose-alanine cycle*). In the presence of acidosis, the kidney also consumes glutamine to provide ammonia for neutralisation.

Munro (1983) has suggested that approximately 300 g of protein are synthesised daily by adult man, whereas the average protein intake in western countries is about 100 g per day. Consequently, there is considerable reutilisation of amino acids released by breakdown of tissue protein and any alteration to muscle protein metabolism due to disease, trauma or malnutrition is likely to have significant effects on the metabolism of free amino acids.

The size of the free amino acid pool is approximately 70 g. This is composed mainly of non-essential amino acids, particularly alanine derived from glucose metabolism, branched chain amino acid metabolism and input, glutamic acid, glutamine and glycine. The essential amino acids constitute about 10 g of the amino acid pool, of which only 200 mg are present in the plasma. The plasma content of non-essential amino acids is approximately 500 mg.

A further amino acid released by the breakdown of myofibrillar protein is 3-methylhistidine. This amino acid is not reutilised, has a low renal clearance, and is excreted rapidly. The content of 3-methylhistidine in muscle has been determined for different age groups, and measurement of its urinary output permits computation of the total breakdown of muscle in man and also the status of protein nutrition.

The amino acid turnover also is influenced by the state of activity of the person and the body's hormonal environment. Present evidence suggests that insulin stimulates protein synthesis in skeletal muscle cells and that it may accelerate amino acid transport and inhibit protein degradation. Insulin also exerts a protein sparing effect on the liver by decreasing hepatic uptake and oxidation of amino acids and inhibits their conversion to glucose. In the isolated perfused liver, it was shown that these effects were mediated through suppression of cAMP, leading to suppression of gluconeogenesis.

Glucagon exerts little or no effect on amino acid metabolism in peripheral tissues. In the liver, glucagon influences amino acid metabolism by stimulating gluconeogenesis.

Increased glucocorticoid secretion has been reported by many workers to affect skeletal muscle in a manner opposite to that of insulin, resulting in loss of body weight, marked atrophy, and decreased rates of protein synthesis. However, contradictory findings have been reported, for example, in burn injuries.

LIPID (FAT) METABOLISM

Lipid (fat) is the main energy substrate in the diet, normally providing approximately 90% of the total body caloric reserve (c. 627 000 kJ or 150 000 kcal). The majority of fat in the diet is in the form of triglycerides, the remainder being primarily phospholipids and cholesterol. Digestion proceeds in the small intestine, mainly under the influence of pancreatic lipase, aided by bile salts which promote aggregation of the liberated free fatty acids, monoglycerides and cholesterol, into micelles. It is from these micelles that fatty acids and monoglycerides enter the intestinal epithelial cells.

During passage through the epithelial cells the fatty acids are resynthesised into triglycerides which, combined with lesser amounts of phospholipid, protein and cholesterol, are released into the circulation as small lipid droplets, the chylomicrons. Plasma lipoprotein lipase hydrolyses triglycerides in the chylomicrons into free fatty acids and glycerol (*lipolysis*). Insulin is required for the synthesis of this lipoprotein lipase and thus plays an important, although indirect, role in the transport of triglycerides across peripheral cell-plasma membranes. Adipose tissue contains a distinct hormone-sensitive cell membrane lipoprotein lipase, which mediates hydrolysis of its triglycerides to free fatty acids and glycerol. This process is activated by catecholamines while insulin effectively inhibits intracellular lipolysis and hence fat mobilisation.

The fatty acids and glycerol then proceed through two separate pathways (see Fig. 5.1). Glycerol is phosphorylated to glycerol-3-phosphate and then enters the Embden-Meyerhoff pathway as dihydroxyacetone phosphate from which point it can proceed into the TCA cycle. Conversely, glucose can provide glycerol required for the synthesis of neutral fats.

The principal route for catabolism of fatty acids, beta-oxidation, occurs in the mitochondria. The beta-carbon atom of the fatty acid is oxidised to a beta-keto acid. Alpha-oxidation of fatty acids occurs in the human brain, and beta-oxidation is a minor pathway found in the liver.

Fatty acids enter the mitochondria after binding to carnitine to produce fatty-acylcarnitine. Once inside, coenzyme A (CoA)-SH displaces carnitine to regenerate fatty-acyl-CoA (Fig. 5.5). Fatty-acyl-CoA then passes through a series of beta-oxidation reactions yielding acetyl-CoA, flavin adenine dinucleotide ($FADH_2$) and NADH. The latter two substances yield

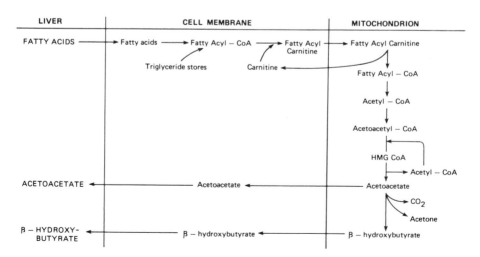

Fig. 5.5 Fatty acid oxidation and ketone body formation. (Adapted from Phillips & Odgers, 1982, with permission of ADIS Press Australasia Pty Ltd)

ATP. Acetyl-CoA subsequently may be oxidised in the TCA cycle, or may be dimerised to acetoacetyl-CoA which, in the liver mitochondria, liberates acetoacetic acid. Acetoacetic acid then may be reduced to beta-hydroxybutyric acid and acetone (*ketogenesis*).

Present evidence suggests that the rate of hepatic fatty acid oxidation is governed by the activity of the carnitine acyltransferase enzyme system. In the fed state malonyl-CoA is a potent inhibitor of carnitine acyltransferase I. During fasting this inhibition is removed through the action of glucagon which lowers the malonyl-CoA concentration of the liver and simultaneously increases the carnitine content.

In the fasting state, extra hepatic tissues such as skeletal muscle and heart muscle utilise ketone bodies as a fuel, via the generation of acetyl-CoA which enters the TCA cycle. The liver overproduces ketones for at least two reasons during severe carbohydrate deficiency. Firstly, carbohydrate deficiency depletes the TCA intermediates and slows the entrance of acetyl-CoA into the cycle. Secondly, the rate controlling enzyme of fatty acid synthesis, acetyl-CoA carboxylase, is inhibited by the absence of citrate, thereby blocking another route of acetyl-CoA metabolism. Thus, under such conditions, acetyl-CoA accumulates in the liver and is excessively converted to ketone bodies.

In humans, the synthesis of saturated fatty acids (*lipogenesis*) proceeds through a series of reactions which are essentially the reverse of fatty acid breakdown. Acetyl-CoA, derived mainly from carbohydrate through pyruvate, and bicarbonate are the necessary precursors of fatty acids, and NADPH, supplied chiefly by the HMP shunt, is required for the conversion to proceed. Ultimately, a 16-carbon compound, palmityl-S-ACP, is generated, and this is cleaved to palmitic acid and acyl carrier protein (ACP–SH). The unsaturated essential fatty acid, linoleic acid, cannot be synthesised by man, and hence must be provided in the diet.

VITAMINS AND INTERMEDIARY METABOLISM

Vitamins are required in the diet for the synthesis, by tissues, of coenzymes that are required in various metabolic pathways. The vitamins of the B complex function in intermediary metabolism in many essential reactions (see Ch 13).

Ascorbic acid functions in a number of biochemical reactions in the body, mostly involving oxidation. These reactions include the conversion of proline to hydroxyproline in collagen synthesis, and the oxidation of lysine side chains of proteins to provide hydroxytrimethyllysine for carnitine synthesis. Ascorbic acid also is required in tyrosine metabolism.

The fat soluble vitamins do not appear to act as coenzymes in intermediary metabolism. Their physiological roles are discussed in Chapter 13.

TRACE ELEMENTS AND INTERMEDIARY METABOLISM

A number of the trace elements are known to serve as cofactors for various enzymes involved in intermediary metabolism (see Ch 12). However, our current knowledge of the metabolic requirements for these elements is limited, particularly in conditions of prolonged malnutrition, critical illness and trauma.

ENERGY REQUIREMENTS

Sufficient energy must be provided to meet the basal or resting metabolic requirement, based on body mass and age, the specific dynamic action (SDA) of food and physical activity. In addition, allowances must be made for the increased energy expenditure and urinary nitrogen loss associated with illness and injury. The nature of the energy source to be used in TPN has been a matter for considerable debate in recent years — glucose alone or a combination of glucose with lipid (fat). Studies such as that of MacFie et al (1983) indicate that inefficient utilisation of energy is most likely to occur when large quantities of glucose are given and that a dual energy system is likely to require fewer calories for nitrogen equilibrium than a glucose only regimen.

BASAL METABOLIC RATE

The basal metabolic rate (BMR) is defined as the energy consumed in performing necessary physiological work at rest, in the post-absorptive state, and in a thermoneutral environment. Harris & Benedict (1919) derived equations to calculate the standard BMR in normal subjects from oxygen consumption measurements. It has been customary to use such BMR values increased by a factor of 10% to arrive at the resting metabolic energy (RME) expenditure, the energy expenditure of a subject at rest under normal environmental conditions.

Energy expenditure can be determined from knowledge of oxygen consumption, carbon dioxide production, and urinary nitrogen excretion. With this data the nonprotein oxygen consumption, nonprotein carbon dioxide production, and, hence the nonprotein respiratory quotient (RQ), can be determined. (The RQ is defined as the ratio of CO_2 produced to O_2 consumed during oxidation of body fuels. It is generally estimated that 1 g of urinary nitrogen represents the metabolism of 6.25 g of protein, utilisation of 5.9 l of O_2, production of 4.76 l of CO_2 and liberation of 110.9 kJ (26.51 kcal)). Energy expenditure then can be calculated by multiplying the litres of oxygen consumed by the caloric value per litre.

The RME expenditure has been determined in critically ill patients by expired air analysis using a continuous gas analyser. The studies of Kinney et al (1970) and Long et al (1979) have demonstrated that the RME is increased above normal by approximately 10% following elective surgery to 80% or more in sepsis and burns. During the period of convalescence, this increased RME returns towards normal as the injury component slowly subsides (see Fig. 6.1).

Long et al developed the following equations to calculate the total daily energy expenditure of their patient groups, taking into consideration the per cent increase above rest due to various degrees of stress, and an activity factor.

$$\text{Daily BMR for men} = (66.47 + 13.75W + 5.0H - 6.76A) \times (\text{activity factor}) \times (\text{injury factor})$$

$$\text{Daily BMR for women} = (655.10 + 9.56W + 1.85H - 4.68A) \times (\text{activity factor}) \times (\text{injury factor})$$

Where: W = weight in kg; H = height in cm; A = age in years,

Activity factor:
Confined to bed: 1.2
Out of bed: 1.3

Injury factor:
Minor operation: 1.20
Skeletal trauma: 1.35
Major sepsis: 1.60
Severe thermal injury: 2.10

These workers suggested that the most reasonable approach to caloric adjustment during convalescence from the injury component would be to maintain a calorie to nitrogen ratio of 150:1. The nitrogen requirement may be determined from the 24 hour urinary urea nitrogen excretion rate (see Ch 9).

Quebbeman has proposed alternate formulae for estimating energy expenditure which were based on indirect calorimetry measurements in 67 patients:

Daily resting energy expenditure
for men = weight (kg) × 12.3 + 754 kcal/day
for women = weight (kg) × 6.9 + 879 kcal/day

He recommends that a caloric input of 20% above the derived resting energy expenditure should be given.

Rainey-MacDonald et al (1982) have published nomograms based on the Harris-Benedict equation (Figs. 5.6 & 5.7) for predicting the resting energy expenditure (or REE) at the patient's bedside.

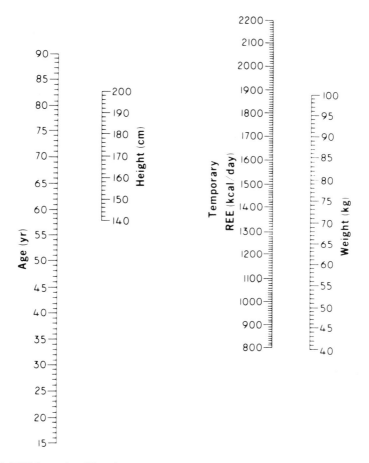

Fig. 5.6 REE for males. Directions:
1. Locate the height and weight on their respective scales, placing a straight edge (ruler) between these points, intersecting the temporary variable line.
2. Holding a pencil at the point of intersection (on temporary variable line), locate the age and pivot ruler to this point on the age scale. The point of intersection on the REE scale is the predicted REE.
(Reproduced with permission of Rainey-MacDonald et al 1982, and the Editor-in-Chief, American Society for Parenteral and Enteral Nutrition)

SPECIFIC DYNAMIC ACTION

The specific dynamic action (SDA) of a foodstuff is the extra heat production, over and above the caloric value of a given amount of food, that is generated when this food is used by the body. Fats, carbohydrates and protein all contribute, with proteins producing the largest increment. Up to 30% more heat can be generated than can be accounted for by the quantity of protein ingested, whereas fat and carbohydrates yield an increment

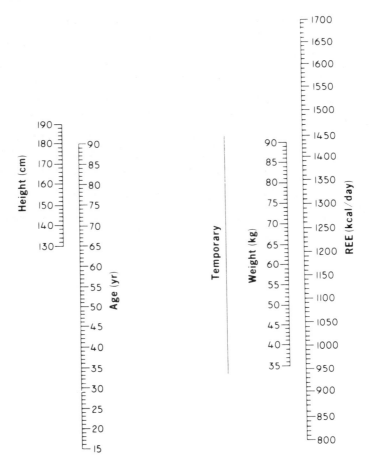

Fig. 5.7 REE for females. For directions see Fig. 5.6. (Reproduced with permission of Rainey-MacDonald et al 1982, and the Editor-in-Chief, American Society for Parenteral and Enteral Nutrition)

of approximately 3% and 5–10%, respectively. The SDA of protein may be reduced by the concomitant administration of carbohydrate and, in addition, nitrogen retention is promoted. The process of lipogenesis from glucose results in a greater increment in the SDA than when glucose is oxidised to carbon dioxide and water.

REFERENCES AND FURTHER READING

Abumrad N N, Miller B The physiological and nutritional significance of plasma-free amino acid levels. JPEN 1983; 7: 163–170
Felig P The glucose-alanine cycle. Metabolism 1973; 22: 179–207

Harris J A, Benedict F G Biometric studies of basal metabolism in man. Carnegie Institute of Washington 1919; Publication 279

Kinney J M, Duke J H Jnr, Long C L, Gump F E Tissue fuel and weight loss after injury. J Clin Path 1970; 23 (Suppl. 4): 65–72

Long C L, Schaffel N, Geiger J W, Schiller W R, Blakemore W S Metabolic response to injury and illness: estimation of energy and protein needs from indirect calorimetry and nitrogen balance. JPEN 1979; 3: 452–456

MacFie J, Holmfield J H M, King R F G, Hill G L Effect of the energy source on changes in energy expenditure and respiratory quotient during total parenteral nutrition. JPEN 1983; 7: 1–5.

Munro H N Metabolism and functions of amino acids in man — overview and synthesis. In: Blackburn G L, Grant J P, Young V R (eds) Amino Acids. Metabolism and Medical Applications. John Wright PSG, Inc., Littleton MA, 1983, p 1–12

Phillips G D, Odgers C L Parenteral nutrition: current status and concepts. Drugs 1982; 23: 276–323

Quebbeman E J, Ausman R K Estimating energy requirements in patients receiving parenteral nutrition. Arch Surg 1982; 117: 1281–1284

Rainey-MacDonald C G, Holliday R L, Wells G A Nomograms for predicting resting energy expenditure of hospitalized patients. JPEN 1982; 6: 59–60

6

Metabolic effects of starvation, sepsis and trauma

Starvation, sepsis, thermal burns and trauma alter intermediary metabolism in different ways. The metabolic and hormonal alterations have implications for the physician in his attempts to provide optimal care for the patient.

STARVATION

In the transition from the fed to the starved state, a sequence of metabolic alterations occurs as the body attempts to maintain glucose homeostasis in the acute phase and to preserve body protein mass in the prolonged phase of starvation.

As glucose absorption from the gut decreases and insulin concentration falls, the liver gradually stops removing glucose from the portal circulation and begins to produce glucose from glycogen. The hepatic glycogen stores, however, are largely exhausted within 24 hours. For a few days thereafter, glucose production is maintained through gluconeogenesis in order to meet the obligatory demand for glucose of the brain, red blood cells and renal parenchyma. Approximately 125–150 g of protein are consumed per day during the first 5–10 days of starvation — the acute phase, to satisfy this obligatory glucose requirement. The fall in insulin concentration which permits increased release of the amino acid alanine from protein while reducing opposition to glucagon-mediated gluconeogenesis, also enhances release of free fatty acids from adipocytes to meet the major portion of the body's energy requirements. Glucagon, by lowering hepatic levels of malonyl-CoA, stimulates hepatic oxidation of free fatty acids.

As the normal individual continues to fast, the ketone bodies substitute for glucose as the major fuel for the brain while the free fatty acids and ketone bodies reduce glucose utilisation in extraneural tissues (the keto-adaptive phase). Recent studies suggest that ketone bodies inhibit the rate of protein degradation in muscle and the rate of alanine release into the blood. The rate of fatty acid mobilisation from adipose tissue also appears to be regulated through the β-hydroxybutyrate concentration in the blood, thus providing a mechanism for integrating the rate of supply of fatty acids from adipose tissue and their conversion to ketone bodies in the liver. The

Table 6.1 Summary of hormone responses in starvation

Hormone	Acute starvation	Chronic starvation
Insulin	↓	↓
Glucagon	→ ↑	→ ↓
Catecholamines	↑	↓
Glucocorticoids	↑	↓
Growth hormone	↑	↓

influences of insulin and the catabolic hormones in the acute and chronic phases of starvation are summarised in Table 6.1.

The decrease in protein catabolism and release of alanine and glutamine, is evidenced by a diminution in urinary nitrogen excretion (Fig. 6.1), decreased hepatic gluconeogenesis, increased formation of ketone bodies and their enhanced oxidation in the brain. A generalised decline in plasma concentrations of amino acids, with a decline in amino acid efflux in muscle and a decrease in splanchnic uptake of amino acids also occur.

The clinical changes that occur with starvation include an initial rapid weight loss which is due largely to diuresis and protein breakdown. Catabolism of body protein results in an increased renal urea load which, together with a substantial loss of body calcium, potassium and magnesium, causes

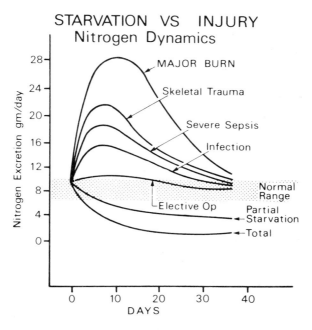

Fig. 6.1 Increase in urinary nitrogen losses in different patient groups with time. (Adapted with permission of Long et al, 1979, and the Editor-in-Chief, American Society for Parenteral and Enteral Nutrition)

a diuresis. The increased glucagon secretion induces a sodium diuresis by its action on the renal tubules. As starvation continues, the rate of weight loss slows after the gluconeogenic phase, and a progressively greater proportion of this is accounted for by the catabolism of fat. Water conservation begins gradually 3–4 days after starvation, and water over-loading of tissues readily occurs.

The basal metabolic rate decreases (see Fig. 6.2) due to the progressively decreasing lean body mass, decreased physical activity and decreased conversion of thyroxine (T_4) to triiodothyronine (T_3). Nitrogen excretion decreases as the need for gluconeogenesis decreases — the brain is preferentially using ketone bodies as fuel. Insulin concentrations continue to be low and glucagon returns to its post-absorptive concentration. However, the ratio insulin:glucagon is still in favour of glucagon. The renal cortex becomes the more important gluconeogenic organ, using glutamine for glucose synthesis. Progressive ketosis and metabolic acidosis are associated with increasing urinary losses of calcium and phosphorus, due to bone dissolution, and increasing serum urate concentration, due to renal retention of uric acid.

The respiratory system is affected adversely as fasting proceeds. The continuing loss of protein results in decreased serum albumin concentration. Interstitial oedema develops together with intra-alveolar accumulation of fluid. The hypoxic ventilatory response diminishes and the patient ultimately progresses into respiratory failure. Also, the starving patient's susceptibility to infection increases as the respiratory muscle function declines, phagocytic activity is impaired and antibody production decreases with the ongoing protein catabolism.

In the absence of sepsis or trauma, the starved patient can usually be converted to the anabolic state by the infusion of moderate amounts of carbohydrate, protein, electrolytes, trace elements and vitamins. A calorie to nitrogen ratio of 150:1 has been suggested with an input of 1 g/kg per 24 hours of amino acids and 105 kJ (25 kcal)/kg per 24 hours, with 60% of the daily caloric load being derived from carbohydrate. Ketone body concentrations fall dramatically, total urinary nitrogen decreases, permitting positive nitrogen balance to be achieved and ultimately fat is gained and the normal body fat stores are replaced.

A more detailed discussion of the regulation of glucose production in starvation may be found in Felig et al (1969) and Cahill (1976).

SEPSIS

Sepsis, a systemic response to an infecting agent involving activation of phagocytosis with mobilisation of white blood cells and increasing body temperature, results in a progressive disorder of intermediary metabolism, which ultimately is reflected in the physiology of sepsis. It runs a spectrum from little clinical significance, in which TPN is well tolerated, to frank metabolic failure, in which TPN is not tolerated and there is a high mortality rate.

The process appears to be one of a progressive inability of the skeletal muscle mass to use carbohydrates appropriately (despite increased glucose uptake by peripheral tissues, hyperglycaemia and variable insulin concentration), and fat, due to an insulin-mediated block in lipolysis. Glucose intolerance is associated with glycosuria and fluid and electrolyte imbalance. Amino acid catabolism is enhanced, leading to protein malnutrition with its overt manifestation of multiple systems organ failure.

There is an enhanced formation of lactic acid, alanine and glutamine in muscle, an enhanced efflux of these substrates from muscle to liver, an acceleration of the synthesis of glucose via the Cori (lactate) and alanine cycles, and accelerated glucose release from the liver (hepatic gluconeogenesis). Amino acids such as phenylalanine and tryptophan, that cannot be catabolised in muscle are released, to be returned to the liver where they are catabolised, releasing ammonia which is used by the liver for ureagenesis. Some of the released glutamine enters the kidney where it is converted into ammonia. These amino acids also contribute to the synthesis of acute phase proteins that are necessary for host resistance, and structural proteins for organ and tissue repair.

There is an increasing reliance on muscle amino acids, particularly the branched chain amino acids, as a fuel source as death approaches. The mitochondria appear to be the target organelles of this process. This mitochondrial dysfunction seems to be one of a failure of effective ATP production resulting in a progressive preference for nonoxidative catabolic pathways and a progressive inability of substrate utilisation as fuel for ATP production.

Proteolysis and gluconeogenesis are accelerated during sepsis by the stimulatory actions of several hormones (Table 6.2). There is a strong neuroendocrine response characterised by an increase in the secretion of the catecholamines, noradrenaline and adrenaline, especially during Gram-negative sepsis. Usually, there is a small increase in the secretion of insulin. Glucagon secretion is increased significantly, with a resulting decrease in the insulin:glucagon ratio. Glucagon and the catecholamines activate hepatic adenylate cyclase which stimulates hepatic glucose production and release. The secretion of adrenal glucocorticoids is increased, augmenting hepatic

Table 6.2 Summary of hormone responses in sepsis

Hormone	Acute sepsis	Overwhelming sepsis
Insulin	↑	↑
Glucagon	↑ ↑	↑ ↑ ↑
Catecholamines	↑ ↑	↑ ↑ ↑
Glucocorticoids	↑ ↑	↑ ↑
Growth hormone	↑ ↑	↑ ↑

gluconeogenesis and stimulating mobilisation of amino acids from the periphery, and also growth hormone, which resets (increases) the peripheral insulin response to glucose. Endogenous pyrogens, leucocyte endogenous mediator (LEM), and other substances released from the site(s) of infection may act directly or indirectly, to stimulate proteolysis and gluconeogenesis. This infection-induced hormone-mediated acceleration of gluconeogenesis is characteristic of the early period of fever, but may not be sustained if the infection becomes overwhelmingly severe. The ensuing hypoglycaemia generally can be explained on the basis of either substrate exhaustion or direct hepatocyte injury.

Sepsis also is associated with an increase in ureagenesis (see Fig. 5.4) as a result of the increased utilisation of amino acids in the liver, particularly alanine, for gluconeogenesis. The amino nitrogen generated from the transamination reactions accounts for approximately 100% of the infection-related increase in urea excretion. Some of the excess amino nitrogen is excreted as ammonia, contributing to the total loss of urinary nitrogen during sepsis.

Some degree of starvation generally is present during sepsis. However, the hormonal responses and substrates available prevent (or reverse) starvation-induced ketosis during sepsis. The release of free fatty acids from adipose tissue is variable, although most body cells continue to metabolise fatty acids as a primary source of energy. Within the liver, free fatty acids are incorporated into triglycerides which contribute to infection-induced hyperlipidaemia. In addition, lipid droplets begin to accumulate within hepatic cells, giving rise to histological changes characteristic of fatty metamorphosis throughout the liver.

Ketone body production is inhibited as the septic state progresses. It is possible that insulin plays a role in inhibiting ketogenesis through its ability to stimulate lipogenesis in hepatic cells and adipocytes.

Studies of the proposed metabolic derangements accompanying the septic state have revealed elevated triglyceride concentrations with decreased triglyceride clearance, and ketogenesis which initially is maintained, but soon becomes abnormal, with an increase in the beta-hydroxybutyrate: acetoacetate (BOHB/AcAc) ratio, principally from a fall in acetoacetate concentration. Increased fat mobilisation and turnover have been reported; and resting metabolic expenditure is generally increased to 125–140% of the normal RME (Fig. 6.2). More recent determinations of the metabolic rate in acutely septic patients suggest that actual requirements may be lower than this.

Eventually the metabolic process leads to hepatic failure which is manifested by increasing concentrations of proline, ornithine and ammonia; of aromatic amino acids; and of threonine, methionine and aminobutyric acid. The clinical changes that accompany this metabolic process include a rapidly decreasing muscle mass with a stable fat mass, a large net negative nitrogen balance (see Fig. 6.1), and a progressive prerenal azotaemia in the

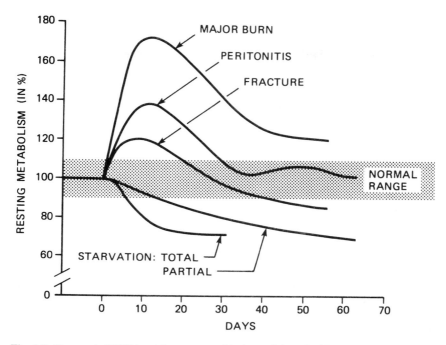

Fig. 6.2 Changes in RME in patient groups with time. (Adapted with permission of Kinney, 1966, and the Harvard University Printing Office)

absence of low cardiac output or hypovolaemia. Stress ulcers and decubitus ulcers, anergy, white blood cell functional failures, recurrent bacteraemias, metabolic encephalopathy and multiple systems organ failure, complete the picture.

Good correlation has been demonstrated between metabolism and physiology in the time course of sepsis. The early physiology is characterised by an elevated cardiac output, a total peripheral resistance that is still reasonably proportionate to the cardiac output, the onset of oxygen extraction failure, and an increased oxygen consumption. The metabolic characteristics include hyperglycaemia, insulin resistance, increased triglycerides, inappropriately increased free fatty acids for the existing glucose concentration, high ketone body concentrations, proportionately elevated lactate and pyruvate concentrations, elevated concentrations of cortisol, insulin and glucagon, and increased secretion of noradrenaline.

As the septic process worsens, the cardiac output increases, peripheral resistance decreases to an inappropriately low level, further oxygen extraction failure, and an increased oxygen consumption. The metabolic characteristics deteriorates further — the BOHB/AcAc ratio increases due to a fall in the concentration of acetoacetate, there are proportional elevations in lactate, pyruvate and alanine, the concentrations of hepatically catabolised amino acids rise, glucagon concentration is very high, and large amounts of noradrenaline are secreted. If adequate myocardial support has not been provided, or if there is a severe degree of myocardial disease, or if advanced septic myocardial depression has occurred, a perfusion-related metabolic deficit can be superimposed on this metabolic deficit.

Although acceleration of gluconeogenesis and ureagenesis and inhibition of ketogenesis appear to be characteristic of the host response to acute sepsis, these responses, and also the hormonal ones, may be modified or abolished if infection develops in a poorly nourished host, in the presence of complicating trauma or other disease, or when the infecting process itself becomes overwhelmingly severe.

A number of studies have been conducted to determine the optimal composition of nutritional support for the septic patient. These have demonstrated that high carbohydrate intake may serve as a physiological stress rather than a nutritional support, and that the infusion of carnitine-independent fats (short and medium chain fatty acids or the ketone bodies) as an energy source, may result in more effective management of the metabolic abnormalities. Normalisation of the plasma amino acid pattern and reversal of encephalopathy have been reported in a small group of septic patients who received an amino acid solution enriched with branched chain amino acids.

The goal of TPN in the hypermetabolic septic patient should be to provide appropriate proportions of the substrates (protein, glucose, fat, vitamins, water and electrolytes) based on the induced metabolic derangements in order to minimise complications and maximise benefit. A calorie to nitrogen ratio of 80:1 has been proposed with an input of 3 g/kg per 24 hours of amino acids and 146 kJ (35 kcal)/kg per 24 hours, with 70% of the total daily calorie load being derived from carbohydrate.

TRAUMA

In the traumatised patient the systemic metabolic and circulatory responses are directed to the support of the healing wound. These responses are proportional to the severity of the injury and are characterised by two phases — the early *ebb* or shock phase, and the subsequent *flow* or hypermetabolic phase.

Cuthbertson (1942) described the separation of these two phases in terms of energy expenditure — the ebb phase being one of depressed energy metabolism to conserve body resources for survival, while the flow phase was considered as a period of resurgence of energy metabolism which had some of the features of increased metabolism seen in inflammation. Cuthbertson also noted that the flow phase was characterised by marked increments in the excretion of nitrogen, sulphur, phosphorus, potassium, magnesium, zinc and creatinine, while the extracellular volume of the body was maintained or even expanded.

Table 6.3   Summary of hormone responses in trauma

Hormone	Ebb phase trauma	Flow phase trauma
Insulin	↓	→ ↑
Glucagon	↑	↑ ↑
Catecholamines	↑	↑ ↑
Glucocorticoids	↑	↑ ↑
Growth hormone	↑	↑ ↑

The ebb phase is characterised by a reduction in body temperature and oxygen consumption. There is an intracellular gain of sodium and water and loss of potassium as a result of alterations to the permeability of cell membranes and impairment of the sodium pump due to hypoxia. This situation is further compounded by an increased release of antidiuretic hormone (ADH) for the first day or so after injury, and secretion of aldosterone, and there may be oliguria. The sympatho-adrenal axis is activated in response to the assault, resulting in increased concentrations of catecholamines, glucocorticoids and glucagon (Table 6.3). There may be a transitory depression in the physiological responses to this hormonal discharge as a result of circulatory inadequacy or neurogenic shock.

The rate of carbohydrate oxidation is decreased in the ebb phase. Wilmore et al (1976) found in patients with burns that, during the ebb phase, total body glucose was elevated, but the mass flow of glucose through the expanded glucose space (extracellular fluid compartment) was only slightly greater than normal. The decrease in the rate of glucose disappearance was considered to be a reflection of impaired translocation of glucose into peripheral tissues as a result of decreased insulin release from the pancreas, mediated through increased sympathetic nervous system activity which is characterised by dominant alpha receptor stimulation of the pancreas during the ebb phase of injury.

If blood volume is restored, adequate oxygenation provided and sufficient circulation re-established, the patient moves from the ebb phase to the flow, or hypermetabolic, phase. This phase is characterised by increased blood concentrations of the catabolic hormones — the catecholamines, glucocorticoids and glucagon (Table 6.3). The insulin:glucagon molar ratio is decreased, despite elevated blood glucose concentration and normal insulin production in response to dominant beta-adrenergic stimulation of the pancreas. Hepatic gluconeogenesis is stimulated by this hormonal milieu to provide an essential supply of glucose for the healing wound. Glucagon acts centrally on the liver, the glucocorticoids induce mobilisation of amino acids which serve as glucose precursors, the catecholamines cause an efflux of lactic acid from muscle which is followed by an outpouring of 3-carbon amino acid fragments that convey carbon intermediates to the liver for conversion to new glucose. The released glucose is converted in muscle to pyruvate which may receive an amino group from the branched chain amino acids, oxidised in muscle, to form alanine. These 3-carbon intermediates are carried back to the liver for reconversion to new glucose via the Cori and alanine cycles. The nitrogen residue is simultaneously processed to urea and the rate of ureagenesis generally correlates with the rate of gluconeogenesis. The nitrogen loss may range from 10 g per day following an uncomplicated elective operation to 28 g or more per day with severe burns (see Fig. 6.1).

This energy shuttle system produces heat, and the rate of 6- to 3-carbon cycling correlates closely with the increased oxygen consumption characteristic of the flow phase of injury. Glucose oxidation is increased and the rate of glucose turnover is similarly increased. The oxidised glucose is replaced primarily from amino acids which are mobilised by skeletal muscle proteolysis and the lean body mass begins to deteriorate. The general increase in RME after multiple fractures is 10–30%, and after major burns it is from 40 to 100% (Fig. 6.2).

Traditionally the hypercatabolic response of thermal injury has been attributed mainly to accelerated evaporative water and heat losses from the wound surface, which impose a cooling load on the thermoregulating mechanisms of the body. However, it has been demonstrated recently that evaporative water loss is not the prime stimulator of the hypermetabolic response in the burn patient, but rather the increased energy production is related to an endogenous reset in metabolic activity which is then influenced by environmental conditions.

In addition to the acceleration of protein catabolism, there is an acceleration of fat catabolism which is stimulated by catecholamines, thyroxine and glucagon. Lipolysis is the major pathway for the supply of free fatty acids which serve as the major nonprotein energy source in traumatised patients. The glycerol released is taken up by the liver as a glucose precursor. There is little or no ketogenesis. Monitoring of all body functions is essential to detect changes in renal or pulmonary function as evidence of organ failure.

The use of parenteral nutrition at the height of the flow phase of injury requires detailed study of the effect of these concentrated nutrients on the altered metabolism. Nitrogen sparing through the use of peripherally administered amino acids has been advocated. Other workers have reported that the pattern of trauma is maintained irrespective of the nutritional regimen used. The role of amino acid solutions enriched with branched chain amino acids requires further evaluation.

Persistent fat oxidation occurs in the hypermetabolic injured patient, in spite of high concentrations of glucose which normally suppress fat oxidation. The infusion of glucose appears to increase hormone production, which in turn stimulates lipolysis. High carbohydrate loads significantly increase minute ventilation and oxygen consumption. The increase in carbon dioxide (CO_2) production is marked. Fat oxidation continues despite increased glucose oxidation — the respiratory quotient (RQ) remains below 1.0. For patients with inadequate respiratory reserves, glucose-induced increases in CO_2 production may precipitate respiratory failure. The replacement of a portion of the carbohydrate calories with fat during parenteral nutrition appears to circumvent the metabolic cost to the patient of converting glucose to fat.

In the acute (ebb) phase of stress, glucose infusion at a rate in excess of 250 mg/kg per hour will lead to lipogenesis rather than enhanced recovery. Glucose tolerance should be assessed by determining plasma and urinary glucose concentrations. Blood glucose concentrations in the range 9–11 mmol/l and in the absence of glycosuria, are acceptable in this altered hormonal state. Higher rates of glucose infusion, together with glucose provided through gluconeogenesis, will result in glycosuria with osmotic diuresis, lipogenesis with an elevated respiratory quotient and anaerobic glucose metabolism with lactate production. The protein requirement during this acute phase may be of the order of 2 g/kg per 24 hours, with a calorie to nitrogen ratio of 100:1 and energy requirement of 125 kJ (30 kcal)/kg per 24 hours, with 40% of the calories derived from carbohydrate.

During prolonged stress, such as is observed with major burns, nutritional support is effective only in preserving protein nutritional status and providing haemodynamic support. Reduction of the burn wound size by aggressive surgical excision and grafting may decrease both urea nitrogen production and dietary nitrogen requirements by reducing the catabolic stress. Restoration must await subsidence of the hypermetabolic phase.

SUMMARY

The metabolic effects of starvation, sepsis and trauma, and the role of parenteral nutrition during prolonged starvation and the hypermetabolic phases of sepsis and trauma are summarised in Table 6.4.

Severe infection and trauma are characterised by hypermetabolism, negative nitrogen balance and accelerated fluxes of substrates among organs. Oxygen consumption is elevated during the hypermetabolic phase, the increase being related to the severity of the insult. The extent of nitrogen loss in patients with normal liver and renal function depends upon the severity of the illness and the nutritional status of the patient, and represents a generalised proteolytic response of skeletal muscle. The increased rate of ureagenesis generally parallels the increased rate of gluconeogenesis.

Kinney has summarised in a Panel Report (1981) those aspects of nutritional support in sepsis or trauma requiring further elucidation. These include:

— a more fundamental understanding of the metabolic responses to trauma and infection, the effects of administration of concentrated nutrient

Table 6.4 Summary of metabolic effects of starvation, sepsis and trauma, and role of TPN

	Primary hormone(s)	Energy substrates	Substrate flux	Active process(es)	Role of TPN
Starvation (↓ BMR)	Glucagon	Glucose → Triglycerides → Alanine, glutamine ← Free fatty acids ← Ketone bodies ←	Storage sites (1° adipocytes) → liver and utilisation sites	Glycogenolysis* Gluconeogenesis* Proteolysis* Lipolysis Ketogenesis	Ketogenesis decreased Urinary nitrogen losses normalised Body cell mass and fat stores replenished
Sepsis (↑ BMR)	Glucagon Catecholamines Glucocorticoids	Glucose ← Triglycerides ← Alanine, glutamine ← †Free fatty acids ↓ BOHB, AcAc ↓ Lactate ←	Storage sites (1° muscle) → liver and utilisation sites	Gluconeogenesis Proteolysis Lipolysis† Ketogenesis* Ureagenesis	Little influence in the absence of control of septic process
Trauma 'flow' phase (↑ BMR)	Glucagon Catecholamines Glucocorticoids	Glucose ← Triglycerides ← Alanine, glutamine ← Free fatty acids ← ‡Ketone bodies ← Lactate ←	Storage sites (1° protein reserves and adipocytes) → liver and utilisation sites	Gluconeogenesis Proteolysis Lipolysis Ureagenesis	Effective in preserving protein status and haemodynamic support during hypermetabolic phase

* These processes are active in the early phase.
† Fat metabolism is altered — hepatic lipogenesis is decreased, lipolysis from adipose tissue is decreased. Free fatty acids are not increased, suggesting increased utilisation both in muscle and liver.
‡ There is little or no ketogenesis.

solutions on such responses, and also the effects of antibiotics, anaesthetics, analgesics and other drugs
— determination of the optimal balance between nitrogen and calorie intake. Additional information is required on protein turnover in individual organs and tissues and also interactions among amino acids within, and rates of their transfer between tissues, to permit interpretation of the altered free amino acid concentrations found in plasma and muscle of traumatised patients and to enable appropriate amino acid solutions to be formulated. Further studies are required to determine the optimal nonprotein caloric source for nutritional support of specific types of trauma, infection or organ dysfunction
— determination of the influence of trauma and infection on vitamin and mineral requirements
— characterisation of the mechanisms of inflammatory aspects of wound healing and the classical inflammation of host defence against infections both in nutritional depletion, and in response to nutritional therapy during various acute catabolic states
— elucidation of improved monitoring methods which will permit better measurement of the effectiveness of nutritional support.

REFERENCES AND FURTHER READING

Askanazi J, Nordenstrom J, Rosenbaum S H, Elwyn D H, Hyman A I, Carpentier Y A, Kinney J M Nutrition for the patient with respiratory failure: glucose vs fat. Anesthesiol 1981; 54: 373–377

Abbott W C, Schiller W R, Long C L, Birkhahn R H, Blakemore W S The effect of major thermal injury on plasma ketone body levels. JPEN 1985; 9: 153–158

Beisel W R, Wannemacher R W Jnr Gluconeogenesis, ureagenesis, and ketogenesis during sepsis. JPEN 1980; 4: 277–285

Birkhahn R H, Border J R Alternate or supplemental energy sources. JPEN 1981; 5: 24–31

Blackburn G L, Flatt J P, Clowes G H A, O'Donnell T E Peripheral intravenous feeding with isotonic amino acid solutions. Am J Surg 1973; 125: 447–454

Cahill G F Jnr Starvation in man. Clin Endocrin Metab 1976; 5: 397–415

Carpentier Y A, Askanazi J, Elwyn D H, Jeevanandam M, Gump F E, Hyman A I, Burr R, Kinney J M Effects of hypercaloric glucose infusion on lipid metabolism in injury and sepsis. J Trauma 1979; 19: 649–654

Cerra F B, Siegel J H, Coleman B, Border J R, McMenamy R R Septic autocannibalism: a failure of exogenous nutritional support. Ann Surg 1980; 192: 570–580

Cerra F B, Mazuski J E, Chute E, Nuwer N, Teasley K, Lysne J, Shronts E P, Konstantinides F N Branched chain metabolic support. A prospective, randomized, double-blind trial in surgical stress. Ann Surg 1984; 199: 286–291

Cuthbertson D P Post-shock metabolic response. Lancet 1942; i: 433–437

Felig P, Owen O E, Wahren J, Cahill G F Jnr Amino acid metabolism during prolonged starvation. J Clin Invest 1969; 48: 584–594

Freund H R, Ryan J A Jnr, Fischer J E Amino acid derangements in patients with sepsis: treatment with branched chain amino acid rich infusions. Ann Surg 1978; 188: 423–430

Kinney J M Energy deficits in acute illness and injury. In: Morgan A P (ed) Proceedings of the Conference on Energy Metabolism and Body Fuel Utilization. Harvard University Printing Office, Cambridge, 1966; p 173

Kinney J M, Duke J H Jnr, Long C L, Gump F E Tissue fuel and weight loss after injury. J Clin Path 1970; 23: (Suppl 4): 65–72

Konstantinidis N N, Teasley K, Lysne J, Shronts E, Olson G, Cerra F B Nutritional requirements of the hypermetabolic patient. Nutr Supp Serv 1984; 4(2): 41–50

Kudsk K A, Mirtallo J M Nutritional support of the critically ill patient. Drug Intell Clin Pharm 1983; 17: 501–506

Long C L, Schaffel N, Geiger J W, Schiller W R, Blakemore W S Metabolic response to injury and illness: estimation of energy and protein needs from indirect calorimetry and nitrogen balance. JPEN 1979; 3: 452–456

Nilsson F, Bake B, Berglin W-O E, Ekroth R, Holm J, Milocco I et al. Glucose and insulin infusion directly after cardiac surgery: effects on systemic glucose uptake, catecholamine excretion, O_2 consumption, and CO_2 production. JPEN 1985; 9: 159–164

Panel report on nutritional support of patients with trauma or infection. Am J Clin Nutr 1981; 34: 1213–1222

Wilmore D W Hormonal responses and their effect on metabolism. Surg Clin N Am 1976; 56: 999–1018

Wilmore D W, Mason A D Jnr, Pruitt B A Jnr Insulin response to glucose in hypermetabolic burn patients. Ann Surg 1976; 183: 314–320

7

Water and electrolytes

The volume and distribution of body water and concentration of electrolytes in the plasma and interstitial fluid and within cells become distorted in disease, trauma, sepsis, and following operation. Thus, to help the patient to maintain normal functional volumes of body fluids, normal concentrations of electrolytes, normal pH of plasma and interstitial fluid, and normal chemical and electrical gradients across cell membranes, careful consideration must be given to the administration of water and electrolytes to accommodate:

— maintenance, or baseline, requirements
— abnormal, ongoing, losses
— deficits or excesses.

WATER

Water is the principal component of the human body, and accounts for more than 50% of the total body weight. The actual total body water (TBW) content varies depending on the subject's fat content, sex, age and body weight. Isotope dilution studies have shown that in the normal adult male, less than 40 years old, the total body water content approximates 60%, whereas it approximates 50% in the normal female of comparative age.

The total body water is divided into two major compartments or fluid spaces — the intracellular fluid (ICF) compartment, and the extracellular fluid (ECF) compartment. In normal healthy adults, approximately 55% of the total body water is intracellular (33% of body weight) and the remaining 45% (27% of body weight) is extracellular. The extracellular fluid compartment is subdivided into the plasma (7.5% of TBW), interstitial fluid (20% of TBW), connective tissue water (7.5% of TBW), bone water (7.5% of TBW) and transcellular water (2.5% of TBW). These various fluid compartments also differ with respect to their electrolyte compositions. The constituents of the extracellular plasma compartment (serum) are measured frequently to diagnose fluid and electrolyte imbalances and to assist determine therapy.

The fluid requirement of an adult varies from patient to patient. While fluid input can be measured accurately, and water of metabolism calculated (see Appendix 4), fluid output is often difficult to estimate, especially in the patient with wound drainage and varying amounts of insensible loss. Weight changes are influenced not only by water gain or loss, but also by the effectiveness of nutrition.

The following explanation is provided to serve as a guide for the determination of daily water requirements. The baseline water requirement may be estimated from the patient's body surface area, allowing 1500 ml/m^2 per 24 hours. This formula provides adequate fluid to compensate for normal urinary excretion and faecal losses (1100–1500 ml/24 hours) and replacement of normal insensible water losses through respiration and sweating (800–1000 ml/24 hours). This formula also assumes that 350–500 ml/24 hours of endogenous water will be produced from the oxidation of fat and proteolysis.

The baseline water requirement may be increased by a number of factors which, essentially, are those that increase the insensible losses:

1. *fever* — results in hyperventilation and increased water evaporation. Endogenous water production also is increased. Allow approximately 110–150 ml/24 hours for each degree C above normal.
2. *excessive sweating* — is dependent on humidity. It is recommended that the baseline water requirement should be increased by 500 ml/24 hours for each 2.8°C (5.0°F) above 29°C (85°F) ambient temperature.
3. *increased metabolism* — for example, when the patient is converted to an anabolic state, additional water is required to substitute for endogenous water production and to provide new intracellular water.

A negative adjustment should be made if the patient is receiving humidified oxygen. The baseline water requirement also should be decreased in situations where there is an excessive amount of body water and the extracellular space is over-expanded as in patients with cardiac failure, renal failure or adult respiratory distress syndrome.

The next consideration in determining the fluid requirement is to allow for the measured external abnormal losses via the gastrointestinal tract, surgical wounds, drains or fistulae, and increased evaporation from the skin and respiratory tract. Consideration must be given to the electrolyte content of these fluids (Table 7.1), the pH and nitrogen content. When these losses are substantial, 1 litre or more per day, samples should be sent to the laboratory for analysis to enable adequate electrolyte replacement to be determined.

Sequestration of extracellular fluids into traumatised areas or infected tissues (third-spacing), or transcellular pooling within the gastrointestinal tract following intestinal obstruction, produce a decrease in the usual distribution of extracellular fluid without any loss of water from the body. If the volume of sequestered fluid is large, it must be replaced and a weight

Table 7.1 Range of electrolyte concentrations of gastrointestinal secretions and sweat. (Adapted from Randall, 1976)

| | *Electrolyte concentration* (mmol/l) | | | | |
	Na$^+$	K$^+$	H$^+$	Cl$^-$	HCO$_3^-$
Gastric Secretions	30–90	4.3–12	90*	52–155	—
Bile	134–156	3.9–6.3	—	83–110	35–50
Pancreatic Fluid	113–153	2.6–7.4	—	55–95	70–110
Small Bowel	72–128	3.5–6.8	—	69–127	10–30
Ileostomy Fluid	112–142	3.0–7.5	—	82–125	15–30
Diarrhoeal Fluid	50	35	—	40	45
Sweat	30–70	0–5	—	30–70	—

* Variable: e.g. achlorhydria

gain generally results. When the third space of sequestered fluid begins to resolve, plasma and intracellular fluid volumes expand, presenting a potential problem of water and electrolyte overloading.

Some patients may have deficits or excesses of some or all of the body compartment fluids prior to the institution of nutrition. For example, in the nutritionally depleted patient the ECF compartment expands while the ICF compartment contracts. These changes are accompanied by a relative increase in the total exchangeable sodium (Na$_e$) and decrease in the total exchangeable potassium (K$_e$). Other patients may develop significant abnormalities of volume, concentration and pH during treatment. The estimation and provision of water needs in dehydration and the recognition of over-expansion of the extracellular fluid volume constitute the third major consideration in determining fluid requirements.

In planning the volume to be used for parenteral nutrition solutions, allowance also must be made for obligatory fluid input separate from TPN, for example, for CVP readings or drug infusions. Fluid input may thus vary from 500 ml per day in the anuric patient, to 6 or more litres per day in the patient with excessive losses. The volume infused in most patients is 2–3 litres per day.

OSMOLALITY

Osmotic changes in the body, which may be induced by the infusion of hypertonic parenteral nutrition solutions, can alter the balance of water between the intracellular and extracellular fluid compartments. For example, a sudden increase in the concentration of glucose or other high molecular weight sugars will result in an increase in the extracellular fluid osmolality. Water shifts from cells into the extracellular fluid, resulting, when maximal renal tubular reabsorption is exceeded, in an osmotic diuresis. Unless sodium intake is maintained, prolonged osmotic diuresis leads to total body sodium depletion, and frank hyperosmolar hyperglycaemic nonketotic dehydration (HHND) will result.

Excessive water administration, particularly in the patient with reduced free renal water clearance, results in reduced extracellular osmolality as the glucose is metabolised, with dilutional overhydration of the cells and extracellular fluid. Inappropriate secretion of antidiuretic hormone (ADH), which may occur following injury, trauma or sepsis, results in water retention and a major alteration of body fluid balance.

The normal serum osmolality is 275–295 mOsm/kg. When the osmolality rises above 300 mOsm/kg due to water deficit, postural hypotension, severe weakness, fainting, CNS changes, stupor and coma occur. If the osmolality falls below 233 mOsm/kg due to water excess, seizures, stupor and coma occur.

ELECTROLYTE REQUIREMENTS

During the early period of nutritional support, the electrolyte requirements may vary considerably. Initially, total body deficits or excesses must be corrected. On conversion to the anabolic state, increased requirements for potassium, magnesium and phosphorus must be met. Once the anabolic state is established and the patient's condition begins to stabilise, electrolyte requirements also become relatively stable. The best estimate of electrolyte requirements is achieved through careful monitoring of losses, estimation of renal function, and regular analysis of serum electrolytes and monitoring of the effects of replacement therapy.

A brief explanation follows of the nutritional requirements for the various electrolytes, their actions, intake, regulation and excretion, and some important abnormalities associated with excesses or deficiencies of each.

SODIUM

The adult body contains approximately 3150 mmol of sodium, the major portion of which is present in the extracellular fluid where its concentration is maintained within the relatively narrow range of 135–145 mmol/l. The sodium concentration in the intracellular fluid is low, 10 mmol/l. This low intracellular concentration is maintained partly through the cell membrane's limited permeability to sodium, and, more importantly, by an active ion pump present in the cell membrane which provides for a tightly coupled sodium-potassium exchange across the cell membrane. Sodium and sodium transport thus play important roles in the establishment and maintenance of the cell membrane potential and in the transmission of neuromuscular impulses. Other important physiological functions of sodium are summarised in Table 7.2.

Sodium is readily absorbed from the gastrointestinal tract and distributed as outlined in Table 7.2. Of the total body sodium content, 60–70% is rapidly exchangeable (Na_e). The remaining 40% is non-exchangeable and is bound to bone matrix and other sites. The principal route of sodium

Table 7.2 Electrolyte summary — Sodium (Na)

Physiological function	Major cation in ECF; regulation of osmotic pressure and water balance in ECF; conductivity/excitability of nerves and muscles; active transport of glucose and amino acids
Absorption site	Small intestine; c. 100% absorption
Distribution	Total body content c. 3150 mmol (70 kg adult) c. 50% in ECF; 40–45% in bone; 5–10% in ICF
Regulation	By kidney — glomerular filtration rate; aldosterone; natriuretic hormone
Excretion	1° in urine; some in body secretions — sweat, gastrointestinal fluids
Recommended dietary intake	
Oral	50–145 mmol/24 h for adult
IV	1–2 mmol/kg per 24 h for adult
Evaluation of nutritional status	
Laboratory	Serum, normal range 135–145 mmol/l
Clinical	Mental status; neuromuscular function; cardiovascular function; renal function; gastrointestinal function; degree of dehydration
Deficiency	
Causes	Gastrointestinal losses, excessive sweating, renal losses, expansion of ECF (water intoxication)
Consequences	In cases of extracellular hypotonicity, cellular overhydration occurs; clinical features are vague and nonspecific — weakness, lethargy, confusion, delirium, convulsions, hypovolaemia leading to circulatory failure, impaired renal function; increased loss of appetite, nausea, vomiting
Toxicity	
Causes	Excessive sodium therapy, dehydration due to water restriction/excessive sweating, steroid therapy
Consequences	Extracellular hypertonicity results in cellular contraction; clinical features include CNS depression — lethargy, coma; hyperreactive reflexes, muscle rigidity, tremor, spasticity; chorea, convulsions, increased CSF protein; brain damage (especially in children); fever; thirst

excretion is via the kidneys. Urinary excretion normally increases or decreases in parallel with the sodium intake.

Sodium homeostasis is complex and involves a balance between intake and output, the maintenance of water balance and ECF osmolality. Alterations in the serum sodium concentration and osmolality are compensated rapidly by the osmotic movement of water. The hormones aldosterone and antidiuretic hormone (ADH) also participate in the regulation of sodium concentration by controlling sodium excretion in the urine and renal excretion of water, respectively.

In spite of these controls over sodium homeostasis, abnormalities of sodium concentration may develop. Some causes and consequences of these abnormalities, hyponatraemia (low sodium concentration) or hypernatraemia (high sodium concentration) are summarised in Table 7.2.

In addition to its role in restoring and/or maintaining extracellular fluid volume and osmolality in the patient receiving nutritional support, sodium plays a major role in the marked weight gain seen with glucose-based TPN. Most of this weight is accounted for by an increased retention of extracellular water (and inferentially, sodium). In the malnourished patient who is fed aggressively using glucose-based TPN, this rapid fluid gain may precipitate congestive heart failure. In addition, interstitial accumulation of sodium and water may interfere with gas exchange and precipitate respiratory failure.

The sodium input may vary from 30 to 40 mmol/24 hours to very high inputs (400–600 mmol/24 hours or more) if there is a high obligatory loss. The usual input is approximately 120 mmol/24 hours. In certain situations, analysis of electrolyte content of urine and gastrointestinal fluid will allow rational replacement.

POTASSIUM

Potassium is the major intracellular electrolyte, where its concentration is estimated to be approximately 140 mmol/l. The extracellular concentration, in contrast, is very low, 3.1–4.8 mmol/l. Potassium plays a major role in the determination of cell membrane resting potential and thus abnormalities of potassium homeostasis impair nerve impulse conduction, neuromuscular conduction and cardiac rhythm. Other important physiological functions of potassium are summarised in Table 7.3.

Potassium is readily absorbed from the gastrointestinal tract, mainly the small intestine, and distributed as outlined in Table 7.3. Normally, there is a small obligatory faecal loss of potassium of approximately 10 mmol/24 hours. However, disturbances such as vomiting, diarrhoea and fistulae cause a significant increase in gastrointestinal potassium losses.

Virtually all of the total body potassium appears to be exchangeable, and approximately 98% of K_e is considered to be intracellular. In healthy individuals, the ratio of $Na_e:K_e$ approximates 0.85 in males and 1.0 in females. In illness, such as trauma, sepsis, prolonged inadequate nutrition, cardiac or renal insufficiency, the ratio $Na_e:K_e$ rises and values of 1.5 or higher are not unusual in debilitated or oedematous individuals.

The major route of potassium excretion is the kidneys. The potassium in the glomerular filtrate is reabsorbed almost totally in the proximal tubule and then secreted in the distal tubule. The major factors regulating urinary potassium excretion are the mineralocorticoid hormone, aldosterone, the activity of the sodium-potassium ATP-ase enzyme, distal tubular flow and acid-base balance which influences urinary potassium and hydrogen ion excretion.

Table 7.3   Electrolyte summary — Potassium (K)

Physiological function	Major cation in ICF; regulation of osmotic pressure, water balance in ICF; regulation of acid-base balance; regulation of nerve and muscle excitability; participation in some enzyme systems, carbohydrate metabolism, protein synthesis
Absorption site	Upper gastrointestinal tract; c. 100% absorption
Distribution	Total body content c. 4000 mmol (70 kg adult); c. 2% in ECF; > 95% in ICF
Regulation	Redistribution across cell membranes — insulin, glucagon, adrenaline, acid-base status; renal excretion — aldosterone; acid-base status; Na/K ATP-ase activity; distal tubular flow rate
Excretion	1° in urine; some in gastrointestinal fluid, faeces
Recommended dietary intake	
Oral	50–145 mmol/24 h for adult
IV	1–2 mmol/kg per 24 h for adult
Evaluation of nutritional status	
Laboratory	Serum, normal range 3.1–4.8 mmol/l; acid-base balance
Clinical	Neuromuscular function; gastrointestinal function; cardiac abnormalities; renal abnormalities; mental status
Deficiency	
Causes	Decreased intake, redistribution, increased losses — gastrointestinal losses; excessive renal losses — diuretics, glucocorticoids, amphotericin; inadequate intake
Consequences	Muscular weakness, paralysis; paralytic ileus; cardiac conduction defects, arrhythmias; decreased renal concentrating ability, chloride-resistant metabolic alkalosis, renal insufficiency; depression, confusion
Toxicity	
Causes	Rapid excessive administration; contraction of volume of ECF; crush injuries, haemolysis, metabolic acidosis; renal failure, Addison's disease
Consequences	Muscular weakness, paraesthesia; conduction defects, arrhythmias, bradycardia; nausea, vomiting, ileus

Abnormalities of potassium homeostasis (hypokalaemia and hyper-kalaemia) are listed in Table 7.3, together with some of their causes and consequences. Acid-base status also influences the distribution of potassium between the ICF and ECF with the serum potassium concentration varying inversely with the pH.

Potassium plays an important role in the cellular uptake of glucose and the administration of glucose-based TPN facilitates an increase in the total body potassium. The addition of insulin further increases the intracellular uptake of potassium. When the patient enters the anabolic phase, his potassium requirement increases to satisfy intracellular utilisation of potassium in protein synthesis (2.7 mmol K/1 g N) and glycogen synthesis

(0.33 mmol K/1 g glycogen). Thus, potassium requirements may be very high in the presence of anabolism or excessive losses, or very low in severe catabolism.

Our usual input is 80–120 mmol/24 hours, but we have had to range from 0 to 600 mmol/24 hours in extreme situations to maintain the serum potassium within the normal range. Frequent measurement of serum potassium concentration is obviously essential if the daily potassium input is high. Determination of total exchangeable potassium (Ke) provides a measure of body cell mass and permits the efficacy of parenteral nutrition to be assessed.

CALCIUM

Calcium is the most abundant electrolyte in the human body, accounting for approximately 2% of the total body weight of adult man. It is deposited in bone and teeth where, with phosphate, it forms the crystal structure hydroxyapatite which provides strength and rigidity. A small portion of the surface crystals provides calcium which is readily exchangeable with the extracellular calcium and tissue calcium. The small pool of calcium in the plasma plays an important role in blood coagulation. Other important physiological functions involving ionised calcium include its roles in neuromuscular and cardiac function and are listed in Table 7.4.

Dietary calcium is absorbed principally in the small intestine. Absorption is stimulated by the vitamin D derivative 1,25-dihydroxycholecalciferol ($1,25(OH)_2 D_3$), which also stimulates the absorption of magnesium and phosphate. Normal gastric acidity also promotes calcium absorption, while decreasing gastric acidity diminishes absorption. Absorption is inhibited by phosphates, oxalates and phytates. The proportion of calcium absorbed is directly related to the body's requirement for calcium. Generally 60–80% of the oral intake appears in the faeces. The remainder is absorbed and excreted in the urine.

The extracellular calcium concentration is maintained within narrow limits by an efficient feedback-control system. In response to a diminished serum calcium concentration parathyroid hormone (PTH) is secreted. PTH acts by stimulating bone resorption and increasing urinary phosphate excretion and renal calcium reabsorption to increase the serum calcium concentration. Increased serum calcium decreases PTH secretion. Calcitonin is secreted in response to an elevated serum calcium concentration and effects lowering of the serum calcium by inhibiting bone resorption, and renal excretion of calcium is increased.

Abnormalities of calcium homeostasis are summarised in Table 7.4, together with common causes and consequences. Increased urinary calcium excretion has been reported in patients receiving TPN. Possible contributing factors include prolonged periods of muscle rest and high parenteral intake of protein or glucose.

Table 7.4 Electrolyte summary — Calcium (Ca)

Physiological function	Mineralisation of bone, teeth; regulation of neuromuscular transmission, muscular contraction; complement activation; fibrinolysis activation; blood clotting mechanisms; activation of some enzymes
Absorption site	Small intestine, particularly ileum, c. 20–40% absorption
Distribution	Total body content c. 32 500 mmol (70 kg adult); c. < 0.1% in ECF (c. 40–50% free ionised Ca^{++}); 1% in soft tissue, teeth; 99% in bone
Regulation	Gastrointestinal tract; kidney; bone; vitamin D, parathyroid hormone, calcitonin
Excretion	1° in urine — 3.75 mmol/24 h; some in faeces — 2.5 mmol/24 h
Recommended dietary intake	
*Oral	20 mmol/24 h for adult
IV	0.1–0.15 mmol/kg per 24 h for adult
Evaluation of nutritional status	
Laboratory	Serum, normal range 2.15–2.55 mmol/l; urine, normal range 2.5–7.5 mmol/day — increases with TPN, immobilisation
Clinical	Neuromuscular function; mental status; cardiovascular function; gastrointestinal function; renal function; bones; eyes; skin
Deficiency	
Causes	Hypoparathyroidism; magnesium depletion; vitamin D deficiency; acute pancreatitis; renal failure; hyperphosphataemia; false hypo-calcaemia-albuminaemia
Consequences	Paraesthesias, tetany, muscle cramps; rickets, osteomalacia; cataracts; seizures, confusion; skin hyperpigmentation; hypotension and cardiac conduction abnormalities
Toxicity	
Causes	Malignancies; 1° hyperparathyroidism; endocrine disorders; immobilisation; hypervitaminosis D or A; thiazides
Consequences	Nausea, anorexia, gastric hyperacidity, vomiting; abdominal pain; pancreatitis; polyuria; confusion, stupor, coma; fatiguability, muscle weakness; ectopic calcification; cardiac arrhythmias

* recommended daily dietary allowance (RDA)

Positive calcium and phosphate balances can be achieved in patients receiving TPN. Calcium intakes reported to produce positive calcium balance range from 4.5 to 12.5 mmol/24 hours with phosphorus intakes ranging from 15 to 40 mmol/24 hours. Our routine maintenance input is 2.2 mmol calcium and 15 mmol phosphate per litre of solution. We omit these electrolytes in renal failure until plasma electrolyte concentrations are available to guide us.

MAGNESIUM

Magnesium is the second most abundant intracellular cation. Approximately 50% of the total body content is located in bone, adsorbed to hydroxyapatite, and 30% of this is readily exhangeable. The tissues of the liver, heart and skeletal muscles contain significant proportions of the remaining 50%. Magnesium is necessary for the synthesis of proteins and nucleic acids and plays an important role in the activation of many enzyme systems, including some involved in the metabolism of glucose for energy. Magnesium often is associated with enzyme systems that require thiamine

Table 7.5   Electrolyte summary — Magnesium (Mg)

Physiological function	Co-factor for many enzyme systems (e.g. ATP-ase); cell permeability regulation; neuromuscular excitability; bone function; DNA function
Absorption site	$1°$ in small intestine; 30–40% absorption
Distribution	Total body content c. 1125 mmol (70 kg adult); c. < 2% in ECF (c. 55% free ionised Mg^{++}); 44% in soft tissue; 54% in bone
Regulation	Hormones — thyroid, growth, parathormone, aldosterone, vasopressin; ion balance across cell membranes; renal excretion
Excretion	$1°$ in faeces; urine
Recommended dietary intake	
*Oral	12.4–14.4 mmol/24 h for adult
IV	0.1–0.2 mmol/kg per 24 h for adult
Evaluation of nutritional status	
Laboratory	Serum, normal range 0.75–1.0 mmol/1; urine, normal range 2.5–5.0 mmol/24 h
Clinical	Neuromuscular function; cardiac function; gastrointestinal function; mental status
Deficiency	
Causes	Decreased intake; malabsorption; prolonged TPN; gastrointestinal losses; acute pancreatitis; hepatic cirrhosis; renal losses; endocrine and metabolic disorders
Consequences	Lethargy, neuromuscular excitability, cramps, tetany; paraesthesias; nausea, vomiting, abdominal pain; cardiac arrhythmias; hypocalcaemia, hypokalaemia; mental status changes
Toxicity	
Causes	Mg^{++} containing medications; acute and chronic renal failure; adrenal insufficiency, hypothyroidism, uncontrolled diabetes mellitus; metabolic acidosis
Consequences	Impaired neuromuscular function; decreased cardiac contraction, hypotension; stupor and coma; respiratory centre depression

* recommended daily dietary allowance (RDA)

pyrophosphate as a co-factor. Other important physiological functions of magnesium are listed in Table 7.5.

Absorption of magnesium occurs principally in the upper small bowel and, under normal conditions, approximately 40% of the dietary intake is absorbed. Magnesium absorption is enhanced by the presence of protein and vitamin D, or its metabolites. PTH and growth hormone appear to facilitate its absorption. High dietary intakes of calcium, phosphorus, fat and phytates appear to inhibit its absorption. The kidney exerts a major influence on magnesium turnover by effectively reabsorbing most of the magnesium filtered in the glomerulus. Renal tubular reabsorption is increased by PTH and when calcium intakes are low. Reabsorption is reduced when calcium or magnesium intakes are high and in the presence of aldosterone, thyroid hormone, growth hormone and antidiuretic hormone.

Magnesium, like calcium, is present in the plasma in two distinct forms — free ionised magnesium and protein bound magnesium. The free ionised form is thought to be the biologically active form and accounts for approximately 60% of the serum magnesium concentration. Abnormalities of the serum magnesium concentration leading to hypomagnesaemia or hypermagnesaemia are summarised in Table 7.5. Many of the important clinical manifestations are related to altered neuromuscular and/or cardiovascular function.

Plasma concentrations of magnesium decrease when TPN is instituted. The insulin stimulated cellular uptake of glucose also is accompanied by an increased uptake of phosphorus and magnesium, as well as potassium. Intracellular magnesium is depleted during malnutrition and, in order to promote nitrogen retention, large quantities of magnesium may be required during refeeding. It has been suggested that approximately 15 mmol should be given per day to replenish body stores and to optimise nitrogen retention. Increased magnesium input also is required in the presence of gastrointestinal fluid losses. Our routine maintenance input in the patient with normal renal function and no additional losses is 2.5 mmol per litre of solution.

PHOSPHATE

Phosphate is the major intracellular anion and is involved in the integrity of the cell wall. Phosphate is an important constituent of bone (Table 7.6), and bone mineralisation is highly dependent on phosphorus and calcium absorption from the gastrointestinal tract. The phosphate buffer system (Na_2HPO_4 and NaH_2PO_4) is biologically important in the maintenance of acid-base balance. Phosphorus also participates in a variety of metabolic reactions, including the phosphorylation of glucose and the production of high-energy phosphate compounds, the most important of which is adenosine triphosphate (ATP), nucleic acid, phosphoprotein and phospholipid

Table 7.6 Electrolyte summary — Phosphate (Inorganic phosphorus)

Physiological function	Major anion in ICF; mineralisation of bone; phosphate buffer system — acid-base balance; high energy bonds — ATP; 2,3-DPG-oxygen carriage, haemoglobin; component of nucleic acids, phosphoproteins, phospholipids
Absorption site	Jejunum, stomach, c. 75% absorption
Distribution	Total body content c. 22 600 mmol (70 kg adult); c. < 0.1% in ECF; 15% in soft tissues, teeth; 85% in bone
Regulation	Parathyroid hormone; 1,25-dihydroxycholecalciferol; calcitonin
Excretion	1° in urine; some in faeces
Recommended dietary intake	
★Oral	25.8 mmol/24 hours for adult; the ratio of Ca: PO_4 being less than 1 in adult and 1–1.5 during periods of growth (e.g. infancy)
IV	0.5–0.7 mmol/kg per 24 h
Evaluation of nutritional status	
Laboratory	Serum, normal range 0.6–1.25 mmol/l
Clinical	Muscular function, haematological abnormalities; skeletal abnormalities, ectopic calcification; acid-base disturbance; impaired renal function
Deficiency	
Causes	1° hyperparathyroidism; vitamin D deficiency or resistance; renal tubular defect; alkalosis; low dietary intake; glucose and insulin administration; chronic alcoholism
Consequences	Impaired cellular energy stores; tissue hypoxia; paraesthesias, weakness; rickets, osteomalacia; haematological abnormalities; skeletal abnormalities; reduced renal tubular bicarbonate reabsorption
Toxicity	
Causes	Hypoparathyroidism; vitamin D toxicity; renal failure; high phosphate intake; malignancies; severe catabolic states; acidosis
Consequences	No specific clinical sequelae, but persistent hyperphosphotaemia influences calcium homeostasis with ectopic calcification; secondary hyperparathyroidism; renal osteodystrophy

★ recommended daily dietary allowance (RDA)

synthesis. An important phosphate containing enzyme is erythrocyte 2,3-diphosphoglycerate (2,3-DPG) which is involved in oxygen carriage and release by haemoglobin.

Dietary phosphate is absorbed principally in the jejunum, with some absorption occurring in the stomach and the remainder in the small intestine. Phosphate absorption is linked to sodium absorption (mmol for mmol) and a decreased pH favours $H_2PO_4^-$ absorption. PTH and vitamin D enhance absorption of phosphate from the jejunum. Phosphate absorption also increases as the amount of phosphate in the diet increases.

The absorbed phosphate is excreted by the kidneys and some is lost in the faeces. A renal threshold exists for phosphate excretion and urinary losses occur only if this threshold is exceeded. PTH increases the renal excretion of phosphate by decreasing its tubular reabsorption. PTH also promotes bone resorption which increases the amount of phosphate released into the ECF. Hyperglycaemia decreases the tubular reabsorption of phosphate. Vitamin D also may positively influence renal phosphate excretion, although some workers claim it decreases phosphate excretion.

As outlined in Table 7.6, the majority of body phosphate is distributed in bone, muscle and other body cells. Much of the intracellular phosphate is sequestered in mitochondria and organelles as amorphous insoluble tricalcium phosphate. An exchangeable phosphate pool of approximately 100 mmol exists in the bone phosphate. Inorganic phosphate also is present and may enter the organic phase by participating in the conversion of glyceraldehyde-3-P to 3-phosphoglycerate, of ADP to ATP and during glycogenolysis with the formation of glucose-3-phosphate.

Although moderate changes in plasma phosphate concentrations can be tolerated without significant effect, hypophosphataemia has been reported as a complication of TPN, due to the various metabolic effects associated with phosphate depletion. Some other causes and consequences of hypophosphataemia, as well as hyperphosphataemia, are summarised in Table 7.6.

Ingestion of high carbohydrate containing diets or infusion of glucose-based TPN, may result in hypophosphataemia and hypomagnesaemia due to increased cellular uptake and utilisation of these electrolytes in response to glucose-mediated insulin release. This rapid decrease in the extracellular fluid concentration of phosphate is associated with a clinical syndrome consisting of disorientation, tremor, convulsions and coma. Hypophosphataemia may be avoided and protein synthesis optimised by administering at least 15 mmol of phosphate per litre of TPN or approximately 15 mmol per 3150–4200 kJ (750–1000 kcal). If the cachetic individual becomes hypophosphataemic during TPN, then the carbohydrate load must be reduced and the phosphate load increased to achieve and maintain a normal serum phosphate concentration.

CHLORIDE

Chloride, the most abundant extracellular anion, is also present in the intracellular fluid, but at a lower concentration of approximately 4 mmol/l. Chloride plays an important role in maintaining the osmotic pressure of the ECF, and its distribution across the cell membrane is determined by the electrical potential. The physiological functions of chloride are summarised in Table 7.7.

Chloride is absorbed readily from the gastrointestinal tract. Excretion occurs principally in the urine, although significant quantities may be lost

Table 7.7   Electrolyte summary — Chloride (Cl)

Physiological function	Major anion in ECF; present in ICF; regulation of osmotic pressure in ECF; acid-base balance; cell membrane electrical potential; gastrointestinal secretions
Absorption site	Gastrointestinal tract, c. 100%
Distribution	Total body content c. 2300 mmol (70 kg adult) predominantly in ECF; small concentration in ICF and bone
Regulation	Associated with regulation of major cations in maintenance of electrical neutrality; reciprocal relationship between chloride and bicarbonate retention/excretion; aldosterone enhances renal tubular reabsorption
Excretion	In gastrointestinal fluids; urine; sweat — closely related to sodium excretion
Recommended dietary intake	
Oral	50–145 mmol/24 h for adult
IV	1.3–1.9 mmol/kg per 24 h
Evaluation of nutritional status	
Laboratory	Serum, normal range 93–103 mmol/l
Clinical	Gastrointestinal function; renal function; acid-base balance; dehydration
Deficiency	
Causes	Gastrointestinal losses; low salt intake; diuretics; potassium depletion and alkalosis; sweating with adequate fluid intake; diabetic ketosis, renal losses
Consequences	Hypochloraemic hypokalaemic alkalosis — consequences are those of 1° disease
Toxicity	
Causes	Excessive chloride intake; dehydration; hyperchloraemic acidosis; excess sodium in advanced renal disease; respiratory alkalosis; drug therapy, e.g. acetazolamide
Consequences	Hyperchloraemic acidosis — appears to have no deleterious effects

in the sweat and gastrointestinal fluids (see Table 7.1). Body balance of chloride is regulated in association with the regulation of the major cations (Na^+ and K^+) in order to maintain electrical neutrality.

Aldosterone enhances renal tubular reabsorption of chloride and sodium present in the glomerular filtrate, while increasing the renal excretion of potassium and hydrogen ions. Chloride also shares a reciprocal relationship with bicarbonate, so that an increase in the concentration of one of these anions is associated with a decrease in the serum concentration of the other (i.e. changes in acid-base balance due to altered bicarbonate may be reflected by changes in the chloride concentration). Abnormalities of chloride balance are listed in Table 7.7.

Table 7.8 Electrolyte content of some amino acid solutions (mmol/l)

Electrolytes	Aminofusin L® 10%	Aminosyn® 7% –elec*	Aminosyn® 7% +elec*	Synthamin® (equivalent to Travasol®)						Vamin N® 7%
				9 (5.5%) +elec†	9 (5.5%) –elec†	13 (8%) +elec†	13 (8%) –elec†	17 (10%) +elec†	17 (10%) –elec†	
Sodium	40	—	70	70	—	70	—	70	—	50
Potassium	30	5.4	66	60	—	60	—	60	—	20
Magnesium	5	—	5	5	—	5	—	5	—	1.5
Calcium	—	—	—	—	—	—	—	—	—	2.5
Acetate	10	88	124	100	45	130	66	150	82	55
Chloride	27.5	—	96	70	22	62	32	70	40	55
Phosphate	—	—	30	30	—	30	—	30	—	—
Malate	5	—	—	—	—	—	—	—	—	—
Sulphate	—	—	—	—	—	—	—	—	—	1.5
Approx mOsm/l	1015	700	1013	850	520	1070	810	1300	1000	690
Approx pH	5.5	5.3	5.3	6.0	6.0	6.0	6.0	6.0	6.0	5.2

* Includes 5.4 mmol K/l from the antioxidant, potassium metabisulphite
† Sodium metabisulphite is present as a stabiliser and provides approximately 3 mmol Na/l

Chloride input may need to be varied during TPN, although often it will be in the range of 120 mmol/24 hours. We have found that when low acetate containing amino acid solutions are used, sodium may be added as the chloride salt, but potassium as acetate or phosphate to maintain a balanced ratio between chloride and acetate. However, when the acetate or phosphate input is already high, potassium is best added as the chloride salt. Regular measurement of plasma chloride and bicarbonate is necessary to detect potential balance problems. Primary hypochloraemia may be the cause of a persisting metabolic alkalosis, which will disappear with adequate sodium, potassium and chloride replacement.

ELECTROLYTE ADDITIVES

The concentrations of electrolytes in the commercially prepared L-amino acid solutions may not provide an adequate electrolyte intake for every patient (see Tables 7.8 & 9.7). It is usually necessary to add electrolytes to the commercial amino acid preparations, or to use an amino acid formulation without electrolytes and tailor the electrolyte content to meet the patient's requirements. Practical problems associated with addition of electrolytes to solutions, for example, calcium phosphate precipitation, are dealt with in Chapter 25.

REFERENCES AND FURTHER READING

Barratt L J Sodium metabolism. Anaesth Intens Care 1977; 5: 305–316
Epstein F H Signs and symptoms of electrolyte disorders. In: Maxwell M H, Kleeman C R (eds) Clinical Disorders of Fluid and Electrolyte Metabolism (3rd edn). McGraw Hill Book Co, New York, 1980, p 499–530
Food and Nutrition Board. Recommended dietary allowances (9th edn). National Academy of Sciences — National Research Council, Washington DC, 1980
Kaminski M V Jnr A review of hyperosmolar hyperglycemic nonketotic dehydration (HHND): etiology, pathophysiology and prevention during intravenous hyperalimentation. JPEN 1978; 2: 690–698
Main A N H, Morgan R J, Russell R I, Hall M J, MacKenzie J F, Shenkin A, Fell G S Mg deficiency in chronic inflammatory bowel disease and requirements during intravenous nutrition. JPEN 1981; 5: 15–19
Pigon J, Lindholm M, Eklund J, Hagelback A Phosphate supplementation in parenteral nutrition. Acta Anaesthesiol Scand 1985; 29: 50–54
Randall H T Fluid, electrolyte, and acid-base balance. Surg Clin N Am 1975; 56: 1019–1058
Shizgal H M Body composition and nutritional support. Surg Clin N Am 1981; 61: 729–741
Sloan G M, White D E, Brennan M F Calcium and phosphorus metabolism during total parenteral nutrition. Ann Surg 1983; 197: 1–6
Starker P M, Askanazi J, Lasala P A, Elwyn D H, Gump F E, Kinney J M The effect of parenteral nutrition repletion on muscle water and electrolytes. Implications for body composition. Ann Surg 1983; 198: 213–217
Stockigt J R Potassium metabolism. Anaesth Intens Care 1977; 5: 317–325
Thomas D W Calcium, phosphorus and magnesium turnover. Anaesth Intens Care 1977; 5: 361–371
Walmsley R N, Guerin M D Disorders of Fluid and Electrolyte Balance. John Wright & Sons Ltd, Bristol, 1984

8

Carbohydrate and other caloric sources

A number of carbohydrate and other caloric sources have been used as energy substrates in parenteral nutrition to facilitate the proper use of nitrogen and to correct energy deficits. The minimum requirement for carbohydrate is difficult to define. For individuals partaking of an average diet, it has been estimated that a minimum of 100 g of carbohydrate (20–25% of the total caloric intake) are required to avoid ketosis, increased protein catabolism and other undesirable metabolic effects. To facilitate the appropriate utilisation of nitrogen sources, at least 30 g of carbohydrate (500 kJ or 120 kcal) should be provided per 1 g of nitrogen administered.

GLUCOSE (Dextrose)

All body cells have the capacity to oxidise glucose, either aerobically via the Embden-Meyerhoff pathway to pyruvate, or anaerobically to lactate. Pyruvate and lactate then can be oxidised further via the tricarboxylic acid cycle to yield energy (see Fig. 5.1). As discussed earlier, the metabolic utilisation of glucose, including oxidation, is dependent on the presence of insulin to facilitate its entrance into body cells.

When insulin synthesis is inhibited, for example in the early post-traumatic state when there is increased secretion of catecholamines, the uptake of glucose into cells is reduced and there is a risk of hyperglycaemia and glycosuria. In this situation it has been reported that up to 21% of the administered glucose, infused at the rate of 500 mg/kg per hour, may be lost through renal overflow.

The infusion of excessive quantities of glucose above that required to meet the basal metabolic rate (BMR), and for the synthesis of lean body tissue, results in lipogenesis with a marked increase in carbon dioxide production (VCO_2) and a lesser increase in oxygen consumption (VO_2). The magnitude of these changes is a function of the patient's clinical state and the glucose load. In the nutritionally depleted patient, lipogenesis occurs and this is associated with a rise in the non-protein respiratory quotient (RQ), often above 1.0 (RQ of glucose is 1.0), an increase in the resting metabolic expenditure (RME) and a greater increase in VCO_2 (Fig. 8.1).

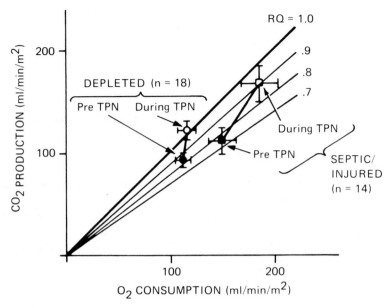

Fig. 8.1 Changes in oxygen (O_2) consumption and carbon dioxide (CO_2) production, induced by glucose based-TPN in depleted and hypermetabolic patients. (Adapted with permission of Askanazi et al, 1980, and the Editor, Annals of Surgery)

In the hypermetabolic patient (for example, after major trauma or sepsis) fat oxidation is suppressed only partially, lipogenesis may be inhibited, RME rises sharply and there appears to be a massive deposition of glycogen. The result of these processes is a large increase in VCO_2 and VO_2, while the total and non-protein RQ usually remain below 1.0 (Fig. 8.1). The effects of glucose loading in excess of energy requirements on patterns of gas exchange in depleted and hypermetabolic patients are summarised in Table 8.1. In both these situations, the increased CO_2 production represents a respiratory load which may become clinically significant, especially in the hypermetabolic patient. Respiratory distress may be precipitated in the patient with borderline respiratory function.

An RQ of greater than 1.0 has been reported with a glucose infusion rate of 9 mg/kg per minute in post-operative patients. If 50% of the non-protein carbohydrate calories are replaced with a fat emulsion, however, there is a significant reduction in VCO_2 in both nutritionally depleted patients and acutely ill patients. In addition, the increase in VO_2 is significantly less in the acutely ill patients.

The effects of increased glucose intake on glucose metabolism in trauma patients may be summarised as:

— plasma glucose concentrations are maintained at the already high level associated with trauma, but are not significantly increased

Table 8.1 Effects of glucose loading on gas exchange, fuel utilisation and storage

	Depleted patient	Hypermetabolic patient
Carbon dioxide production	↑	↑ ↑
Oxygen consumption	sl ↑	↑
Respiratory quotient (RQ)	> 1	< 1
Lipogenesis	↑ ↑	? →
FFA oxidation	↓ ↓ ↓	↓
Glycogen deposition	↑	↓ ↓

sl = slight increase

— rates of glucose oxidation and non-oxidative metabolism increase proportionately with intake
— there is an abnormally high rate of glycogen deposition which is proportional to glucose intake
— gluconeogenesis from protein is abnormally high, but can be completely suppressed with an intake of approximately 600 g of glucose per day
— glucose recycling with glycogen, glycerol or both, is increased with increasing intake.

Fatty infiltration of the liver and the development of liver function abnormalities (including elevated SGOT, SGPT, bilirubin and alkaline phosphatase) appear to be correlated with the infusion of excess calories as glucose both in malnourished and hypermetabolic patients. However, these derangements also have been reported during the administration of TPN using lipids as the primary caloric source. The use of cyclic parenteral nutrition has been proposed as a means of minimising this problem. Investigations to determine the maximal rate of glucose infusion beyond which physiologically significant increases in protein synthesis and direct oxidation of glucose no longer occur, indicate that there is little increase when the infusion rate exceeds 5 mg/kg per minute in burn patients, and 6–7 mg/kg per minute in general surgical patients.

Concentrated solutions of glucose are hypertonic, the osmolality of a 20% solution being 1250 mOsm/kg water. In addition, the pH of these solutions is low, 3–5, hence they should be administered via the central venous route to prevent phlebitis. One gram of anhydrous glucose provides 15.7 kJ (3.76 kcal) of energy on complete oxidation.

If solutions containing glucose and amino acids or peptides are sterilised by autoclaving, the content of available amino acids is lowered. This loss begins with the Maillard reaction — an amino group on a free amino acid or on the side chain of a protein-bound amino acid combines with the carbonyl carbon of the reducing sugar to form an N-glycosylamino derivative (Fig. 8.2). The Amadori rearrangement then converts this derivative to a 1-amino-1-deoxy-2-ketose derivative, and the browning reaction with the formation of complex polymers then proceeds along complex pathways.

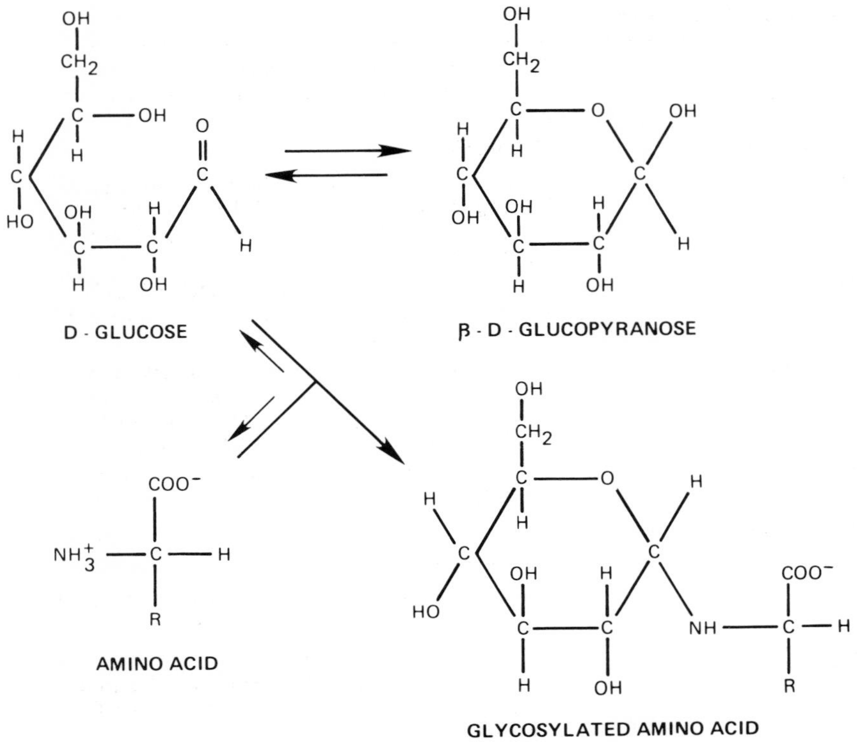

Fig. 8.2 Formation of N-glycosylated amino acid.

Browning also will occur during ordinary storage of glucose-amino acid solutions sterilised by filtration.

Mild dehydration in infants has been reported in association with the infusion of these compounds. Excessive excretion of zinc and other trace metals has been observed in infants and adults.

Glucose has been used extensively in parenteral nutrition and is the preferred caloric source. Its principal properties are summarised in Table 8.2. To minimise the adverse effects associated with excessive infusion, the balance of the caloric requirements may be infused as lipid. In some countries, extra calories are supplied as fructose, sorbitol or xylitol.

Fourth-hourly urinalysis and daily blood sugar usually are adequate monitors of the infused glucose load, but in the difficult patient, fourth-hourly blood sugars may be necessary. Rebound hypoglycaemia may be avoided by reducing glucose input over a 24 hour period prior to cessation, and by impressing on staff the danger of allowing the infusion to stop.

INSULIN

Patients vary in their tolerance to glucose. Provided the load is increased

Table 8.2 Glucose summary

Physiological function	Principal energy source of cellular metabolism; stored in cells as glycogen; converted to triglycerides in adipose tissue
Absorption site	1° in proximal small bowel
Distribution	Blood and tissue fluids — c. 15% of ingested glucose (10–20 g in adults); in tissues, 1° liver, muscle — as glycogen, c. 85% of ingested glucose; adipose tissue — as triglyceride
Metabolism	Aerobic to pyruvic acid yielding NADH and ATP; anaerobic to lactic acid yielding ATP; ultimately to CO_2 and H_2O via TCA cycle
Regulation	Elevated blood glucose stimulates insulin release, which stimulates tissue uptake, promoting glycogenesis; decreased blood glucose suppresses insulin release; glucagon maintains blood concentration via glycogenolysis
Excretion	In urine; renal threshold — (adult): 1.8 ± 0.4 mmol (323 ± 64 mg)/min
Recommended dietary intake	
Oral	Minimum intake: 100 g/24 h
IV	4–7 mg/kg per min, maximum IV rate; for appropriate nitrogen utilisation, 30 g glucose/1 g nitrogen
Evaluation of nutritional status	
Laboratory	Blood glucose (fasting): 3–5.5 mmol/l; blood glucose (during TPN): < 7 mmol/l; urine glucose (normal): 0.06–0.84 mmol/l
Clinical	Fluid volume; mental status; thirst; urinary frequency
Deficiency	
Causes	Insulin excess; deficiency in available glycogen; immaturity; renal glycosuria; reactive hypoglycaemia with sudden cessation of TPN
Consequences	Sweating, tremor, anxiety, palpitations; depressed consciousness, coma, seizures
Toxicity	
Causes	Increasing circulating adrenaline, e.g. in stressed patient; decreased insulin output, insulin resistance; pituitary, adrenal disorders; pancreatic disease; vitamin B_1 deficiency; diabetic ketoacidosis; hyperglycaemic nonketotic coma
Consequences	Hyperosmolality, volume depletion, metabolic acidosis; polyuria, polydipsia; weight loss; lethargy, twitching, seizures, coma.

slowly, most patients will tolerate 300–400 g per 24 hours. Some will not tolerate this without exogenous insulin, while others will tolerate more.

If insulin is required, it should be added to the parenteral nutrition solution. The availability of insulin from these solutions has been the subject of a number of controversial reports in the literature. Insulin loss is associated with adsorption to plastic and glass containers with attached administration tubing and to inline filters. Reports of the extent of insulin adsorption vary considerably, with some workers claiming that 44–47% of 30 units of insulin added to amino acids and protein hydrolysates in glucose is lost and that the loss is greater if inline filters or polyvinyl chloride bags are used. Other workers have described much lower losses than this. The percentage loss, however, is irrelevant since, provided the insulin is always added to the same solution, increasing the dose will eventually control hyperglycaemia. Addition of albumin is not necessary. Continuous insulin infusion in the feed is a more satisfactory and safer method of controlling hyperglycaemia due to TPN than subcutaneous administration. If the infusion stops following subcutaneous insulin, hypoglycaemia may occur.

One method for determining the amount of soluble insulin to be added initially to the parenteral nutrition solution is based on the patient's blood glucose concentration when receiving 5% glucose. If the blood glucose concentration ranges between 7.2 and 8.3 mmol/l, add 6–10 units of soluble insulin per 250 g of glucose infused. If the blood glucose ranges from 8.3 to 11.1 mmol/l, add 12–18 units of soluble insulin per 250 g of glucose. If the blood glucose is greater than 11.1 mmol/l, 25 units or more of soluble insulin are required per 250 g of glucose. Regular monitoring of blood and urine glucose concentrations is essential to determine response to this exogenous insulin and to permit further adjustments to be made. Exogenous insulin should be administered only if the serum potassium concentration is normal and if adequate potassium supplementation is provided. The addition of exogenous insulin to the nutritional regimen results in a gain in total body potassium. There are many situations when it is preferable to reduce the amount of glucose infused than to increase the amount of insulin necessary to control hyperglycaemia.

FRUCTOSE

The introduction of alternate energy sources, including fructose, was based on two major objections to the use of glucose, namely, the vascular irritation resulting from peripheral infusions of glucose, and the metabolic complications associated with its use. It was argued that fructose was rapidly utilised, was not dependent on insulin for its metabolism and would not stimulate insulin secretion. The reasons behind these arguments have been proven questionable. The pathways for the metabolism of fructose in the liver, its main site of metabolism, are illustrated in Figure 5.1. Other sites of fructose metabolism include muscle, adipose tissue, kidney and gut. Fructose, as such, is not utilised by the brain.

Although fructose enters cells independently of insulin, under normal conditions approximately 30% of the fructose load is converted to lactate and pyruvate, and the remainder (approximately 70%) is converted to glucose. This glucose then requires the presence of insulin for its further metabolism. Acute administration of fructose has been shown to result in rapid accumulation of fructose-1-phosphate in the liver and kidney with simultaneous depletion of cell ATP and intracellular sequestration of inorganic phosphate. This is followed by depression of protein synthesis in the liver.

Hyperuricaemia and increased urinary uric acid excretion may accompany the use of intravenous fructose. This has been shown to be due to increased adenine nucleotide breakdown in the liver, leading to adenine nucleotide depletion.

Another adverse effect associated with rapid infusion of fructose is metabolic acidosis due to accumulation of the intermediary metabolites pyruvate and lactate. Severe, and even fatal cases of lactic acidosis have been reported, particularly in children. Rapid and/or large infusions of fructose are contraindicated in dehydrated or acidotic patients, or patients with impaired liver function. The concurrent use of ethanol with fructose may increase the risk of lactic acidosis.

If fructose is infused into patients with hereditary fructose intolerance, fructose-1-phosphate rapidly accumulates in the liver, renal cortex and intestinal mucosa. The metabolic consequences of such an infusion may result from an accumulation of fructose-1-phosphate, which is toxic in excess, or from the sequestration of inorganic phosphate as fructose-1-phosphate, with resulting intracellular phosphate deficiency. The clinical manifestations include hypoglycaemia, hypophosphataemia, lactic acidosis, fructosuria, proteinuria (with an impairment of resorption of bicarbonate, phosphate, amino acids and uric acid, resembling the Fanconi syndrome), coma and shock.

The maximum infusion rate of fructose tolerated in the post-operative period has been reported to be between 250 and 500 mg/kg per hour. A maximum infusion rate of 200 mg/kg per hour has been recommended, provided frequent biochemical monitoring is carried out. Increased infusion rates involve the risks of metabolic acidosis and depletion of ATP and total adenine nucleotides in the liver. The loss through renal overflow at an infusion rate of 500 mg/kg per hour in the early post-traumatic state has been determined to be approximately 9%.

A 10% solution of fructose has an osmolality of approximately 555 mOsm/kg and a pH of 3–6. Thus, there is a risk of inducing phlebitis if concentrated solutions are infused peripherally. 1 g of fructose provides an equivalent amount of energy as 1 g of glucose on complete oxidation. Solutions containing fructose and amino acids may undergo the Maillard reaction.

SORBITOL

Sorbitol, a polyol, is converted predominantly in the liver by sorbitol dehydrogenase to fructose, which is then metabolised as outlined in Figure

5.1. Only the conversion of sorbitol to glucose via fructose is independent of insulin.

Because sorbitol is converted to fructose, similar disadvantages are associated with its infusion, including an effect on hepatic purine nucleotide metabolism leading to a temporary depletion of ATP and a rise in serum uric acid levels and lactic acidosis. The risk of lactic acidosis may be increased when sorbitol is infused concurrently with ethanol and/or fructose. In addition, sorbitol imposes the same risks to fructose intolerant patients and patients with an hereditary deficiency of fructose-1,6-diphosphatase.

Observations based on studies in dogs have revealed that infusions of sorbitol result in hyperosmolality of the extracellular fluid compartment, suggesting that intracellelar movement of sugar alcohols is, in some way, partially restricted. In addition, there appears to be a greater urine output than that required for the obligatory excretion of solute. With administration rates of 500 mg/kg per hour the urinary loss of sorbitol in humans has been reported to be approximately 11%. Urinary losses of sorbitol range from 4 to 25% in paediatric patients.

Sorbitol does not appear to have any advantages over fructose and certainly not over glucose as a caloric source in parenteral nutrition.

XYLITOL

Xylitol, a five carbon polyol, is metabolised first to xylulose-5-phosphate, which enters the hexose monophosphate shunt to be converted to fructose-6-phosphate and glyceraldehyde-3-phosphate (see Fig. 5.3), intermediary metabolites of the Embden-Meyerhoff pathway. The major site for the metabolism of xylitol is the liver, although many other tissues, including gut, testis and brain possess polyol dehydrogenase activity, and hence can convert xylitol to D-xylulose. The subsequent metabolism of glucose derived from xylitol metabolism is insulin dependent. 60–75% of the administered xylitol is converted to glucose in the liver.

Initially, xylitol was considered to be a suitable energy source for parenteral nutrition, and capable of inhibiting gluconeogenesis more efficiently than glucose. However, a number of adverse effects, some fatal, have been associated with its use. These adverse effects include abdominal distress, nausea, diarrhoea, hyperuricaemia, uricosuria, polyuria, lactic acidosis, oliguria and azotaemia, and hepatic and cerebral disturbances.

A syndrome of adverse reactions was described in 22 patients following infusions of xylitol at rates ranging from an average of 230 $\pm$ 20 mg/kg per hour to 490 $\pm$ 30 mg/kg per hour. The most striking adverse effect noted on autopsy was the precipitation of calcium oxalate crystals within the renal tubules and mid-brain arterioles. It was postulated that glycolaldehyde may be released under certain circumstances during the metabolism of xylitol and subsequently may be metabolised to oxalic acid. Later observations of the increased production of oxalate in vitamin B_6-deficient rats infused with xylitol were consistent with this proposed mechanism.

As a result of these observations, the use of intravenous xylitol has been prohibited in Australia, Great Britain, North America and some European countries.

ETHANOL

Ethanol has a high caloric value, 29 kJ (7 kcal) per 1 g, and was used widely as an energy source prior to the introduction of hyperosmolar carbohydrate solutions and the acceptance of fat emulsions. Its rate of utilisation is limited by its pharmacological effects.

Ethanol is metabolised principally in the liver to acetaldehyde and acetyl-CoA utilising the enzyme nicotinamide adenine dinucleotide, NAD, as the coenzyme (see Fig. 5.1). This coenzyme also is required for the oxidation of lactate to pyruvate.

The use of ethanol, particularly in patients with hepatic dysfunction, results in an increase in the NADH:NAD ratio, which in turn inhibits gluconeogenesis from lactate, causing an increase in the lactate:pyruvate ratio, and lactic acidosis may supervene. Other adverse effects of ethanol include toxicity to organs such as the heart, muscle and brain, impaired leucocyte migration and phagocytosis and impaired function of the respiratory mucosal cilia. There appears to be no justification for the use of ethanol in modern parenteral nutrition.

MALTOSE

The disaccharide maltose has been considered by a number of workers as a possible energy substrate for parenteral nutrition. Although intravenously administered maltose can be metabolised by man (see Fig. 5.1), the ability to retain maltose for utilisation appears to be dependent on the concentration of the solution and the rate of delivery. At present this substrate would appear to have little place in parenteral nutrition. Its eventual role depends on the further elucidation of its metabolic pathways and its ability to produce the desired effects on nitrogen utilisation and body weight.

GLUCOSE OLIGOSACCHARIDES

Short-term parenteral infusions of a glucose oligosaccharide mixture in human subjects have been studied recently. The glucose oligosaccharide mixture contained less than 5% glucose units, and was prepared by fractionation of hydrolysed corn starch. No adverse effects were reported with infusions delivered over a 12 hour period at the rates of 1.75, 2.5 or

5.0 mg/kg per minute. The amount of oligosaccharides oxidised to carbon dioxide ranged from 7 to 15% for the higher infusion rates. Serum glucose and insulin concentrations were not observed to change during the infusions and the plasma free fatty acid concentration decreased at the 2.5 and 5.0 mg/kg per minute rates. The percentage of infused oligosaccharides retained by the body was found to be dose related, with 79.5% being retained at the lowest infusion rate and 34% being retained at the highest infusion rate.

Although it is proposed that the use of oligosaccharides as a carbohydrate substrate in parenteral nutrition would significantly decrease the infused osmotic load compared to an iso-osmotic solution of glucose, and would permit use of the peripheral route, the findings from this study suggest that the ability of normal subjects to metabolise infused glucose oligosaccharides is limited.

REFERENCES AND FURTHER READING

Andersson G, Brohult J, Sterner G Increasing metabolic acidosis following fructose infusion in two children. Acta Paediat Scand 1969; 58: 301–304

Askanazi J, Carpentier Y A, Elwyn D H, Nordenstrom J, Jeevanandam M, Rosenbaum S H, Gump F E, Kinney J M Influence of total parenteral nutrition on fuel utilization in injury and sepsis. Ann Surg 1980; 191: 40–46

Askanazi J, Weissman C, Rosenbaum S H, Hyman A I, Milic-Emili J, Kinney J M Nutrition and the respiratory system. Crit Care Med 1982; 10: 163–172

Baker J P, Detsky A S, Stewart S, Whitwell J, Marliss E B, Jeejeebhoy K N Randomised trial of total parenteral nutrition in critically ill patients: metabolic effects of varying glucose-lipid ratios as the energy source. Gastroenterol 1984; 87: 53–59

Batstone G F, Alberti K G M M, Dewar A K Reversible lactic acidosis associated with repeated intravenous infusions of sorbitol and ethanol. Postgrad Med J 1977; 53: 567–569

Bergstrom J, Hultman E, Roch-Norlund A E Lactic acid accumulation in connection with fructose infusion. Acta Med Scand 1968; 184: 359–364

Burke J F, Wolfe R R, Mullany C J, Mathews D E, Bier D M Glucose requirements following burn injury. Parameters of optimal glucose infusion and possible hepatic and respiratory abnormalities following excessive glucose intake. Ann Surg 1979; 190: 274–285

Ellis GP The Maillard reaction. Adv Carbohyd Chem 1959; 14: 63–134

Elwyn D H, Kinney J M, Jeevanandam M, Gump F E, Broell J R Influence of increasing carbohydrate intake on glucose kinetics in injured patients. Ann Surg 1979; 190: 117–127

Fry L K, Stegink L D Formation of Maillard reaction products in parenteral alimentation solutions. J Nutr 1982; 112: 1631–1637

Georgieff M, Moldawer L L, Bistrian B R, Blackburn G L Xylitol, an energy source for intravenous nutrition after surgery. JPEN 1985; 9: 199–209

Lowry S F, Brennan M F Abnormal liver function during parenteral nutrition: relation to infusion excess. J Surg Res 1979; 26: 300–307

MacFie J, Smith R C, Hill G L Glucose or fat as a nonprotein energy source? A controlled clinical trial in gastroenterological patients requiring intravenous nutrition. Gastroenterol 1981; 80: 103–107

MacFie J, Yule A G, Hill G L Effect of added insulin on body composition of gastroenterologic patients receiving intravenous nutrition — a controlled clinical trial. Gastroenterol 1981; 81: 285–289

Miller M, Craig J W, Drucker W R, Woodward H Jnr The metabolism of fructose in man. Yale J Biol Med 1956; 29: 335–360

Narins R G, Weisberg J S, Myers A R Effects of carbohydrates on uric acid metabolism. Metabolism 1974; 23: 455–465

Petty C, Cunningham N L Insulin adsorption by glass infusion bottles, polyvinylchloride infusion containers, and intravenous tubing. Anesthesiol 1974; 40: 400–404

Principi N, Reali E, Rivolta A Sorbitol in total parenteral nutrition in pediatric patients. Helv Paediat Acta 1973; 28: 621–627

Schumer W Adverse effects of xylitol in parenteral alimentation. Metabolism 1971; 20: 345–347

Sprandel U, Heuckenkamp P-U, Zollner N Evaluation of maltose as intravenous nutrient in man. Nutr Metab 1977; 21: (Suppl 1): 112–114

Tate J T, Cowan G S M Jnr Insulin kinetics in hyperalimentation solution and routine intravenous therapy. Am Surg 1977; 43: 811–816

Thomas D W, Edwards J B, Gilligan J E, Lawrence J R, Edwards R G Complications following intravenous administration of solutions containing xylitol. Med J Aust 1972; 1: 1238–1246

Thomas D W, Edwards J B, Edwards R G Side effects of sugar substitutes during intravenous administration. Nutr Metab 1975; 18 (Suppl 1): 227–241

Wagner W H, Lowry A C, Silberman H Similar liver function abnormalities occur in patients receiving glucose-based and lipid-based parenteral nutrition. Am J Gastroenterol 1983; 78: 199–202

Weber S S, Wood W A, Jackson E A Availability of insulin from parenteral nutrient solutions. Am J Hosp Pharm 1977; 34: 353–357

Wilson N M, Brown P M, Juul S M, Prestwich S A, Sonksen P H Glucose turnover and metabolic and hormonal changes in ethanol-induced hypoglycaemia. Br Med J 1981; 282: 849–853

Wolfe R R, O'Donnell T F Jnr, Stone M D, Richmand D A, Burke J F Investigation of factors determining the optimal glucose infusion rate in total parenteral nutrition. Metabolism 1980; 29: 892–900

Woods H F, Alberti K G M M Dangers of intravenous fructose. Lancet 1972; ii: 1354–1357

Young E A, Fletcher J T, Cioletti L A, Hollrah L A, Weser E Metabolism of parenteral glucose oligosaccharides in man. JPEN 1981; 5: 369–377

9

Protein

Since Rose and his colleagues performed their extensive studies, commencing in the early 1930s, on the essential nature of amino acids in human nutrition, and Elman reported in 1937 that infusions of protein hydrolysates and glucose stimulated regeneration of plasma proteins in blood volume depleted dogs, our knowledge of amino acid requirements and metabolism has progressed significantly. Likewise, the sources of amino acids and methods of preparing these solutions have changed dramatically (Table 9.1).

Table 9.1   Generations of amino acid solutions (adapted from Winters et al, 1984)

Generation	Composition	Clinical usefulness, problems
1st	Hydrolysate bovine serum proteins casein fibrin human serum albumin lactalbumin	Satisfied adult requirements — not infants Amino acid composition dependent on protein $\uparrow$ NH_4^+, hyperammonaemia, $\downarrow$ cystine, tyrosine, $\uparrow$ aspartate, glutamate Peptides, Maillard reaction products $\downarrow$ utilisation Variable trace element contamination
2nd	Crystalline D, L-amino acids	As effective as commercial protein hydrolysates Only L-isomers utilised
3rd	Crystalline L-amino acids	Satisfied adult essential amino acid requirements — not infants Hyperammonaemia (infants) Hyperchloraemic acidosis Plasma amino acid abnormalities
4th	Specific L-amino acid formulations renal failure (EAA) hepatic failure ($\uparrow$ BCAA, $\downarrow$ AAA) trauma ($\uparrow$ BCAA) growth in infants	 Correct specific abnormalities of uraemia Correct specific abnormalities of hepatic failure Minimise protein catabolism Augment protein anabolism

EAA = essential amino acids; AAA = aromatic amino acids; BCAA = branched chain amino acids

The first part of this chapter is directed towards elucidating the essential amino acids and their requirements. Then, some of the reasons for the various developments leading to the third and fourth generation solutions that are currently in use are presented. Major differences in these amino acid solutions are highlighted in order to assist the reader to select an appropriate solution for most common clinical situations.

ESSENTIAL (INDISPENSABLE) AMINO ACIDS AND THEIR REQUIREMENTS

Of the 20 amino acids required for protein synthesis, Rose concluded that 8 amino acids were essential (indispensable) for the attainment and maintenance of nitrogen equilibrium in man. These amino acids are isoleucine, leucine, lysine, methionine, phenylalanine, threonine, tryptophan and valine. Rose's recommendations for the minimum amount of each of these essential amino acids required in the diet per day are listed in Table 9.2.

Table 9.2 Minimum amounts of essential amino acid requirements in daily diet (after Rose, 1957)

	Minimum daily requirements (g)
Isoleucine	0.7
Leucine	1.1
Lysine	0.8
Methionine	1.1
Phenylalanine	1.1
Threonine	0.5
Tryptophan	0.25
Valine	0.8

However, further work has suggested that the differentiation between essential and non-essential (dispensable) amino acids is not clear cut. Histidine is considered essential in infants and in uraemic patients because of impaired renal synthesis of this amino acid. Cysteine and taurine may be essential in premature infants who cannot convert methionine into these amino acids — or can do so only in inadequate amounts. Also, the ability of the premature infant to synthesise tyrosine has been questioned. The current recommended daily requirements of essential amino acids in relation to body mass for infants and adults are summarised in Table 9.3.

The recommended protein intake, based on high biological value protein (milk, egg) is 2.2 g/kg body weight for an infant (0–6 months), and 0.6 g/kg body weight for the healthy adult. Therefore, the recommended essential amino acid requirement expressed on a kilogram body weight basis, can be expressed as a percentage of the total protein intake per kilogram body weight, i.e.

D

Table 9.3 Recommended requirements for essential amino acids (mg/kg body weight) (adapted from Food and Nutrition Board, USA, 1980)

Amino acids (mg/kg body weight)	Infant (4–6 months)	Adult*
Histidine	33	
Isoleucine	83	12
Leucine	135	16
Lysine	99	12
Methionine + Cystine	49	10
Phenylalanine + Tyrosine	141	16
Threonine	68	8
Tryptophan	21	3
Valine	92	14
Total essential amino acids	*721*	*91*

* Minimum requirement + 30% to cover individual variations

— for an infant (4–6 months) essential/total amino acids (%) = 38
— for an adult (healthy) essential/total amino acids (%) = 15.2

This percentage is often reported as grams of essential amino acids per grams of total nitrogen (E:T ratio). The E:T ratio of body proteins or other proteins with high biological value is 3. An amino acid solution with an E:T ratio of 3 is considered to be optimal for growing infants, and also for restoration of body protein in the adult. These recommended protein and amino acid intakes are conditional on:

— the protein intake being of high biological value. If proteins of a lower value are consumed, then the intake must be increased
— the required energy requirements being met (480 kJ (115 kcal)/kg body weight per day for infants 0–6 months, 145–170 kJ (35–40 kcal)/kg body weight per day for healthy adults), otherwise the protein consumed will be used for energy production and not for protein synthesis.

A source of energy should be administered simultaneously with the amino acids. The optimal ratio of energy (kilojoules or kilocalories) to nitrogen for the most effective utilisation of nitrogen, has been variously estimated from 630 kJ (150 kcal) to 1046 kJ (250 kcal) per 1 g of nitrogen. Recent studies suggest that the provision of approximately 630 kJ per 1 g of nitrogen (150 kcal/1 g N) would be a more reasonable approach. A lower energy to nitrogen ratio, possibly as low as 502 kJ (120 kcal) per 1 g of nitrogen may be required in severe hypercatabolic conditions. In fact, one group has proposed a ratio of just 80:1 for septic patients with an input of 3 g/kg per 24 hours of amino acids and 146 kJ (35 kcal)/kg per 24 hours.

If the amounts of amino acids (essential and non-essential) administered exceed the amounts required for protein synthesis, then the excesses will be degraded and used for energy. During their degradation, a series of inter-relationships occur between the essential and non-essential amino acids in connection with:

— nitrogen removal from the essential amino acids as the initial step in forming carbon skeletons which can be used in gluconeogenesis, lipogenesis, ketogenesis or direct oxidation

— nitrogen transfer, intracellularly from one amino acid to another to form compounds that participate in the interorgan transport of nitrogen and, ultimately, transport to the liver

— released amino acid nitrogen incorporation into urea, a nontoxic substance, which is transported from the liver to the kidneys where it is excreted in the urine.

Also it has been determined that, for optimal utilisation of an amino acid mixture, the amino acids should be supplied as the laevo-isomers. The body can utilise only these L-forms for protein synthesis. A summary of the major products of amino acid metabolism, together with a classification of the amino acids, is presented in Table 9.4.

DEVELOPMENT OF AMINO ACID SOLUTIONS

Over the last 40 years a number of important developments have occurred in the preparation of amino acid solutions and, in particular, in the composition of the amino acid sources used to prepare these solutions. These developments may be classified into generations according to the amino acid sources and are summarised in Table 9.1.

Protein hydrolysates

Protein hydrolysates derived from protein by partial enzymatic hydrolysis of casein or partial acid hydrolysis of fibrin were used extensively from the early 1940s until the middle 1970s. The profiles of amino acids presented in these protein hydrolysate solutions reflected those naturally occurring in milk or beef blood, and were markedly different from the normal serum amino acid pattern. Also, the manufacturing process used to prepare these products influenced the amino acid profile. For example, the first hydrolysate solutions were prepared using an acid hydrolysis process which destroyed most of the tryptophan and required addition of this amino acid. When alkaline hydrolysis was used, the tryptophan content of the solution was preserved, but extensive racemisation of the amino acids resulted, with a lowering of their nutritional value. Partial enzymatic hydrolysis, coupled with dialysis to remove large polypeptides proved to be a more successful method for preparing these solutions.

These solutions suffered from a number of deficiencies, including the amino acid composition of the hydrolysate being determined by the structure of the protein hydrolysed. Large quantities of ammonium ion were released during the hydrolysis process, thus increasing the potential for these solutions to produce hyperammonaemia. In addition, the arginine intake delivered by the hydrolysates was low, which possibly led to a

Table 9.4 Classification of amino acids

Amino acid	Classification and charge at pH7	Nutritional value and metabolism (some physiologically significant products)
Isoleucine	Monoaminomonocarboxylic (branched chain) acid — neutral[†]/[*]	Essential — degraded to alpha-keto acid and catabolised to propionyl-CoA and acetyl-CoA
Leucine	Monoaminomonocarboxylic (branched chain) acid — neutral[*]	Essential — degraded to alpha-keto acid and catabolised to acetyl-CoA and acetoacetic acid
Lysine	Diaminomonocarboxylic (aliphatic) acid — basic[†]	Essential — degraded to alpha-ketoglutaric acid and glutamic acid
Methionine	Monoaminomonocarboxylic (aliphatic) acid — neutral (S-containing)[†]	Essential — precursor of cysteine; acts as methyl donor. Participates in synthesis of creatine/creatinine, choline
Phenylalanine	Monoaminomonocarboxylic (aromatic) acid — neutral[†]/[*]	Essential — transformed to tyrosine; participates in synthesis of hormones listed under tyrosine; excess converted via tyrosine to tyramine, octopamine
Threonine	Monoaminomonocarboxylic (aliphatic) acid — neutral (polar-OH gp)[†]/[*]	Essential — degraded to glycine and acetyl-CoA
Tryptophan	Monoaminomonocarboxylic (heterocyclic) acid — neutral[†]	Essential — metabolised to provide part of nicotinic acid requirement; precursor of serotonin
Valine	Monoaminomonocarboxylic (branched chain) acid — neutral[†]	Essential — degraded to alpha-keto acid and catabolised to propionyl-CoA and succinyl-CoA
Alanine	Monoaminomonocarboxylic (aliphatic) acid — neutral[†]	Non-essential — required for optimal amino acid utilisation; deaminated to pyruvic acid
Arginine	Diaminomonocarboxylic (aliphatic) acid — basic[†]	Non-essential — required for optimal amino acid utilisation; protects against hyperammonaemia; participates in synthesis of creatine/creatinine; yields glutamic acid
Aspartic Acid	Monoaminodicarboxylic (aliphatic) acid — acidic[†]	Non-essential — source of non-specific nitrogen; excess may lower pH and cause metabolic complications; participates in synthesis of purines, pyrimidines; deaminated to oxaloacetic acid
Cystine (di-Cysteine)	Diaminodicarboxylic (aliphatic) acid — neutral (S-containing)[†]	Non-essential (adult) — inadequately synthesised in foetus and new-born; participates in formation of mercapturic acids for detoxification; metabolised in liver, via cysteine sulphinic acid, to taurine

Table 9.4 Classification of amino acids

Amino acid	Classification and charge at pH7	Nutritional value and metabolism (some physiologically significant products)
Glutamic Acid	Monoaminodicarboxylic (aliphatic) acid — acidic[†]	Non-essential — required for optimal amino acid utilisation; excess lowers pH and may result in metabolic complications; readily converted to glutamine; degraded to alpha-ketoglutaric acid
Glycine	Monoaminomonocarboxylic (aliphatic) acid — neutral (polar)[†]	Non-essential — source of non-specific nitrogen; excess may cause imbalance especially in new-born; participates in synthesis of creatine/creatinine; purines/pyrimidines and haeme; interconverted to serine
Histidine	Monoaminomonocarboxylic (heterocyclic) acid — basic[†]	Non-essential (adult) — essential for infants and uraemic patients; stimulates protein synthesis; transformed to histamine
Ornithine	Diaminomonocarboxylic (aliphatic) acid — basic[†]	Non-essential — intermediate in urea cycle, converted to arginine; convertible to proline, glutamic acid
Proline	Monoaminomonocarboxylic (heterocyclic) acid — neutral[†]	Non-essential — required for optimal amino acid utilisation; yields glutamic acid
Serine	Monoaminomonocarboxylic (aliphatic) acid — neutral (polar-OH gp)[†]	Non-essential — source of nitrogen; can be synthesised from glycine; participates in synthesis of cysteine
Taurine	Monoaminosulphonic (aliphatic) acid — (S-containing)	Non-essential — in new-born, synthesis from cysteine is inadequate, possibly due to decreased enzyme activity. Conjugates with bile acid to form taurocholic acid
Tyrosine	Monoaminomonocarboxylic (aromatic) acid — neutral (polar-OH gp)[†]/[*]	Non-essential — in new-born, synthesis from phenylalanine is inadequate; metabolised to fumaric and acetoacetic acids; utilised in formation of the neuro-transmitter noradrenaline, thyroxine and melanin

[†] = glucogenic (glycogenic) Glucogenic amino acids, by definition, are potentially convertible to glucose.
[*] = ketogenic amino acids, by definition, yield acetyl-CoA or acetoacetyl-CoA on catabolism, both of which can be converted to ketogenic bodies.

deficiency of arginine in the urea cycle, thus interfering with the conversion of ammonia to urea (see Fig. 5.4), and an augmented excretion of orotic acid. Cystine and tyrosine, liberated during the hydrolysis process, precipitated out of solution because of their low solubilities while large amounts of glutamate and aspartate were liberated into the solution. The resulting imbalances in the concentrations of these amino acids were of concern, particularly in infants as it had been shown that the dicarboxylic acids glutamate and aspartate were potentially neurotoxic in large amounts in the infant rodent.

A significant percentage, up to 40%, of the total nitrogen content of these hydrolysate solutions was bound in di- and tri-peptides which were considered to be of inferior biological value compared to free amino acids, and appeared to be poorly utilised. However, many of these solutions were terminally heat sterilised with glucose which resulted in the formation of Maillard reaction products (glycosylated amino acids) which behave analytically like peptides and are excreted, unchanged, in the urine. The hydrolysates contained significant quantities of trace elements (zinc, copper, selenium, manganese, chromium) as contaminants, which no doubt were advantageous in preventing trace element deficiencies. Other trace element contaminants such as aluminium, have been reported to produce deleterious effects with long term administration.

Racemic crystalline amino acids

The first complete mixture of crystalline amino acids was used by Shohl & Blackfan in 1940. This and other early crystalline amino acid solutions were racemic mixtures containing both D- and L-isomers of the amino acids. Although these isomers have similar chemical properties, in vivo enzyme systems readily differentiate between the isomers such that in humans the L-isomers are used almost exclusively. Subsequently, it was demonstrated that solutions of pure crystalline L-amino acids were more efficiently utilised than racemic mixtures of the amino acids. Racemic mixtures are no longer recommended.

Crystalline L-amino acids

The development of methods to prepare synthetic crystalline L-amino acids has enabled a variety of solutions to be formulated which are used extensively today. These solutions permit more efficient utilisation of nitrogen for protein synthesis than either the protein hydrolysates or racemic amino acid mixtures. Their profiles of amino acids vary considerably. Some have been designed to reflect that of normal serum, while others have been based on the amino acid composition of egg protein (Table 9.5). More recently, solutions have been formulated specifically to fulfill the known requirements for amino acids and nitrogen in certain diseases such as renal failure or hepatic failure (Table 9.6).

A number of metabolic complications were reported with some of the earlier crystalline L-amino acids formulations, including the development of hyperammonaemia in infants during prolonged parenteral nutrition. Although the precise aetiology of the elevated blood ammonia concentration is not known, this complication was reversed by the infusion of arginine hydrochloride or arginine glutamate. It has been postulated that the amount of infused arginine was insufficient to replace that lost to protein or creatine synthesis and that this deficiency of arginine could thus interfere with the conversion of ammonia to urea via the urea cycle. It is possible that the large amount of glycine present in some of these solutions may also have contributed to the hyperammonaemia.

Hyperchloraemic acidosis was a particular problem during the administration of an early crystalline L-amino acid solution to infants. The proposed mechanisms delineating this complication and also the role of acetate salts of potassium or sodium in its prevention or correction are:

1. The cationic (basic) amino acids arginine, histidine, and lysine, were included as the hydrochloride salts which resulted, on catabolism of these amino acids, in a large amount of preformed acid being delivered in the solution. As plasma chloride and bicarbonate concentrations demonstrate an inverse relationship due to reciprocal tubular reabsorption, an increase in the plasma chloride would be expected to result in a decrease in the plasma bicarbonate, leading to hyperchloraemic acidosis. The inclusion of acetate in the solutions would presumably decrease the renal reabsorption of chloride, thus combating the development of hyperchloraemic acidosis. Subsequently, the addition of these amino acids as the hydrochloride salts has been avoided in most formulations.

2. These solutions had a deficit of the anionic (dicarboxylic) amino acids, aspartate and glutamate, which accept a proton during their metabolism. Thus the metabolism of the cationic amino acids led to production of hydrogen ion in excess of the solution's buffering capacity. Consequently, the inclusion of a metabolisable organic acid anion such as acetate in the solution, which would partially offset this imbalance, was promoted (see Table 9.8).

The newer L-amino acid solutions have been modified to eliminate this source of excess hydrogen ions and acidosis is now an infrequent complication. However, there have been some recent reports of these solutions causing alkalosis in infants.

The inappropriate balance of amino acids in some solutions, particularly the non-essential amino acids, has resulted in plasma amino acid imbalances. Some manufactures have excluded the dicarboxylic amino acids glutamic acid and aspartic acid, which have been demonstrated to cause brain damage and retinal damage in experimental animals. In their place, they have substituted large quantities of glycine to serve as the major source

Table 9.5 Some general amino acid solutions and amino acid content of egg protein (amino acid content expressed as grams per 16 g of nitrogen)

L-amino acids	Aminofusin L10 (J. Pfrimmer) gAA/ 16gN	% of Total	Aminoplex 12 (Geistlich) gAA/ 16gN	% of Total	Aminosyn 10% (Abbott Labs) gAA/ 16gN	% of Total	Freamine III 8.5% (Am. McGaw) gAA/ 16gN	% of Total
Isoleucine	3.26	3.10	4.90	4.75	7.34	7.30	7.26	7.16
Leucine	4.62	4.40	7.48	7.25	9.59	9.53	9.47	9.33
Lysine	4.20	4.00	7.02	6.80	7.34	7.30	7.63	7.52
Methionine	4.41	4.20	6.19	6.00	4.08	4.06	5.54	5.46
Phenylalanine	4.62	4.40	8.88	8.60	4.49	4.46	5.90	5.82
Threonine	2.10	2.00	4.13	4.00	5.30	5.27	4.18	4.12
Tryptophan	0.95	0.90	1.81	1.75	1.63	1.62	1.60	1.58
Valine	3.15	3.00	5.78	5.60	8.16	8.11	6.89	6.79
Cystine (Cysteine)	—	—	—	—	—	—	(<0.20)	(<0.20)
Tyrosine	—	—	—	—	0.45	0.45	—	—
Alanine	12.60	12.00	12.90	12.50	13.06	12.98	7.38	7.27
Arginine	8.40	8.00	11.87	11.50	10.00	9.94	9.96	9.82
Aspartic acid	—	—	—	—	—	—	—	—
Glutamic acid	18.90	18.00	2.58	2.50	—	—	—	—
Glycine	21.00	20.00	5.68	5.50	13.06	12.98	14.64	14.43
Histidine	2.10	2.00	2.84	2.75	3.06	3.04	2.96	2.92
Ornithine-L-Aspartate	—	—	2.58	2.50	—	—	—	—
Proline	14.70	14.00	15.48	15.00	8.77	8.72	11.69	11.52
Serine	—	—	3.10	3.00	4.28	4.25	6.15	6.06
Calculated totals	105.01	100.00	103.22	100.00	100.61	100.00	101.45	100.00
Essential AA %		26.00		44.75		47.65		47.78
Aromatic AA %		4.40		8.60		4.91		5.82
Branched chain AA %		10.50		17.60		24.94		23.28
Nitrogen %		15.24		15.50		15.90		15.77
E = Total essential AA	27.31		46.19		47.93		48.47	
AA:Nitrogen ratio	6.56		6.45		6.29		6.96	
E:T ratio	1.71		2.89		3.00		3.03	

Figures in parentheses refer to stated amounts of cysteine included in formulations

of dispensable amino acid nitrogen (see Table 9.5). As a consequence, gross elevations of plasma glycine concentrations have been reported by a number of workers. It is not known whether sustained gross elevation of plasma glycine has a deleterious effect on humans, particularly infants. However, it is known that inborn errors of metabolism leading to accumulation of phenylalanine, glycine and other amino acids can result in deleterious effects on human growth and development. It would seem appropriate to reduce the amount of glycine present in these formulations.

Recent studies in infants with an amino acid solution (Neopham® — Table 9.7) containing significant amounts of aspartate and glutamate (which are present in dietary protein) and a reduced amount of glycine, have demonstrated that low birth weight infants can adequately metabolise

Novamine 11.4% (Cutter Labs)		Synthamin 10% (Travenol Labs)		Travasol 10% (Travenol Labs)		Vamin N 7% (KabiVitrum AB)		EGG protein	
gAA/16gN	% of Total	gAA/16gN	% of Total	gAA/16gN	% of Total	gAA/16gN	% of Total	gAA/16gN	% of Total
5.07	5.00	5.82	6.07	5.82	6.07	6.63	5.56	6.6	5.87
7.02	6.92	7.08	7.39	7.08	7.39	9.01	7.55	8.8	7.83
8.00	7.89	5.63	5.87	5.63	5.87	6.63	5.56	6.4	5.69
5.07	5.00	3.88	4.05	3.88	4.05	3.23	2.71	3.1	2.76
7.02	6.92	5.43	5.67	5.43	5.67	9.35	7.83	5.8	5.16
5.07	5.00	4.07	4.25	4.07	4.25	5.10	4.27	5.1	4.54
1.69	1.67	1.75	1.83	1.75	1.83	1.70	1.42	1.6	1.42
6.49	6.40	4.46	4.65	4.46	4.65	7.31	6.13	7.3	6.49
(0.53)	(0.52)	—	—	—	—	(2.38)	(1.99)	(2.4)	(2.14)
0.27	0.27	0.38	0.40	0.38	0.40	0.85	0.71	4.2	3.74
14.13	13.93	20.08	20.95	20.08	20.95	5.10	4.27	7.4	6.58
9.96	9.82	11.16	11.64	11.16	11.64	5.61	4.70	6.1	5.43
2.93	2.89	—	—	—	—	6.97	5.84	9.0	8.01
5.07	5.00	—	—	—	—	15.30	12.82	16.0	14.23
7.02	6.92	9.99	10.42	9.99	10.42	3.57	2.99	3.6	3.20
6.04	5.96	4.66	4.86	4.66	4.86	4.08	3.42	2.4	2.14
—	—	—	—	—	—	—	—	—	—
6.04	5.96	6.60	6.89	6.60	6.89	13.77	11.54	8.1	7.21
4.00	3.94	4.85	5.06	4.85	5.06	12.75	10.68	8.5	7.56
101.42	100.00	95.84	100.00	95.84	100.00	119.34	100.00	112.4	100.00
	44.80		39.78		39.78		41.03		39.76
	5.27		6.07		6.07		8.54		8.90
	18.32		18.11		18.11		19.24		20.19
	15.77		16.69		16.69		13.41		14.23
45.43		38.12		38.12		48.96		44.7	
6.34		5.99		5.99		7.46		7.03	
2.84		2.38		2.38		3.06		2.79	

aspartate and glutamate. It would appear that these amino acids can be used as alternative sources of dispensable amino acid nitrogen.

Most of the general purpose amino acid solutions listed in Table 9.5 are lacking cystine and the tyrosine content is low in those solutions containing this amino acid. Both these amino acids have low solubilities in aqueous solutions, and hence it is difficult to formulate parenteral nutrition solutions that will contain adequate amounts. Some workers have suggested using the N-acetyl-derivatives of these amino acids to increase their content in solution (Table 9.7).

Plasma amino acid imbalance also may be related to hepatic complications and renal function. It has been suggested that a completely normal plasma amino acid pattern during parenteral nutrition should be the optimal end point for defining the safety and efficacy of amino acid solutions.

Table 9.6 Special purpose amino acid solutions for use in renal failure* and hepatic failure† (amino acid content expressed as grams per 16 g of nitrogen)

L-amino acids	Aminess* 5.2% (KabiVitrum AB)		Aminosyn RF* 5.2% (Abbott Labs)		Nephramine* 5.4% (American McGaw)		Renamin* 6.5% (Travenol Labs)		Aminosteril† Hepa 8% (Fresenius)		F080† (Fischer et al 1976)		Hepatamine† 8% (American McGaw)	
	gAA/16gN	% of Total	gAA/16gN	% of Total	gAA/16gN	% of Total	gAA/16gN	% of Total	gAA/16gN	% of Total	gAA/16gN	% of Total	gAA/16gN	% of Total
Isoleucine	12.73	10.14	9.24	8.77	13.67	10.48	7.97	7.69	12.90	13.00	11.79	11.26	11.78	11.25
Leucine	20.01	15.94	14.66	13.90	21.48	16.46	9.56	9.23	16.23	16.36	14.41	13.76	14.40	13.75
Lysine	14.55	11.59	10.84	10.28	15.62	11.97	7.17	6.92	8.53	8.60	7.96	7.60	7.98	7.62
Methionine	20.01	15.94	14.66	13.90	21.48	16.46	7.97	7.69	1.36	1.37	1.31	1.25	1.31	1.25
Phenylalanine	20.01	15.94	14.66	13.90	21.48	16.46	7.81	7.54	1.09	1.10	1.31	1.25	1.31	1.25
Threonine	9.09	7.24	6.63	6.29	9.76	7.48	6.06	5.85	5.46	5.50	5.90	5.64	5.89	5.63
Tryptophan	4.56	3.63	3.41	3.24	4.88	3.74	2.55	2.46	0.87	0.88	1.00	0.96	0.86	0.83
Valine	14.55	11.59	10.64	10.09	15.62	11.97	13.07	12.61	12.50	12.60	11.00	10.51	11.00	10.51
Cystine (Cysteine)	—	—	—	—	(<0.40)	(<0.31)	—	—	(0.64)	(0.65)	(0.36)	(0.34)	(<0.26)	(<0.25)
Tyrosine	—	—	—	—	—	—	0.64	0.62	—	—	—	—	—	—
Alanine	—	—	—	—	—	—	8.93	8.62	5.75	5.80	9.83	9.39	10.08	9.63
Arginine	—	—	12.05	11.43	—	—	10.04	9.69	13.29	13.40	7.86	7.51	7.85	7.50
Aspartic acid	—	—	—	—	—	—	—	—	—	—	—	—	—	—
Glutamic acid	—	—	—	—	—	—	—	—	—	—	—	—	—	—
Glycine	—	—	—	—	—	—	4.78	4.61	7.22	7.28	11.79	11.26	11.78	11.25
Histidine	9.99	7.96	8.64	8.20	6.10	4.67	6.69	6.46	3.47	3.50	3.14	3.00	3.14	3.00
Proline	—	—	—	—	—	—	5.58	5.38	7.11	7.17	10.48	10.01	10.47	10.00
Serine	—	—	—	—	—	—	4.78	4.61	2.78	2.80	6.55	6.26	6.55	6.26
Calculated totals	125.50	100.00	105.43	100.00	130.49	100.00	103.60	100.00	99.20	100.00	104.69	100.00	104.66	100.00
Essential AA %		92.04		80.37		95.02		59.99		59.41		52.23		52.09
Aromatic AA %		15.94		13.90		16.47		8.16		1.10		1.25		1.25
Branched chain AA %		37.67		32.76		38.91		29.53		41.96		35.53		35.51
Nitrogen %		12.75		15.12		12.27		15.40		16.13		15.28		15.32
E = Total essential AA	115.51		84.74		123.99		62.16		58.94		54.68		54.53	
AA:Nitrogen ratio	7.84		6.59		8.16		6.48		6.20		6.54		6.53	
E:T ratio	7.22		5.30		7.75		3.89		3.68		3.42		3.40	

Figures in parentheses refer to stated amounts of cysteine included in formulation

Table 9.7 Special purpose amino acid solutions for use in trauma and hypermetabolic conditions* and infants† (amino acid content expressed as grams per 16 g of nitrogen)

L-amino acids	Aminoplasmal* PO 10% (B. Braun)		Freamine* HBC 6.9% (American McGaw)		Aminoplasmal† PED 5% (B. Braun)		Aminovenos† PAD 10% (Fresenius)		Neopham† 6.5% (Cutter Medical)		Human milk	
	gAA/16gN	% of Total	gAA/16gN	% of Total	gAA/16gN	% of Total	gAA/16gN	% of Total	gAA/16gN	% of Total	gAA/16gN	% of Total
Isoleucine	4.90	4.73	12.46	11.30	3.04	2.79	7.09	6.37	5.35	4.77	5.4	4.5
Leucine	8.57	8.28	22.47	20.37	5.43	4.99	11.91	10.70	12.08	10.76	11.9	9.9
Lysine	7.62	7.36	6.72	6.09	6.97	6.40	7.86	7.06	9.67	8.62	9.6	8.0
Methionine	2.04	1.97	4.10	3.72	1.74	1.60	5.12	4.60	2.24	2.00	2.2	1.8
Phenylalanine	4.28	4.13	5.25	4.76	4.12	3.78	5.06	4.55	4.66	4.15	4.7	3.9
Threonine	4.90	4.73	3.28	2.97	6.51	5.98	5.71	5.13	6.21	5.53	6.2	5.1
Tryptophan	2.04	1.97	1.48	1.34	1.30	1.19	2.03	1.82	2.42	2.16	2.3	1.9
Valine	6.53	6.31	14.43	13.08	3.47	3.19	7.86	7.06	6.21	5.53	6.2	5.1
Cystine (Cysteine)	—	—	(<0.26)	(<0.24)	(2.19)	(2.01)	(0.42)	(0.38)	(1.73)	(1.54)	(1.8)	(1.5)
Tyrosine	—	—	—	—	0.65	0.60	6.08	5.46	0.86	0.76	3.7	3.1
Alanine	12.65	12.22	6.56	5.95	12.59	11.56	7.93	7.13	10.87	9.69	5.5	4.6
Arginine	8.77	8.47	9.51	8.62	4.77	4.38	7.09	6.37	7.08	6.31	5.5	4.6
Aspartic acid	0.92	0.89	—	—	4.12	3.78	—	—	7.08	6.31	9.7	9.7
Glutamic acid	9.18	8.87	—	—	21.27	19.53	—	—	12.26	10.92	20.3	16.9
Glycine	7.14	6.90	5.41	4.91	10.63	9.76	4.59	4.12	3.63	3.24	3.6	3.0
Histidine	5.51	5.32	2.62	2.37	6.51	5.98	4.59	4.12	3.63	3.24	3.6	3.0
Ornithine	1.89	1.83	—	—	1.94	1.78	—	—	—	—	—	—
Proline	7.14	6.90	10.33	9.37	5.86	5.38	17.94	16.12	9.67	8.62	9.6	8.0
Serine	3.26	3.15	5.41	4.91	2.17	1.99	10.01	9.00	6.56	5.85	6.5	5.4
Asparagine	0.92	0.89	—	—	1.74	1.60	—	—	—	—	—	—
N-Acetyl-L-Tyrosine	2.51	2.42	—	—	1.74	1.60	—	—	—	—	—	—
N-Acetyl-L-Cysteine	2.75	2.66	—	—	1.87	1.72	—	—	—	—	—	—
Calculated totals	103.52	100.00	110.29	100.00	108.89	100.00	111.29	100.00	112.21	100.00	120.3	100.0
Essential AA %	39.49		63.63		29.92		47.29		43.52		40.3	
Aromatic AA %	6.55		4.76		5.86		10.01		4.91		7.0	
Branched chain AA %	19.32		44.75		10.97		24.13		21.06		19.5	
Nitrogen %	15.46		14.51		14.69		14.38		14.26		13.3	
E = Total essential AA	40.88		70.19		32.58		52.64		48.84		48.5	
AA:Nitrogen ratio	6.47		6.89		6.81		6.96		7.01		7.5	
E:T ratio	2.56		4.39		2.04		3.29		3.05		3.0	

Figures in parentheses refer to stated amounts of cysteine included in formulations

The present trend in the development of new amino acid mixtures is to formulate solutions that have amino acid patterns which will correct specific metabolic abnormalities. For example, solutions have been developed specifically for the treatment of renal failure (based on essential amino acids only and relying on the in vivo utilisation of urea to provide nonessential amino acids) and hepatic failure (containing increased quantities of branched chain amino acids and decreased quantities of aromatic amino acids) (see Table 9.6). A number of workers are investigating the use of amino acid solutions containing increased quantities of branched chain amino acids to counter the metabolic abnormalities of trauma and other hypermetabolic states. Other workers are investigating the value of amino acid solutions with profiles based on human milk protein and postprandial plasma amino acid patterns following enteral feeding, in relation to anabolism in infants. However, the true value and roles of these specific formulations have yet to be proven in clinical trials. Examples of these solutions are presented in Table 9.7.

Specific amino acid formulations

Two distinct approaches have evolved in the nutritional management of patients with renal failure. Proponents of the first approach, based on a number of studies performed between 1970 and 1980, maintain that mortality is reduced in those patients who are fed on essential amino acids only. Also, it has been proposed that protein restriction providing only essential amino acids favours the recycling of urea nitrogen as a nitrogen source for protein synthesis (a theory which now has been discredited). In some countries, solutions of essential amino acids have been marketed specifically for use in renal failure (see Table 9.6).

Proponents of the second approach, based on more recent studies, maintain that there is no specific advantage to be derived by infusing essential amino acids only. In fact, it is argued that, while protein restriction is appropriate when providing nutritional support to patients with renal failure to limit accumulation of nitrogenous waste, the administration of a percentage of the protein intake as nonessential amino acids may decrease the need for de novo amino acid synthesis and thus patient stress is decreased. Renamin® (see Table 9.6) has been marketed as an amino acid solution containing both essential and nonessential amino acids, which is indicated for the nutritional management of patients with renal failure. However, it should be noted that patients with renal failure have been nourished satisfactorily using some of the general purpose amino acids listed in Table 9.5.

Recent recommendations for the provision of protein (as essential and nonessential amino acids) to patients with renal failure include:

1. restriction of fluid volume

2. provision of adequate calories generally in the range 150–200 kJ (35–50 kcal)/kg per 24 hours
3. restriction of amino acids to provide in the form of essential and nonessential amino acids:
   — 0.4–0.5 g/kg per 24 hours if GFR < 25 ml/minute and dialysis not contraindicated
   — 1–1.5 g/kg per 24 hours if receiving peritoneal dialysis
   — 1–1.2 g/kg per 24 hours if receiving treatment with haemodialysis.

For some years, it was maintained that the use of alpha-ketoanalogues of the essential amino acids in renal failure or liver disease would result in reduced urea nitrogen appearance, while improving nitrogen balance. These claims have been largely discredited.

Controversy also has existed regarding the efficacy of branched chain amino acid (BCAA) enriched solutions in stressed patients. Freund proposed that the BCAA provided substrates for muscle fuel metabolism and amino groups to produce alanine for hepatic gluconeogenesis, and also blocked amino acid efflux from muscle.

More recently, crystalline amino acid solutions, supplemented with branched chain amino acids, have been marketed for sustaining protein synthesis in the presence of injury, infection and sepsis (Table 9.7). Initial studies with BCAA-enriched solutions appeared to confirm these proposals. Results of more recent studies suggest that the ratio of the individual BCAA is more critical than the total amount present, and that there appears to be a critical concentration of leucine required in these solutions to achieve a significant reduction in the rate of whole body protein catabolism. For patients undergoing major elective operations, this concentration appears to be 0.13 g/kg per 24 hours of leucine.

BCAA-enriched solutions also have been shown to promote normalisation of plasma aminograms in patients with hepatic encephalopathy, and, recently, this ability has been related directly to the leucine concentration. Investigations of the specific amino acid patterns in the plasma of patients and experimental animals with hepatic insufficiency and hepatic encephalopathy, have revealed marked abnormalities. The concentrations of the BCAA isoleucine, leucine and valine are decreased, and the concentrations of the aromatic amino acids phenylalanine and tyrosine are increased, as well as free tryptophan, methionine, histidine, glutamate and aspartate. It has been suggested that these alterations result in an imbalance in brain neurotransmitters, leading to a decreased concentration of noradrenaline and possibly dopamine, and an increase in serotonin and the beta-hydroxylated amines such as octopamine and phenylethanolamine.

Fischer hypothesised that hepatic encephalopathy resulted from an accumulation of aromatic amino acids in the brain when the plasma concentration of BCAA was decreased. It had been demonstrated previously that a competitive transport mechanism into the central nervous system operated between the branched chain amino acids and the aromatic amino acids. Fischer also noted that the molar ratio of the plasma branched chain amino acids to the aromatic amino acids was 3–3.5 in normal man, whereas in patients with hepatic encephalopathy it was 1–1.5.

On the basis of these and other observations, these workers compounded an amino acid solution, F080 (see Table 9.6), that was enriched with branched chain amino acids and deficient in aromatic amino acids. The infusion of this solution, together with hypertonic glucose (23%) resulted in improvement in encephalopathy both in animals and humans. This solution, however, did not appear to benefit those patients with hepatic encephalopathy due to acute hepatic necrosis where the plasma concentrations of the branched chain amino acids were normal and those of all other amino acids were raised. The solution has been marketed commercially as Hepatamine® (see Table 9.6).

A number of research groups have addressed the problem of developing an amino acid solution that will specifically promote anabolism in parenterally nourished infants. Only a few of these solutions have reached the marketing phase (Table 9.7). One such solution, Neopham® (also marketed under the trade mark of Vaminolac® in Europe) has been formulated to provide amino acids resembling those in mature breast milk protein. From the results of a limited number of studies, this solution appears to be safe and efficacious in both preterm and term infants.

SELECTING A GENERAL PURPOSE AMINO ACID SOLUTION

If one examines the composition of some of the solutions that are currently in general use (see Table 9.5) in the light of:

— similarity to egg potein
— essential amino acids as a percentage of total protein
— balance of non-essential amino acids
— concentration of branched chain amino acids

then the following observations can be made to assist in selection:

Aminofusion L® contains no aspartic acid, cystine, serine or tyrosine, and has a high content of glutamic acid and glycine. Essential amino acids constitute 26% of the total, and branched chain amino acids constitute 11% of the total. The total content of L-amino acids per litre of Aminofusin L® 10% is 100 g, providing 15.2 g of utilisable nitrogen. Other strengths available in the Aminofusin L® series include Aminofusin L® 5% containing 50 g amino acids per litre and providing 7.6 g nitrogen.

Aminoplex® contains no aspartic acid, cystine or tyrosine. Essential amino acids constitute 45% of the total and branched chain amino acids constitute 18% of the total. The total content of L-amino acids per litre of Aminoplex 12® is 80 g, providing 12.4 g of utilisable nitrogen. Other strengths available — Aminoplex 5® containing 32.2 g amino acids per litre, and providing 5 g of utilisable nitrogen; Aminoplex 14® containing 82 g amino acids per litre, and providing 13.4 g of utilisable nitrogen.

Aminosyn® contains no aspartic acid, cystine or glutamic acid, and has a high content of glycine. Essential amino acids constitute 47% of the total, and branched chain amino acids constitute 25% of the total. The total L-amino acid content in Aminosyn® 10% is 100 g per litre, providing 15.7 g of utilisable nitrogen. Other strengths available — Aminosyn® 7% containing 70 g amino acids per litre and providing 11 g nitrogen; Aminosyn® 5% containing 50 g amino acids per litre and providing 7.9 g nitrogen; Aminosyn® 3.5% M containing 35 g amino acids per litre and providing 5.5 g nitrogen.

Freamine III® contains no aspartic acid, glutamic acid or tyrosine, and has a high content of glycine. The essential amino acids constitute 48% of the total and branched chain amino acids constitute 23% of the total. The total L-amino acid content is 82.5 g per litre, providing 13.0 g of utilisable nitrogen.

Novamine® is a complete formulation of essential and non-essential amino acids. The essential amino acids constitute 45% of the total, and branched chain amino acids constitute 18% of the total. The total amino acid content in Novamine® 11.4% is 114 g per litre, providing 18 g of utilisable nitrogen. Novamine® also is available as an 8.5% solution, providing 13.5 g of utilisable nitrogen per litre.

Travasol® & **Synthamin**® contain no aspartic acid, cystine or glutamic acid, have a high content of alanine, and the content of glycine has been reduced. Essential amino acids constitute 40% of the total, and branched chain amino acids constitute 18% of the total. The total amino acid content in the 10% solution is 100 g per litre, providing 16.8g of utilisable nitrogen. Other strengths available — Travasol® 8.5% containing 85 g amino acids per litre and 14.2 g nitrogen; Synthamin® 8% containing 80 g amino acids per litre and 13.5 g nitrogen; Travasol® (Synthamin®) 5.5% containing 55 g amino acids per litre and 9.26 g nitrogen; Travasol® 3.5% M containing 35 g amino acids per litre and providing 5.88 g nitrogen.

Vamin N® was the first complete formulation to be marketed. Essential amino acids constitute 41% of the total, and branched chain amino acids constitute 19% of the total. The total amino acid content in Vamin N® 7% is 70.2 g per litre, providing 9.4 g of utilisable nitrogen.

Studies by the authors have been directed at examining nitrogen balances and plasma amino acid concentrations during administration of Vamin N®, Synthamin®, Aminosyn®, and Aminofusin L® to critically ill patients without liver or renal failure. Preliminary results have shown that the main deviations from normal amino acid concentrations in plasma were explicable on the composition of the solution administered. Thus, plasma threonine, valine and isoleucine were lower with Aminofusin L®, glycine was higher with the previous formulation of Synthamin®, and phenylalanine higher with Vamin N®. Plasma concentrations of cystine, glutamic acid, serine and tyrosine were normal, even when these amino acids were absent from the infusion.

Although the glycine content of Synthamin® and Aminofusin L® was similar, plasma glycine was not elevated in the patients infused with Aminofusin L®, presumably because the different composition of the two solutions allowed better metabolism of glycine with Aminofusin L®. Urinary excretion of amino acids, and nitrogen balance depended more on nitrogen and energy input relative to the degree of catabolism of the patient than on the composition of the infused solution.

For routine short-term administration in adults, there is no clear cut argument for selecting one solution above another, and it would seem reasonable to base selection in part on factors such as cost, supply and convenience. The electrolyte content also should be borne in mind, particularly with regard to phosphate and acetate. Contents are listed in Table 9.8. In selected patients, especially premature infants and uraemic patients, closer examination of the arguments presented is advisable.

PROTEIN REQUIREMENTS

Whichever amino acid solution is used, amino acid requirements are of the order of 1–2 g/kg per 24 hours, although this may increase in catabolic states to 3 g/kg per 24 hours or more. Calorie:nitrogen ratio should be approximately 150:1 unless the patient is severely hypercatabolic, when it should be lowered to 120:1 or even 80:1. Thus, for the majority of patients requiring 16 g of nitrogen daily, 10 040 kJ (2400 kcal) of energy should be provided using a mix of glucose and lipid.

The amount of nitrogen required to meet the changing metabolic needs of the stressed or septic patient can be adjusted quantitatively in accordance with the results of nitrogen balance determinations. Nitrogen balance is determined by measuring the 24 hour urinary urea nitrogen excretion. The value obtained is adjusted by approximately 20% to account for other forms of urinary nitrogen loss, including urinary ammonia, purine derivatives and creatinine. Further adjustments are made by allowing for any rise in the patient's blood urea over the preceding 24 hours and also non-urinary losses. Nitrogen balance then is determined by relating nitrogen input to nitrogen loss. Measurement of urinary 3-methylhistidine enables the contribution of increased muscle catabolism to the negative nitrogen balance to be determined.

REFERENCES AND FURTHER READING

Abel R M Parenteral nutrition in the treatment of renal failure. In: Fischer J E (ed) Total Parenteral Nutrition. Little, Brown and Company, Boston, 1976; 143–170
Anderson T L, Heird W C, Winters R W Clinical and physiological consequences of total parenteral nutrition in the pediatric patient. In: Greep J M, Soeters P B, Wesdorp R I C,

Table 9.8 Electrolyte content of some general amino acid solutions (mmol/l)

Electrolyte	Aminofusin L10 (J. Pfrimmer)	Aminoplex 12 (Geistlich)	Aminosyn 10% (Abbott Labs)	Freamine III 8.5% (American McGaw)	Novamine 11.4% (Cutter Medical)	Travasol 10% (Synthamin) with elec. (Travenol Labs)	w/out elec.	Vamin N 7% (KabiVitrum AB)
Sodium	40	35	—	10	—	70[1]	—[1]	50
Potassium	30	30	5.4[2]	—	—	60	—	20
Magnesium	5	2.5	—	—	—	5	—	1.5
Calcium	—	—	—	—	—	—	—	2.5
Acetate	10	5	148	74[3]	114	150	87(82)[4]	—
Chloride	27.5	67.2	—	<2.0	—	70	40	55
Phosphate	—	—	—	10.0	—	30	—	—
Malate	5	34.3	—	—	—	—	—	—
Sulphate	—	—	—	—	—	—	—	1.5
Approx. mOsm/l	1015	NS	1000	810	1049	1300	1000	720
Approx. pH	5.5	7.4	5.3	6.6	5.6	6.0	6.0	5.2

1. Sodium metabisulphite is present as a stabiliser and provides approximately 3 mmol Na/l
2. Includes 5.4 mmol K/l from the antioxidant, potassium metabisulphite
3. Provided as acetic acid and lysine acetate
4. Travasol® contains c. 87 mmol/l acetate; Synthamin® 82 mmol/l acetate
NS. Not stated in product literature

Phaf C W, Fischer J E (eds) Current Concepts in Parenteral Nutrition. Martinus Nijhoff, The Hague, 1977; 111–127

Bell E F, Filer L J Jnr, Wong A P, Stegink L D Effects of a parenteral nutrition regimen containing dicarboxylic amino acids on plasma, erythrocyte, and urinary amino acid concentrations of young infants. Am J Clin Nutr 1983; 37: 99–107

Bonau R A, Ang S D, Jeevanandam M, Daly J M High-branched chain amino acid solutions: relationship of composition to efficacy. JPEN 1984; 8: 622–627

Cerra F B, Mazuski J, Teasley T, Nuwen N, Lysne J, Shronts E, Konstantinides F Nitrogen retention is proportionate to branched chain load: a randomised double blind prospective study. Crit Care Med 1983; 10: 775–778

Elia M, Carter A, Bacon S, Winearls C G, Smith R Clinical usefulness of urinary 3-methylhistidine excretion in indicating muscle protein breakdown. Br Med J 1981; 282: 351–354

Fischer J E, Baldessarini R J Pathogenesis and therapy of hepatic coma. In: Popper H, Schaffner F (eds) Progress in Liver Diseases. Grune and Stratton, New York, 1976; 363–397

Food and Nutrition Board, Recommended Dietary Allowances (9th edn). National Academy of Sciences, Washington DC, 1980

Freund H, Hoover H C Jnr, Atamian S, Fischer J E Infusion of the branched chain amino acids in postoperative patients: anticatabolic properties. Ann Surg 1979; 190: 18–23

Geggel H S, Ament M E, Heckenlively J R, Martin D A, Kopple J D Nutritional requirement for taurine in patients receiving long-term parenteral nutrition. New Engl J Med 1985; 312: 142–146

Giordano C Amino acids and ketoacids — advantages and pitfalls. Am J Clin Nutr 1980; 33: 1649–1653

Heird W C, Nicholson J F, Driscoll J M Jnr, Schullinger J N, Winters R W Hyperammonemia resulting from intravenous alimentation using a mixture of synthetic L-amino acids: a preliminary report. J Pediatr 1972; 81: 162–165

Heird W C, Dell R B, Driscoll J M Jnr, Grebin B, Winters R W Metabolic acidosis resulting from intravenous alimentation mixtures containing synthetic amino acids. New Engl J Med 1972; 287: 943–948

Hill G L, Church J Energy and protein requirements of general surgical patients requiring intravenous nutrtion. Br J Surg 1984; 71: 1–9

Kinney J M Energy requirements for parenteral nutrition. In: Fischer J E (ed) Total Parenteral Nutrition. Little Brown and Company, Boston, 1976; 135–142

Klein G L, Alfrey A C, Miller N L, Sherrard D J, Hazlet T K, Ament M E, Coburn J W Aluminium loading during total parenteral nutrition. Am J Clin Nutr 1982; 35: 1425–1429

Peters C, Fischer J E Studies on calorie to nitrogen ratio for total parenteral nutrition. Surg Gynecol Obstet 1980; 151: 1–8

Rose W C The amino acid requirements of adult man. Nutrition Abstracts and Reviews 1957; 27: 631–647

Shenkin A, Wretlind A Parenteral nutrition. Wld Rev Nutr Diet 1978; 28: 1–111

Stegink L D Amino acids in pediatric parenteral nutrtion solutions infused — lessons learned. Am J Dis Child 1983; 137: 1008–1018

Walser M Principles of keto acid therapy in uremia. Am J Clin Nutr 1978; 31: 1756–1760

Walser M Therapeutic aspects of branched-chain amino and keto acids. Clin Sci 1984; 66: 1–15

Winters R W, Heird W C, Dell R B History of parenteral nutrition in pediatrics with emphasis on amino acids. Fed Proc 1984; 43: 1407–1411

10

Lipid

There are two major reasons for administering lipid in total parenteral nutrition. Firstly, because it provides 38 kJ (9 kcal) per gram, it is a useful energy source in low volume. Secondly, it provides essential fatty acids, without which a deficiency syndrome occurs. Administration of lipid daily is, by definition, essential in total parenteral nutrition. While this is practised in many centres, some workers prefer to administer lipid only in sufficient quantity to prevent essential fatty acid deficiency, either because of technical difficulties in administration, or because they have fears of complications.

The emulsions currently available are derived from soybean, safflower or cottonseed oils, with egg yolk phospholipid, soybean phospholipid or lecithin as emulsifying agents. Isotonicity with blood is obtained by addition of glucose, sorbitol, xylitol or glycerol. Particle size is of the order of that of chylomicrons, and they are processed metabolically by the same processes involving lipoprotein lipase used for endogenous lipid. Basic intermediary metabolism of lipid has been described in Chapter 5. Lipid is present in plasma in a number of forms (Table 10.1), and the function and metabolism of the various types is the subject of ongoing research.

Chylomicrons are spheres of triacylglycerol and cholesterol, surrounded by cholesterol, and phospholipid, and then by aproproteins. The triacylglycerol is broken down in the bloodstream with the aid of lipoprotein lipase, found in the endothelium of capillaries in many tissues. Free fatty acids thus released either enter cells or are bound to albumin for further

Table 10.1 Circulating lipids

Type	Function	Protein %	Lipid %	Size (nm)
Chylomicron	Triglyceride transport	2	98	100–1000
Very low density lipoprotein	Triglyceride transport	8	92	30–80
Intermediate density lipoprotein	Cholesterol transport	12	88	25–30
Low density lipoprotein	Cholesterol transport	21	79	20–25
High density lipoprotein	Cholesterol esterification	50	50	10–20
Non-esterified fatty acids	Energy source	Bound to albumin		

transport. Free fatty acids are either oxidised, or converted into adipose tissue, or are synthesised into very low density lipoprotein for further transport. Clearance of lipid is dependent on the presence of lipoprotein lipase. Normal lipid clearance has a maximum rate of 3.8 g/kg per 24 hours, but this is increased after trauma, sepsis, and during starvation. Clearance may be decreased in immature infants.

The compositions of available preparations are shown in Table 10.2, and the fatty acid patterns in Table 10.3. Different manufacturers quote slightly different fatty acid compositions of the same oil. Hansrani has described the preparation of sterile intravenous emulsions.

ROLE OF LIPID

The use of lipid in TPN regimens appeared logical to early workers, because lipid was an integral part of the normal diet, and lipid storage and breakdown an integral part of intermediary metabolism, being particularly valuable for energy storage during times of plenty, and energy delivery during starvation. However, there were many mishaps associated with some of the early lipid emulsions, which fell into disrepute.

When Intralipid® became established as a safe intravenous lipid preparation, a variety of studies aimed at determining the relative merits of lipid versus carbohydrate calories was undertaken. One prominent group in the USA spearheaded a school which advocated glucose without lipid on the grounds that lipid calories were not as effective as glucose calories at nitrogen sparing. More recent studies have shown that both substrates are of equal value in nitrogen sparing at high protein and energy intakes (Fig. 10.1). When traumatised or septic patients were given TPN containing non-protein energy as glucose alone, or as half glucose, half lipid to a total energy input of 150–160 kJ (36–38 kcal)/kg per 24 hours, with 280–290 mg N/kg per 24 hours, there was no significant difference in nitrogen sparing between the two systems.

The next issue addressed was whether or not administration of excessive amounts of glucose was harmful. A situation was reached in the early 1970s when it was believed that, in order to obtain positive nitrogen balance, it was necessary to provide up to 33 500 kJ (8000 kcal)/24 hours or more in some patients, giving large doses of insulin to force them to tolerate the glucose.

Now there is considerable evidence which indicates that there is a maximum glucose load tolerated. In normal subjects this is 4 mg/kg per minute rising to some 7 mg/kg per minute in post-operative patients.

The Columbia-Presbyterian University group has provided most of the evidence for the harmful effects of excess glucose, and the advantages of providing a proportion (50%) of nonprotein calories as lipid. In 1979 and 1980, evidence was published that patients with chronic nutritional depletion given some 8400 kJ (2000 kcal)/24 hours as 50% from glucose and 50%

Table 10.2 Lipid emulsion compositions (content per 500 ml)

	Intralipid (KabiVitrum AB)	Lipiphysan (Egic)	Lipofundin S (B. Braun)	Liposyn (Abbott Labs)	Liposyn II (Abbott Labs)	Soyacal (Alpha Therapeutic)	Travamulsion (Travenol)†
Soybean Oil	50 or 100 g	—	50 or 100 g	—	25 or 50 g	50 or 100 g	50 g or 100 g
Safflower Oil	—	—	—	50 or 100 g	25 or 50 g	—	—
Cottonseed Oil	—	75 g	—	—	—	—	—
Egg Yolk Phospholipids	6 g	—	—	6 g	6 g	6 g	6 g
Soybean Phospholipids	—	—	3.75 or 7.5 g	—	—	—	—
Lecithin	—	10 g	—	—	—	—	—
Glycerol	11.25 g	—	12.5 g*	12.5 g	12.5 g	11 g	11.25 g
Sorbitol	—	25 g	25 g*	—	—	—	—
Xylitol	—	—	—	—	—	—	—
DL-α-tocopherol	—	0.25	—	—	—	—	—
Water to-	500 ml	500 ml	500 ml	500 ml	500 ml	500 ml	500 ml

Intralipid contains 15 mmol P/litre. Soybean oil contains vitamin E
* Lipofundin S is optionally available with xylitol instead of glycerol.
† In Australia, Travenol markets the Green Cross Corporation product under the name Travenol Fat Emulsion

Table 10.3   Lipid emulsion fatty acid patterns

Fatty acid		Soybean oil %	Cottonseed oil %	Safflower oil %
Myristic	C14:0	0.035	—	—
Palmitic	C16:0	9.18	25.0	7.0
Palmitoleic	C16:1	0.026	—	—
Stearic	C18:0	2.87	2.8	2.5
Oleic	C18:1	26.41	17.1	13.0
Linoleic	C18:2ω6	54.27	52.7	77.0
Linolenic	C18:3	7.81	—	—
Arachidic	C20:0	0.12	—	—
Arachidonic	C20:4	—	—	—
Behenic	C22:0	0.059	—	—

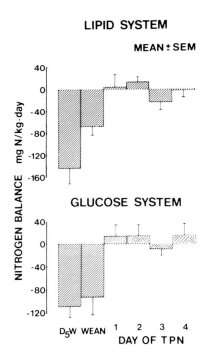

Fig. 10.1 Lipid versus glucose. Nitrogen balance of acutely ill patients weaned from 5% glucose to a glucose-based TPN system providing 29 kcal/kg per 24 hours from glucose plus 281 mg N/kg per 24 hours, or to a lipid-base TPN system providing 17 kcal/kg per 24 hours from glucose, and 14.5 kcal/kg per 24 hours from lipid, plus 292 mg N/kg per 24 hours. No significant difference in N balance was demonstrated between the two systems. (Reproduced with permission from Nordenstrom et al 1983, and Annals of Surgery).

from lipid, plus amino acids, had a 20% decrease in CO_2 production compared to those given the same number of calories as glucose. In acutely ill patients there was a similar but less marked effect. It was noted that, whereas the depleted patient given excess glucose channelled this into lipogenesis, with a minimal rise in energy expenditure, excess infusion of glucose in the hypermetabolic patient resulted in a greater increase in energy expenditure and continuing fat oxidation. It was suggested that high glucose loads which resulted in increased CO_2 production, may embarrass the respiratory function of some patients, particularly during weaning from artificial respiration.

A further problem which arose from these studies was the question of the differences in handling of lipid by nutritionally depleted patients compared to hypermetabolic patients. In a further study of glucose versus lipid calories, depleted patients had a 29% increase in CO_2 production, a 2% increase in O_2 consumption, and an increase in respiratory quotient from 0.77 to 0.97 while receiving glucose/protein TPN, compared to glucose/lipid/protein TPN. Hypermetabolic patients on the same regimen had a 44% increase in CO_2 production, a 15% increase in O_2 consumption, and an increase in RQ to 0.9. It was noted that exogenous glucose is less effective in suppressing fat mobilisation in hypermetabolic patients compared with depleted patients. Whereas depleted patients utilise glucose, decrease lipid oxidation, and increase lipogenesis, acutely ill patients do not utilise glucose appropriately, and there is continued lipid oxidation, due in part to plasma free fatty acid oxidation.

Finally, there has been concern about whether or not lipid clearance is adequate in the hypermetabolic patient. In one study, septic patients given up to 1.4 g lipid/kg per 24 hours as part of their TPN regimen, did not have elevated blood concentratons of total lipids, triglycerides, cholesterol, phospholipids or free fatty acids. Pancreatitis does not preclude administration of lipid provided clearance is monitored, and infusion does not produce hyperlipidaemia. The rate of lipid clearance is reduced in premature infants, possibly due to the fact that they have immature enzyme systems and small adipose tissue mass.

MONITORING

The simplest method of monitoring lipid clearance is to spin down a sample of plasma prior to the next period of lipid infusion and inspect for turbidity. Alternatively, plasma cholesterol, free fatty acids, and triglycerides can be measured.

At very low concentrations of lipid emulsion, the rate of removal of lipid from plasma is dependent on lipoprotein lipase concentration. As the rate of infusion is increased, a maximum elimination capacity is reached. This may be up to 3.8 g lipid/kg per 24 hours.

It should be remembered that hyperlipidaemia interferes with some laboratory measurements and results in spurious hyperbilirubinaemia, hyponatraemia, and hypocalcaemia.

INTRALIPID®

Intralipid®, the most widely used intravenous lipid preparation, has a long and respectable history, in contrast to some of the other early lipid emulsions. It is available as a 10% and a 20% emulsion of soybean oil, with 2.25% glycerol in the aqueous phase and 1.2% egg yolk phosphatides as the emulsifying system. It is relatively expensive, and care should be taken to prevent cracking of the emulsion, for example, by freezing or mixing with other solutions (see chapter 25). The recommended infusion rate for Intralipid® is 2 g/kg per 24 hours, or approximately 50% of nonprotein caloric input given over 6–8 hours. The administration of amounts higher than this, especially for long periods, requires careful monitoring, and establishment of the fact that plasma lipids have returned to normal prior to the next infusion. The pH of the emulsion is approximately 7.0 (range 5.5–9.0) and the osmolarity is stated as 280 mOsm/l for the 10% emulsion and 330 mOsm/l for the 20% emulsion.

In recent years, a number of soybean oil emulsions with formulations similar to Intralipid have been marketed, e.g. Travamulsion®, Soyacal®, Intrafat®.

LIPOSYN®

Liposyn® is a safflower oil emulsion which contains glycerol and egg yolk phosphatides, and differs from Intralipid® in that it has a higher linoleic acid content, and negligible linolenic acid. In several studies it has been shown to be safe and effective, and to have as few complications as the soybean oil emulsion. However, there has been a suggestion that essential fatty acid deficiency may develop with prolonged use, and this has been attributed to the negligible linolenic acid content. The manufacturer now has modified the formulation of Liposyn so that the linolenic acid content is increased — Liposyn II (Table 10.2). The pH of Liposyn II is approximately 8.0 and the osmolarity is 320 mOsm/l and 340 mOsm/l for the 10% and 20% emulsions, respectively. Mild deviation in liver function tests may occur, but several studies in surgical patients have shown no deleterious effects from the emulsion. Abnormal liver functions tests have been shown to occur with Intralipid® and with fat-free TPN.

COMPLICATIONS

Although complications with early lipid emulsions were numerous, Intralipid® and Liposyn® are considered to cause few complications, and are contraindicated only in patients with hyperlipidaemia, hepatocellular disease and acute pancreatitis in the hyperlipidaemic phase. Febrile reactions have been reported with both emulsions.

The fat overload syndrome, with pyrexia, irritability, hyperlipidaemia, gastrointestinal disturbances, hepatosplenomegaly with impaired liver function, anaemia, thrombocytopaenia, prolonged clotting time, elevated prothrombin time, and spontaneous bleeding, has been reported, as have haematological abnormalities. Intrapulmonary lipid accumulation in the lungs of severely ill premature infants has been described, although a recent study concluded that the fat globules may be postmortem artefacts. In jaundiced infants, free fatty acids may displace unconjugated bilirubin from albumin binding sites.

In adults, acute hyperlipidaemia may result in deposition of lipid particles in pulmonary capillaries, with a fall in pulmonary diffusion capacity and arterial hypoxaemia.

The presence of an abnormal lipoprotein, similar to lipoprotein-X, has been identified in the plasma of patients receiving Intralipid®. Its significance is uncertain, but lipoprotein-X is found in the plasma of patients with obstructive jaundice, and those with familial lecithin-cholesterol acyltransferase deficiency.

ESSENTIAL FATTY ACID DEFICIENCY (EFAD)

Essential fatty acid deficiency was recognised in infants in 1958. The effect of essential fatty acid deficiency is shown in Figure 10.2. Normally linoleic

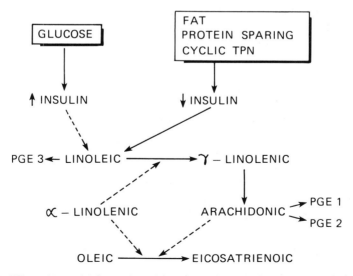

Fig. 10.2 Effect of essential fatty acid deficiency (see text). (Adapted from Phillips & Odgers, 1982, with permission of ADIS Press Australasia Pty, Ltd).

acid ($18:2\omega6$) is desaturated to form γ-linolenic acid ($18:3\omega6$), which is then converted to arachidonic acid ($20:4\omega6$). In the absence of $\omega6$ fatty acids, oleic acid ($18:1\omega9$) is converted to eicosatrienoic acid ($20:3\omega9$). Since $\omega6$ and $\omega9$ families are not interconvertible, the relative decrease of plasma $20:4\omega6$ and increase of $20:3\omega9$ acids is a useful indicator of decreased linoleate metabolism. The triene/tetraene ratio is used as an index of EFAD although the content of eicosatrienoic acid in tissues can be depressed by fatty acids other than linoleic. The upper limit of normal for the ratio is often regarded as 0.4, although Holman regards 0.3 as the upper limit of normal, the average being closer to 0.1. Arachidonic acid is normally the precursor of biologically active prostaglandins, although essential fatty acids probably have other roles. It has been demonstrated that they are necessary for a variety of physiological functions including platelet function, prostaglandin synthesis, wound healing, and integrity of the skin hair and nerve. Clinical manifestations of fatty acid deficiency usually occur 1–3 weeks after the occurrence of the biochemical changes. These include a scaly dermatitis, alopecia, hepotomegaly, growth retardation in infants, diminished skin pigmentation and fatty liver. Cases of linolenic acid deficiency with neurological abnormalities have now been reported, following TPN with linolenic acid-deficient lipid emulsions. However, it has been pointed out that in one of these cases, improvement followed several changes in therapy, including change from safflower to soybean oil emulsion, increased lipid administration and addition of trace elements and biotin. High glucose, lipid free infusions cause hyperinsulinaemia, and mobilisation of linoleic acid is blocked. Essential fatty acid deficiency may be prevented by administration of approximately 1000 ml of 10% emulsion weekly intravenously, by protein-sparing therapy, by cyclic hyperalimentation, or by dermal application of oil. A stable, acceptable oil in water lotion has been described. It contains safflower seed oil, acacia, vitamin E, rose soluble, benzoic acid and water.

CARE

Intralipid® should be stored below 25°C. Liposyn® may be stored below 30°C. It has been accepted practice that nothing should be added directly to the emulsion except heparin, if required. However, heparin should be added to lipid emulsions only if plasma clearance, as determined by inspection of centrifuged blood prior to the next infusion, is inadequate. Care must be taken that the emulsion does not come into contact with other solutions, except close to the site of entry to the patient.

Although several workers have mixed lipid emulsions with amino acid, carbohydrate and electrolyte solutions, and compatibility of Intralipid® with a number of drugs has been demonstrated, these practices are not universally recommended at present. The question of the stability of lipid emulsions when mixed with other nutrients is still being investigated (see

Table 10.4   Lipid/protein/carbohydrate mixtures

	Trive 1000 (Egic)	Nutrafundin (B. Braun)
Soybean oil	19 g	19 g
Egg yolk phospholipids	3.5 g	1.9 g
Glycerol	50 g	—
Sorbitol	—	50 g
DL-tocopherol	0.2 g	—
Amino acid	30 g	30 g
Water to-	500 ml	500 ml

Chapter 25). There are at least two lipid-protein-carbohydrate mixtures available (Table 10.4).

REFERENCES AND FURTHER READING

Abbott W C, Grakauskas A M, Bistrian B R, Rose R, Blackburn G L Metabolic and respiratory effects of continuous and discontinuous lipid infusions. Arch Surg 1984; 119: 1367–1371

Adamkin D H, Gelke K N, Andrews B F Fat emulsions and hypertriglyceridemia. JPEN 1984; 8: 563–567

Askanazi J, Nordenstrom J, Rosenbaum S H, Elwyn D H, Hyman A I, Carpentier Y A, Kinney J M Nutrition for the patient with respiratory failure: glucose vs fat. Anesthesiol 1981; 54: 373–377

Berge Hvd, de Jong P C M, Soeters P B, Greep J M Clearance of fat emulsions in severely stressed patients. Nutr Supp Serv 1984; 4(12): 18–26

Bivins B A, Bell R M, Rapp R P, Griffen W O Jnr Linoleic acid versus linolenic acid: what is essential? JPEN 1983; 7: 473–478

Elwyn D H, Kinney J M, Gump F E, Askanazi J, Rosenbaum S H, Carpentier Y A Some metabolic effects of fat infusions in depleted patients. Metabolism 1980; 29: 125–132

Goodgame J T, Lowry S F, Brennan M F Essential fatty acid deficiency in total parenteral nutrition: time course of development and suggestions for therapy. Surgery 1978; 84: 271–277

Hansrani P K, Davis S S, Groves M J The preparation and properties of sterile intravenous emulsions. J Parent Sci Technol 1983; 37: 145–150

Heyman M B, Storch S, Ament M E The fat overload syndrome. Report of a case and literature review. Am J Dis Child 1981; 135: 628–630

Holman R T The deficiency of essential fatty acids. In: Kunau W H, Holman R T (eds) Polyunsaturated Fatty Acids. American Oil Chemists' Society, Champaign, Illinois, 1977; 163–182

Holman R T, Johnson S B, Hatch T F A case of human linolenic acid deficiency involving neurological abnormalities. Am J Clin Nutr 1982; 35: 617–623

Jeejeebhoy K N, Anderson G H, Nakhooda A F, Greenberg G R, Sanderson I, Marliss E B Metabolic studies in total parenteral nutrition with lipid in man: comparison with glucose. J Clin Invest 1976; 57: 125–136

Lindor K D, Fleming C R, Abrams A, Hirschkorn M A Liver function values in adults receiving total parenteral nutrition. JAMA 1979; 241: 2398–2400

Long J M III, Dudrick S J, Duke J H Jnr A rationale for glucose as primary calorie source. In: Richards J R, Kinney J M (eds) Nutritional Aspects of Care in the Critically Ill. Churchill Livingstone, Edinburgh, 1977; 331–344

Martin D J Topical lotion for essential fatty acids. Nutr Supp Services 1981; 1(7): 40

Mascioli E A, Smith M F, Trerice M S, Meng H C, Blackburn G L Effect of total parenteral nutrition with cycling on essential fatty acid deficiency. JPEN 1979; 3: 171–173

Miyahara T, Fujiwara H, Yae Y, Okano H, Okochi K, Torisu M Abnormal lipoprotein appearing in plasma of patients who received a ten percent soybean oil emulsion infusion. Surgery 1979; 85: 566–574

Nanni G, Siegel J H, Coleman B, Fader P, Castiglione R Increased lipid fuel dependence in the critically ill septic patient. J Trauma 1984; 24: 14–29

Nordenstrom J, Askanazi J, Elwyn D H, Martin P, Carpentier Y A, Robin A P, Kinney J M Nitrogen balance during total parenteral nutrition: glucose vs fat. Ann Surg 1983; 197: 27–33

Phillips G D, Odgers C L Parenteral nutrition: current status and concepts. Drugs 1982; 23: 276–323

Robin A P, Nordenstrom J, Askanazi J, Carpentier Y A, Elwyn D H, Kinney J M Influence of parenteral carbohydrate on fat oxidation in surgical patients. Surgery 1984; 95: 608–618

Schroder H, Paust H, Schmidt R Pulmonary fat embolism after Intralipid therapy — a post-mortem artefact? Acta Paediatr Scand 1984; 73: 461–464

Silberman H, Dixon N P, Eisenberg D The safety and efficacy of a lipid based system of parenteral nutrition in acute pancreatitis. Am J Gastroenterol 1982; 77: 494–497

Solassol C, Joyeux H, Serrou B, Pujol H, Romieu C Nouvelles techniques de nutrition parenterale a long terme pour suppleance intestinale. Chirurgie 1973; 105: 15–24

Steginck L D, Freeman J B, Wispe J, Connor W E Absence of the biochemical symptoms of essential fatty acid deficiency in surgical patients undergoing protein sparing therapy. Am J Clin Nutr 1977; 30: 388–393

Wretlind A Development of fat emulsion. JPEN 1981; 5: 230–235

11

Newer substrates

A number of metabolic substrates are currently being investigated in the search for alternate or supplementary nutritional sources that will optimise nutritional support in the critically ill patient. Protein metabolism is altered drastically in these patients and there is a progressive inability of skeletal muscle to use carbohydrates and fat as energy sources for ATP production (see Chapter 6).

GLYCEROL

Glycerol is a naturally occurring sugar alcohol in foods and living tissues. In the mammalian species glycerol is made available from adipose tissues by lipolysis (see Fig. 5.1) and from dietary fats. On oxidation, this 3-carbon sugar alcohol enters the glycolytic pathway through phosphorylation to alpha-glycerophosphate, to be utilised as an energy substrate in the TCA cycle. Alternatively, glycerol can be utilised to form glucose and glycogen via gluconeogenesis. Exogenous glycerol also may participate in lipogenesis through conversion to triglyceride (Fig. 11.1).

Because glycerol possesses a number of important metabolic properties, its use as a potential nutrient to serve as an energy source and to conserve body protein is currently being investigated. Tao et al (1983) have reviewed the literature concerning glycerol metabolism in mammalian species and its possible adverse effects and concluded that:

— glycerol is gluconeogenic and can be metabolised under hypocaloric conditions to generate energy, 18 kJ (4.32 kcal) per 1 g, and conserve body proteins
— the insulin response to exogenous glycerol is small and inconsistent and appears to be dependent on the route of administration. Intravenous administration of 1 g/kg body weight did not result in increased serum insulin concentrations in humans; thus they postulated that fat mobilisation should occur during nutritional therapy with glycerol
— transport of glycerol across cell membranes appears to be independent of insulin

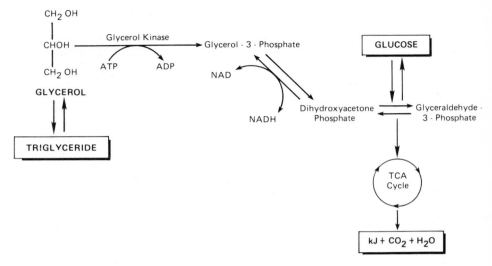

Fig. 11.1 Metabolism of glycerol.

— addition of glycerol to the postoperative protein sparing regimen may reduce ketosis (i.e. glycerol has antiketogenic properties)
— the undesirable effects reported, including haemolysis, haemoglobinuria and renal damage, are highly dose and route dependent with the incidence of adverse effects being relatively low with intravenous administration
— the turnover rate is of the order of 0.74 g/kg per hour
— a solution of amino acids, glycerol and electrolytes is chemically compatible and can be heat sterilised.

A recent multicentre study comparing the safety and efficacy of a commercially prepared amino acid-glycerol-electrolyte solution (Procal-Amine® — Table 11.1) with an isonitrogenous amino acid control solution in patients undergoing elective gastrointestinal or vascular surgery, demonstrated that the glycerol containing solution was safe and contributed to an improvement in nitrogen homeostasis.

SYNTHETIC GLYCERIDES

Preliminary investigations have been undertaken in rats to ascertain whether synthetic glycerides of short and medium chain fatty acids (C_{10} or less), and the so-called ketone bodies acetoacetic acid and beta-hydroxybutyric acid can support weight gain and be considered as potential alternatives to glucose in parenteral nutrition.

The reasons for investigating these substances have been based on a number of considerations, including:

Table 11.1 Composition of peripheral amino acid-glycerol-electrolyte solution (amino acid content expressed as grams per 16 g of nitrogen)

L-Amino acids	ProcalAmine 3% (American McGaw) gAA/16g N	% of total
Isoleucine	7.30	7.14
Leucine	9.39	9.18
Lysine	7.65	7.48
Methionine	5.56	5.44
Phenylalanine	5.91	5.78
Threonine	4.17	4.08
Tryptophan	1.60	1.56
Valine	6.96	6.80
Cystine (Cysteine)	(<0.70)	(<0.68)
Tyrosine	—	—
Alanine	7.30	7.14
Arginine	10.09	9.86
Aspartic acid	—	—
Glutamic acid	—	—
Glycine	14.61	14.28
Histidine	2.96	2.89
Proline	11.83	11.57
Serine	6.26	6.12
Calculated totals	102.29	100.00
Essential AA %		47.46
Aromatic AA %		5.78
Branched chain AA %		23.12
Nitrogen %		15.64
E = Total essential AA	48.54	
AA:Nitrogen ratio	6.39	
E:T Ratio	3.03	
Glycerol g/16g N	104.34	—

— the shorter chain fatty acids are more water soluble, and hence complications associated with emulsifiers are avoided
— short chain fatty acid esters are hydrolysed by hydrolases and esterases located throughout the body water space
— oxidation of these fatty acids can occur independently of the intracellular carnitine transport system
— carnitine-independent fats provide substrates for tissues such as skeletal muscle, which have an obligatory need for fats, either as fatty acids or as ketogenic amino acids and ketone bodies
— even chain fatty acids are ketogenic, and ketone bodies have been shown to be an important facet of protein sparing accompanying uncomplicated starvation in obese man
— ketone bodies can readily replace glucose as the major energy substrate in many tissues, including the brain, although the liver does not oxidise ketones

— synthetic glycerides provide glucose by releasing glycerol for hepatic gluconeogenesis
— thermodynamic data indicate that, if they are fully oxidised to carbon dioxide and water, the water-soluble monoglycerides, monobutyrin and monoacetoacetin provide 23.8 kJ (5.7 kcal) per 1 g and 18.4 kJ (4.4 kcal) per 1 g, respectively.

The concept of a carbohydrate, carnitine independent fat energy system would appear to merit further investigation as a potential energy substrate in parenteral nutrition.

MEDIUM CHAIN TRIGLYCERIDES

Medium chain triglycerides (MCTs) are components of certain dietary fats and have been used for some years as fat and caloric sources in enteral nutrition. MCTs are a mixture of medium chain saturated fatty acids containing 6–12 carbon atoms — C6:0 (1–2%), C8:0 (65–75%), C10:0 (25–35%) and C12:0 (1–2%). They are obtained by the hydrolysis of coconut oil followed by the fractionation of the fatty acids. Esterification with glycerol results in the formation of triacylglycerols. Medium chain fatty acids (MCFAs) have a lower molecular weight than the long chain fatty acids and are relatively soluble in water. As weak electrolytes, MCFAs are highly ionised at neutral pH, thus increasing their solubility in biological fluids. MCTs are a concentrated source of energy, providing 34.7 kJ (8.3 kcal) per gram.

MCTs, administered enterally, are hydrolysed quickly and more completely than long chain triglycerides in the presence of pancreatic lipase to MCFAs, which are absorbed mainly as the free fatty acids. However, because the enzyme acyl-CoA synthetase which is present in the mucosa and which facilitates conversion of long chain fatty acids to triacylglycerol (the major component of chylomicrons), is specific to fatty acids with more than 12 carbon atoms, MCFAs are not incorporated to any significant degree into chylomicrons. Unlike the long chain fatty acids, the MCFAs do not stimulate the flow of lymph. Instead, they are transported to the liver via the portal venous system, bound to serum albumin.

The majority of the MCFAs are retained in the liver. They are not incorporated into the acids synthesised in the liver, but rather cross rapidly into the mitochondria where they are acylated by octanoyl-CoA synthetase, then undergo beta-oxidation with the production of excess amounts of acetyl-CoA. Many hydrogen ions are produced during the process which, together with the excess acetyl-CoA, reduce the amount of oxaloacetate available to the TCA cycle (see Fig. 5.2). As a consequence, a large part of the acetyl-CoA is redirected towards the synthesis of ketone bodies, i.e. MCTs are ketogenic.

MCFA transport across the mitochondrial membrane and their subsequent oxidation, can occur independently of the intracellular carnitine transport system, which is essential to the hepatic metabolism of long chain fatty acids. The hepatic metabolism of MCFAs and long chain fatty acids is depicted in Figure 11.2. The role of extrahepatic tissues in the metabolism of MCTs is small, except for the utilisation of ketone bodies.

Although MCTs have been used successfully for many years as a source of energy and lipid precursors in enteral nutrition, it was argued that their incorporation into parenteral nutrition regimens was inappropriate because they would be 'absorbed too rapidly'. In fact, it has been demonstrated that the clearance of MCFAs by extrahepatic tissues is increased considerably when MCTs are infused intravenously. Also, it has been shown in animals that excessive intravenous doses of MCTs will induce metabolic acidosis due to hyperketonaemia and hyperlacticacidaemia. MCTs do not satisfy the requirement for essential fatty acids.

It has been proposed that mixtures of MCTs and long chain fatty acids,

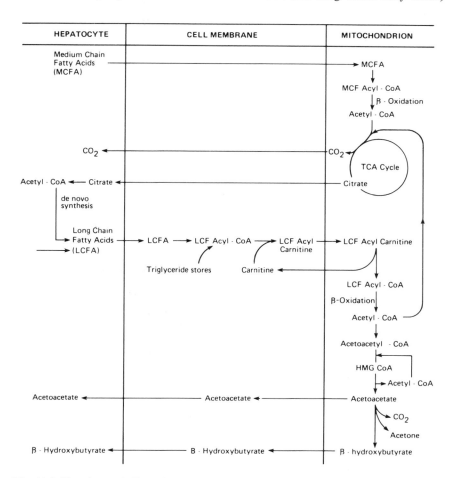

Fig. 11.2 Hepatic metabolism of medium chain fatty acids and long chain fatty acids.

E

or mixtures of MCTs with linoleic acid, would ensure the presence of essential fatty acid for nutritional needs, while slowing down the absorption of the balance of the triglyceride. The results of some of the studies published using fat emulsions containing a high percentage of medium chain triglycerides indicate that they are rapidly oxidised, at least in part. Some metabolic changes have been reported in patients infused with a soybean oil-medium chain triglyceride emulsion, and these include increased blood glucose concentration and signs of impaired hepatic function. However, the specific cause(s) of these disturbances has not been determined. An increase in the leucocyte count also has been observed during infusion, although this increase was significantly less than when the subjects were receiving Lipofundin® S 10%.

CARNITINE

The principal route for catabolising fatty acids is beta-oxidation, which occurs in the mitochondria. Long chain fatty acids enter the mitochondria after binding of the activated fatty acid, fatty-acyl-CoA to L-carnitine to produce fatty-acyl-carnitine. Once inside the mitochondria, CoA-SH displaces carnitine to regenerate fatty-acyl-CoA and then acetyl-CoA is produced by beta-oxidation. This acetyl-CoA is either oxidised via the TCA cycle or leaves the matrix space as acetyl carnitine (Fig. 11.2). It has been suggested that carnitine serves a dual function in ketone metabolism, stimulating both hepatic ketogenesis and utilisation of ketones by extrahepatic tissues. These suggestions have been based on investigations in rats. Other investigations, using animal models with induced myocardial ischaemia, have reported decreased fatty acid oxidation and low carnitine concentrations in cardiac tissues. Exogenous carnitine increased oxygen uptake and contractile forces of cardiac muscle, and stimulated oxidation of branched chain amino acids. Systemic carnitine deficiency (low plasma and tissue carnitine concentrations with multiple system involvement), presenting as a familial cardiomyopathy, has been reported recently in 4 of 5 children.

Carnitine, beta-hydroxy-γ-trimethylaminobutyric acid, can be synthesised endogenously by mammalian species from two essential amino acids, lysine and methionine, and man can synthesise 16–20 mg daily. Carnitine is present in foods of animal origin. Carnitine concentrations have been correlated with an increased glucagon:insulin ratio, increased catecholamine concentration and increased metabolic utilisation of fat. Although a classical carnitine deficiency resulting from dietary manipulation has not been observed, it has been suggested that the endogenous synthesis of carnitine may be insufficient to meet total body needs under certain disease conditions.

Decreasing blood and urine concentrations of carnitine have been reported in premature infants receiving carnitine-free parenteral nutrition. Limited intakes of lysine and/or methionine have been shown from animal studies to result in low tissue carnitine concentrations, and to lead to retarded growth and fatty liver. Measurements of tissue concentrations of carnitine in premature infants receiving TPN for periods greater than 15 days revealed low concentrations in the liver and heart, whereas the carnitine content of skeletal muscle was not significantly lower than that in term infants.

Adult patients receiving TPN appear to be able to maintain normal plasma carnitine concentrations for considerable periods of time. However, endogenous synthesis may not be sufficient to maintain stable concentrations for more than 20–40 days. Low concentration of plasma carnitine and reduced urinary carnitine excretion with persistently elevated plasma bilirubin concentration, reactive hypoglycaemia and generalised muscle weakness, have been described in an adult patient requiring long-term TPN. Plasma values were corrected by the infusion of L-carnitine 400 mg/24 hours for 7 days, and subsequently maintained with a daily infusion of 60 mg of L-carnitine. Bilirubin concentration returned to normal, reactive hypoglycaemia was no longer present, and muscle strength improved.

Tao & Yoshimura (1980) hypothesised that exogenous carnitine can enhance fat utilisation in patients supported by parenteral nutrition by several mechanisms, including:

— increasing utilisation of endogenous fat to conserve body proteins in post-operative patients on protein sparing therapy
— eliminating fat deposition in the liver of patients receiving concentrated glucose solutions
— enhancing utilisation of fat emulsions.

Tao has reported since that hepatic fatty infiltration induced in rats by hypercaloric infusions of glucose was ameliorated but not eliminated by high doses of carnitine.

Both the free carnitine, acyl-carnitine and hence total blood carnitine concentrations, were demonstrated to be significantly lower in premature infants maintained on solutions commonly used for intravenous feeding (Intralipid® and Travasol®) compared to when they were fed orally with expressed milk or a proprietary formula known to contain carnitine. Although no clinical problem was ascribed to the low concentrations of total carnitine, it was hypothesised that some of the toxic effects of Intralipid® in very small infants may, at least in part, have been due to the lack of carnitine and hence a relative inability of these infants to utilise lipids.

Schmidt-Sommerfeld et al (1983) have reported that an infusion of L-carnitine over approximately 5 hours at the rate of 10 mg/kg body weight per 24 hours improved the ability of immature infants to oxidise fatty acids. However, they recommend that further investigations be carried out to determine whether this represents a clinically significant contribution to parenteral nutrition.

These studies and others emphasise the need to elucidate further the morphologic and metabolic changes associated with low tissue concentrations of carnitine and the potential therapeutic benefit of supplementing carnitine during the course of parenteral nutrition for premature infants in particular.

REFERENCES AND FURTHER READING

Bach A C, Babayan V K Medium-chain triglycerides: an update. Am J Clin Nutr 1982; 36: 950–962

Birkhahn R H, Border J R Alternate or supplemental energy sources. JPEN 1981; 5: 24–31

Bohmer T, Rydning A, Solberg H E Carnitine levels in human serum in health and disease. Clin Chim Acta 1974; 57: 55–61

Boudin G, Mikol J, Guillard A, Engel A G Fatal systemic carnitine deficiency with lipid storage in skeletal muscle, heart, liver and kidney. J Neurol Sci 1976; 30: 313–325

Eckart J, Adolph M, Muhlen U van der, Naab V Fat emulsions containing medium chain triglycerides in parenteral nutrition of intensive care patients. JPEN 1980; 4: 360–366

Freeman J B, Fairfull-Smith R, Rodman G H Jnr, Bernstein D M, Gazzaniga A B, Gersovitz M Safety and efficacy of a new peripheral intravenously administered amino acid solution containing glycerol and electrolytes. Surg Gynecol Obstet 1983; 156: 625–631

Penn D, Schmidt-Sommerfeld E, Pascu F Decreased tissue carnitine concentrations in newborn infants receiving total parenteral nutrition. J Pediatr 1981; 98: 976–978

Penn D, Schmidt-Sommerfeld E, Wolf H Carnitine deficiency in premature infants receiving total parenteral nutrition. Early Hum Dev 1980; 4: 23–34

Rovamo L Postheparin plasma lipases and carnitine in infants during parenteral nutrition. Pediatr Res 1985; 19: 292–296

Rudman D, Sewell C W, Ansley J D Deficiency of carnitine in cachetic cirrhotic patients. J Clin Invest 1977; 60: 716–723

Sailer D, Muller M Medium chain triglycerides in parenteral nutrition. JPEN 1981; 5: 115–119

Schmidt-Sommerfeld E, Penn D, Wolf H Carnitine deficiency in premature infants receiving total parenteral nutrition: effect of L-carnitine supplementation. J Ped 1983; 102: 931–935

Sherwin R S, Hendler R G, Felig P Effect of ketone infusions on amino acid and nitrogen metabolism in man. J Clin Invest 1975; 55: 1382–1390

Tao R C, Yoshimura N N Carnitine metabolism and its application in parenteral nutrition. JPEN 1980; 4: 469–486

Tao R C, Kelley R E, Yoshimura N N, Benjamin F Glycerol: its metabolism and use as an intravenous energy source. JPEN 1983; 7: 479–488

Tripp M E, Katcher M L, Peters H A, Gilbert E F, Arya S, Hodach R J, Shug A L Systemic carnitine deficiency presenting as familial endocardial fibroelastosis. A treatable cardiomyopathy. New Engl J Med 1981; 305: 385–390

Worthley LIG, Fishlock R C, Snoswell A M Carnitine deficiency with hyperbilirubinemia, generalized skeletal muscle weakness and reactive hypoglycemia in a patient on long-term total parenteral nutrition: treatment with intravenous L-carnitine. JPEN 1983; 7: 176–180

12

Trace elements

Trace elements in human and animal metabolism have been investigated extensively for many years, but it is only in recent years that clinical interest has accelerated.

CRITERIA

A trace element may be classified as essential if it fits certain criteria:

— it is present in all healthy tissues of all living things
— its concentration from one animal to the next is fairly constant
— its withdrawal from the body induces reproducibly the same physiological and structural abnormalities regardless of the species studied
— its addition either reverses or prevents these abnormalities
— the abnormalities induced by deficiency are always accompanied by pertinent, specific biochemical changes
— these biochemical changes can be prevented or cured when the deficiency is prevented or cured.

Trace elements proven essential for man are zinc (Zn), copper (Cu), manganese (Mn), iodine (I), chromium (Cr), iron (Fe), cobalt (Co), selenium (Se) and molybdenum (Mo). Other trace elements proven essential for animals, but not yet for man, include nickel (Ni), silicon (Si), tin (Sn), and vanadium (V). Some of the roles of trace elements in physiological processes are listed in Table 12.1. In this chapter, current knowledge about zinc is reviewed in some detail, while the other elements are dealt with much more briefly, since their deficiency is a problem only in long-term TPN.

Zinc

Kay & Tasman-Jones, in a letter to the Lancet in 1975, reported zinc deficiency in 4 patients receiving intravenous feeding. These patients were all cachectic due to gastrointestinal disease or complications of abdominal surgery. All were commenced on intravenous feeding with glucose, sorbitol,

Table 12.1 Role of trace elements in enzymes

Element	Dependent enzymes	Deficiency effects
Zinc	RNA polymerase	
	DNA polymerase	
	Carbonic anhydrase	Growth retardation
	Alkaline phosphatase	Alopecia
	Alcohol dehydrogenase	Dermatitis
	Superoxide dismutase	Diarrhoea
	Glyceraldehyde-3-P dehydrogenase	Decreased wound healing, depression
	Procarboxypeptidase	Ileus
	Retinene reductase	Infertility
Copper	Cytochrome-c-oxidase	Neutropenia
	Dopamine-β-hydroxylase	Anaemia
	Monoamine oxidase	Subperiosteal haematomas
	Superoxide dismutase	Hypotonia
	Tyrosinase	Psychomotor retardation
	Lysyl oxidase	Apnoea
	Urate oxidase	
Manganese	Cholinesterase	
	Pyruvate carboxylase	Vitamin K deficiency
	Glycosyl transferase	(one preliminary report)
	Arginase	
	Superoxide dismutase	
Chromium	Glucose tolerance factor	Neuropathy
		Diabetes
Molybdenum	Xanthine oxidase	
	Aldehyde oxidase	See text
Selenium	Glutathione peroxidase	Myositis
		Cardiomyopathy

fat emulsion and crystalline amino acid solutions. At times varying from 2 to 5 weeks following the institution of TPN, they developed a syndrome of mental apathy, depression, irritability, tremor, poor concentration, diarrhoea, alopecia and a rash. The rash usually started as a moist eczematoid area in the nasolabial folds and progressed to crusting, followed by bullous or pustular lesions on other parts of the face, in the groins, and on the hands and feet, which in some cases coalesced to form large erosive areas (Fig. 12.1).

It was noted that there was a high urinary zinc loss (up to 23.6 mg/24 hours), and that the plasma zinc concentration fell when the patients became anabolic. It was speculated that the severe plasma zinc deficiency resulted from the avid demands for zinc during new protein formation and enzyme synthesis in the anabolic phase. Administration of zinc reversed the lesions — mental changes in a few hours, diarrhoea and skin lesions in a few days, and alopecia in a few weeks. The syndrome was likened to swine parakeratosis and acrodermatitis enteropathica, both known to be due to zinc deficiency.

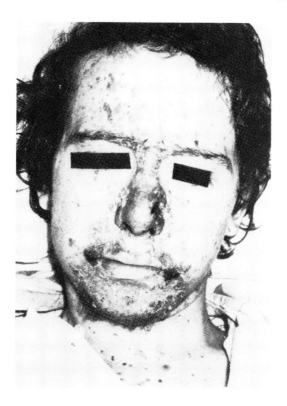

Fig. 12.1 Facial lesions induced by zinc deficiency. (Reproduced with permission of Kay et al, 1976, and Annals of Surgery)

Other reports of the clinical zinc deficiency syndrome appeared in quick succession, and they indicated that a zinc deficiency syndrome developed in some patients receiving TPN; that the deficiency was associated with gastrointestinal disease and diarrhoea; and that low concentrations of serum zinc and alkaline phosphatase were sometimes present. The syndrome occurred in patients receiving crystalline amino acid solutions but not in those receiving protein hydrolysates. The clinical features were reversed by administration of zinc.

There have been several balance studies of zinc in patients receiving TPN. Wolman et al studied 24 patients receiving a standard intravenous mixture of crystalline amino acids, glucose and fat emulsion. Additional zinc was added to provide 0.0, 1.5 and 3 mg, or 6.0, 12.0 and 23 mg per day for 1 week, during each of the 3 week study periods. They found that in the absence of excess zinc loss, 3 mg/day ensured a positive balance, whereas, if patients with significant diarrhoea were included, 6 mg/day was required to achieve zinc balance (Fig. 12.2). A formula was proposed to allow for zinc loss in gastrointestinal fluid:

$$\text{zinc requirements (mg/24 hours)} = 2 + 17.1a + 12.2b$$

where: a = mass (kg) of stool or ileostomy output in a patient with intact small bowel; b = mass (kg) of small bowel fluid loss via fistula/stoma or duodenojejunocolostomy; and 2 = urinary losses. They observed that urine zinc loss was not related to zinc input, that plasma zinc concentrations increased as the amount of zinc infused increased, but that plasma zinc concentrations did not correlate with zinc balances. There was a relationship between achieving positive zinc balance and improving nitrogen retention.

In a study of 8 critically ill patients, one of the authors reported positive

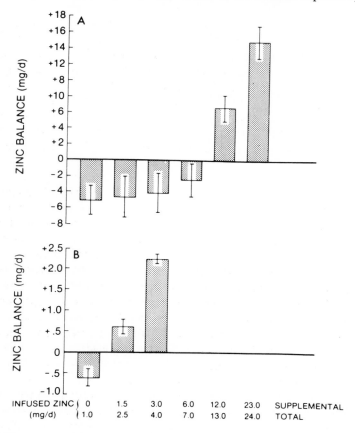

Fig. 12.2 Zinc balance almost achieved in 24 patients receiving 6 mg of zinc/day, with positive balance readily achieved with 12 mg/day (A). If patients without significant diarrhoea are considered separately, positive balance (with one exception) was achieved with addition of 3 mg zinc/day (B). (Reproduced with permission of Wolman et al, 1979, and Gastroenterology)

zinc balance in 4 of 8 patients receiving 1–1.25 mg zinc/day over a 7 day period. Serum zinc concentrations increased in all patients, irrespective of zinc balance. There was no consistent pattern of loss in urine or gastrointestinal fluid.

Although balance studies have a number of potential problems, including collection errors, sample quantitation and analytical difficulties, they do indicate the likelihood of whole body trace element deficiency occurring over a period of time in the absence of supplementation. They have demonstrated that negative balances occur either due to excess zincuria, or to excess zinc loss in gastrointestinal fluid.

Zincuria is known to occur in the catabolic state, and in conditions in which the relative proportions of protein bound and low molecular weight complexed zinc in plasma is altered. Heat sterilisation of solutions of glucose and amino acids may result in urinary zinc excretion up to four-times control concentrations, because of the formation of sugar-amine compounds which bind zinc and are then excreted in the urine. There appear to be many complex factors controlling serum and urine zinc.

It is clear that zinc should be administered to all patients receiving total parenteral nutrition, although caution is needed in the presence of impaired renal function. The American Medical Association recommendations of 2.5–4 mg (38–61 μmol) elemental zinc/24 hours for adults, plus an additional 2 mg if there is a catabolic state, meet most patients' requirements. If there is intestinal loss it is recommended that Wolman's formula be followed.

The AMA recommendation for premature infants up to 3 kg is 300 μg/kg per 24 hours, and for children up to 5 years is 100 μg/kg per 24 hours. The recommendations for premature infants have been challenged, and a figure of 488 μg/kg per 24 hours suggested by James. Therapeutic doses of zinc for an established deficiency state have varied. In the original series, 40–220 mg/24 hours were given, but toxicity clearly must be avoided.

It is now well established that zinc is present as a contaminant in significant amounts in protein hydrolysates, but not in synthetic amino acid solutions, glucose or fat emulsions. In view of the varying report of zinc content of intravenous solutions, there should be a requirement for manufacturers of amino acid solutions to state their zinc content so that more accurate zinc supplementation is possible. Administration of plasma or blood cannot supply adequate amounts of zinc.

Detection of zinc deficiency and monitoring of zinc status is difficult, since plasma or serum zinc concentrations are unreliable guides to zinc status. Other indicators of zinc status have been proposed, including the zinc containing enzymes serum alkaline phosphatase and red blood cell carbonic anhydrase and leucocyte zinc concentrations — there are conflicting views about the value of these. Clinical awareness remains the best guide to detection of zinc deficiency, and urine zinc excretion the best indicator of requirements.

Essential fatty acid deficiency produces a clinical picture difficult to distinguish from zinc deficiency. It has been suggested that zinc deficiency blocks a step in the formation of γ-linolenic acid and the subsequent synthesis of series 2 prostaglandins from arachidonic acid. Use of plasma prostaglandin concentrations as an index of zinc deficiency is complicated by the fact that the primary prostaglandins E2 and F2α, and their plasma concentrations, show wide diurnal variations.

Copper

Copper, like zinc, is present in a number of enzymes, including cytochrome-c-oxidase, and also is of known importance in erythropoiesis. A deficiency state, with neutropenia and anaemia responding to copper administration, was described in 1972 in a neonate on long-term parenteral nutrition. Development of subperiosteal haematomas in an infant has been attributed to copper deficiency, which may result in defective kinetics of lysyl oxidase and ascorbic acid oxidase, producing a scurvy-like lesion.

In a study of 24 patients reported in 1981, copper requirements were found to be 0.3 mg/24 hours, increasing to 0.5 mg/24 hours in patients with excess gastrointestinal fluid loss. As with zinc, plasma copper concentrations do not reflect copper balance.

Chromium

Chromium deficiency during prolonged parenteral nutrition has resulted in glucose intolerance and neuropathy, reversed by chromium administration. Chromium acts as a cofactor with insulin at the cellular level, promoting glucose oxidation, lipogenesis and muscle glycogenesis. Chromium deficiency can best be assessed by demonstrating an abnormal glucose clearance responding to chromium supplementation.

Manganese

Manganese deficiency has been observed in man in association with a vitamin K deficiency, although this was an isolated preliminary report in 1977.

Iodine

Iodine metabolism is relatively well understood, and its administration is necessary in long-term parenteral nutrition to prevent the development of hypothyroidism with goitre, secondary to decreased synthesis of the iodine-containing hormones thyroxine and triiodothyronine.

Iron

Iron metabolism likewise is well understood. Iron is not included in many regimens, since iron deficiency anaemia develops slowly. A dilute iron dextran formulation has been used, added to the TPN solution, but many are reluctant to administer this because of the risk of adverse reactions.

Cobalt

Cobalt is an integral part of vitamin B_{12} and requirements are met if vitamin B_{12} is administered in appropriate doses.

Selenium

Van Rij et al have described a 37 year old woman from a known selenium deficient area of New Zealand who developed severe muscle pain and tenderness 30 days after commencing TPN following surgery and radiotherapy. Serum and red blood cell selenium concentrations, and that of glutathione peroxidase, were all low. Daily administration of 100 μg selenomethionine intravenously resulted in resolution of the muscle pain and tenderness within a week.

There have been several case reports of patients receiving home TPN developing a cardiomyopathy similar to that of Keshan disease, an endemic cardiomyopathy responsive to selenium, and occurring in parts of China. Thus evidence is accumulating of TPN-related selenium deficiency.

Molybdenum

A recent case report indicates that molybdenum deficiency may cause a defect in sulphur amino acid and uric acid metabolism. A patient who developed tachycardia, tachypnoea, central scotomas, night blindness, irritability and coma while receiving prolonged TPN, improved on administration of 300 μg/24 hours of ammonium molybdate.

TOXICITY

Zinc toxicity has occurred. A death has been reported from inadvertent administration of 46 mmol (7.4 g) of zinc sulphate over 60 hours. The serum zinc was 640 μmol/l (4184 μg %). The patient developed hypotension, pulmonary oedema, vomiting, diarrhoea, jaundice and oliguria.

Another patient given 150 μmol zinc sulphate intravenously over 1 hour developed sweating, vomiting, blurred vision, decreased level of consciousness, tachycardia, and hypothermia. Of 7 patients inadvertently given a solution containing 100 mg zinc sulphate per litre, equivalent to 22.7 mg elemental zinc, 6 developed high serum amylase concentrations, which decreased when the dose was reduced.

REQUIREMENTS

Several authors have reported the trace element content of intravenous solutions, noting that while trace elements are present to a varying degree as contaminants, the quantities are not enough to provide daily requirements.

Maintenance requirements in adults have been variously estimated. Table 12.2 sets out the recommendations of Shenkin and also the American Medical Association.

Table 12.2 Maintenance requirements for trace elements per 70 kg (adult intravenous administration)

Element μmol/day (μg/day)	Shenkin 1977*		A.M.A. 1979*	
Cr	1	(50)	0.19–0.29	(10–15)
Cu	5–70	(300–4500)	7.9–23.6	(500–1500)
Fe	21–70	(1170–3900)	NR	
Mn	7–35	(380–1900)	2.7–14.5	(150–800)
Zn	49–210	(3200–13700)	38–61	(2500–4000)
F	21	(400)	NR	
I	1–7	(130–910)	NR	
Mo	0.2	(20)	NR	
Se	0.4	(30)	NR	

* Range of recommendations allows for increased requirements, as in catabolism, but see text for special circumstances, especially for zinc.
NR = no specific recommendations.

STABILITY

Various companies have developed commercial solutions of trace elements and market these either as single element solutions or multiple element solutions. In spite of initial concern regarding the stability of the sulphate salts of trace elements when solutions are autoclaved, a number of companies are using the sulphate salts of zinc, copper and manganese in their solutions; others are using the chloride salts. The physical and chemical stability of combinations of heavy metals and organonitrogenous moieties requires further elucidation. It has been suggested that when heavy metals such as iron and iodides are combined with organonitrogenous moieties such as protein hydrolysates, less soluble protein-metal complexes may be formed.

SUMMARY

Trace element deficiency is most unlikely during short-term TPN, but can occur particularly in patients with long-standing enteropathies. Administration of trace elements as contaminants in intravenous fluids is inadequate to prevent deficiency. No complications have been reported from administration of recommended doses of trace elements intravenously. Serum zinc and copper concentrations can be measured in major laboratories, but do not necessarily reflect whole body status. The most common deficiency state in the absence of supplementation is that of zinc.

Wolman et al have proposed, following studies in 24 patients with gastrointestinal disease receiving TPN, that administration of zinc improves nitrogen retention by influencing the insulin response and utilisation of glucose and amino acids.

REFERENCES AND FURTHER READING

Abumrad N N, Schneider A J, Steel D, Rogers L S Amino acid intolerance during prolonged total parenteral nutrition reversed by molybdate therapy. Am J Clin Nutr 1981; 34: 2551–2559

Beisel W R Metabolic balance studies — their continuing usefulness in nutritional research. Am J Clin Nutr 1979; 32: 271–274

Brocks A, Reid H, Glazer G Acute intravenous zinc poisoning. Br Med J 1977; 2: 1390–1391

Chen X, Wen Z, Ge K Studies on the relations of selenium and Keshan disease. Biol Trace Element Res 1980; 2: 91–107

Expert Panel, AMA Department of Foods and Nutrition. Guidelines for essential trace element preparations for parenteral use. JAMA 1979; 241: 2051–2054

Fleming C R, McCall J T, O'Brien J F, Forsman R W, Ilstrup D M, Petz J Selenium status in patients receiving home parenteral nutrition. JPEN 1984; 8: 258–262

Freund H, Atamian S, Fischer J E Chromium deficiency during total parenteral nutrition. JAMA 1979; 241: 496–498

Jacobson S, Wester P-O Balance study of twenty trace elements during total parenteral nutrition in man. Br J Nutr 1977; 37: 107–126

James B E, Hendry P G, MacMahon R A Total parenteral nutrition of premature infants. 2: Requirements for micronutrient elements. Aust Paediat J 1979; 15: 67–71

Jeejeebhoy K N, Chu R C, Marliss E B, Greenberg G R, Bruce-Robertson A Chromium deficiency, glucose intolerance, and neuropathy reversed by chromium supplementation, in a patient receiving long-term total parenteral nutrition. Am J Clin Nutr 1977; 30: 531–538

Karpel J T, Peden V H Copper deficiency in long-term parenteral nutrition. J Pediatr 1972; 80: 32–36

Kay R G, Tasman-Jones C, Pybus J, Whiting R, Black H A syndrome of acute zinc deficiency during total parenteral alimentation in man. Ann Surg 1976; 183: 331–340

Phillips G D Zinc in total parenteral nutrition. In: Prasad A S, Hetzel B S, Dreosti I (eds) Clinical Application of Recent Advances in Zinc. Alan Liss, New York, 1982

Prasad A S (ed) Trace elements in human health and disease. Vols. I and II. Academic Press, New York, 1976

Shenkin A, Wretlind A. Complete intravenous nutrition including amino acids, glucose and lipids. In: Richards J R, Kinney J M (eds) Nutritional Aspects of Care in the Critically Ill. Churchill Livingstone, Edinburgh, 1977; 345–365

Shils M E, White P L Trace element conference report. Bull NY Acad Med 1984; 60: 115–212

Underwood E J Trace elements in human and animal nutrition. 4th edition. Academic Press, New York, 1977

Van Rij A M, Thomson C D, McKenzie J M, Robinson M F Selenium deficiency in total parenteral nutrition. Am J Clin Nutr 1979; 32: 2076–2085

Wolman S L, Anderson G H, Marliss E B, Jeejeebhoy K N Zinc in total parenteral nutrition: requirements and metabolic effects. Gastroenterol 1979; 76: 458–467

13

Vitamins

The role of vitamins is summarised in Table 13.1, together with the classical deficiency states which develop from their dietary omission. The vitamins of the B complex function in a number of the essential reactions of intermediary metabolism:

Thiamine

Thiamine's physiologically active form, thiamine pyrophosphate (TPP), functions in carbohydrate metabolism as a coenzyme in the decarboxylation of alpha-keto acids such as pyruvate and alpha-keto-glutarate and in the utilisation of pentose in the HMP shunt.

Thiamine deficiency impairs carbohydrate metabolism in neurones and, with severe deficiency, carbohydrate metabolism in the heart and blood vessels is impaired. Signs of thiamine deficiency may occur when the carbohydrate intake is disproportionately high compared with the thiamine intake.

Wernicke's encephalopathy and death have been reported in association with prolonged intravenous feeding, in spite of thiamine supplementation. It has been suggested recently that in long-term parenteral nutrition, a polyneuropathy may develop, which is due to relative thiamine deficiency.

Riboflavine

Riboflavine's physiologically active forms, flavin mononucleotide (FMN) and flavin adenine dinucleotide (FAD), function as coenzymes in the oxidative deamination of amino acids, the beta-oxidation of fatty acids, oxidative phosphorylation, tissue respiration, and also purine catabolism.

Niacin (nicotinic acid)

Niacin's physiologically active forms, nicotinamide adenine dinucleotide (NAD) and nicotinamide adenine dinucleotide phosphate (NADP), function as coenzymes in numerous oxidation-reduction reactions including those of the TCA cycle, HMP shunt and beta-oxidation of fatty acids.

Table 13.1   Role of vitamins

Vitamin	Role	Deficiency state
Thiamine (B₁)	Coenzyme of: pyruvate decarboxylase alpha-ketoglutaric decarboxylase transketolase Structural component of neural membranes	Cardiomyopathy Neuropathy Encephalopathy
Riboflavine (B₂)	Flavin mononucleotide (constituent of: cytochrome-c-reductase l-amino acid dehydrogenase) Flavin adenine dinucleotide (constituent of: glycine oxidase xanthine oxidase acyl CoA dehydrogenase)	Stomatitis Cheilosis
Pantothenic acid	Coenzyme A	
Niacin	Constituent of: nicotinamide adenine dinucleotide nicotinamide adenine dinucleotide phosphate	Pellagra
Pyridoxine (B₆)	Constituent of coenzyme of: amino acid transaminases amino acid carboxylases	Dermatitis Cheilosis Glossitis Neuropathy
Biotin	Coenzymes in carboxylation reactions	Dermatitis Alopecia
Folic acid	Coenzymes in amino acid metabolism and DNA synthesis	Anaemia
Cyanocobalamin (B₁₂)	Coenzymes in amino acid metabolism and DNA synthesis	Anaemia Neuropathy
C	Connective tissue formation Oxidation/reduction reactions	Scurvy
A	Retinal pigment formation Epithelial integrity	Xerophthalmia Keratomalacia Night blindness
D	Calcium and phosphate absorption and metabolism	Rickets Osteomalacia
E	Antioxidant	
K	Synthesis of prothrombin factors VII, IX, X, II, IV	Haemorrhage

Pyridoxine

Pyridoxal phosphate functions as a coenzyme for a variety of reactions in intermediary metabolism. It is required to transfer amino groups in transamination reactions (for example, the conversion of alanine to pyruvate), then donates the amino group to another alpha-keto acid to transform it into an amino acid. It also participates in the decarboxylation and racemisation of amino acids and in the conversion of tryptophan to 5-hydroxytryptamine and of methionine to cysteine.

Pyridoxine deficiency causes convulsions, perhaps due to interference with the conversion of glutamic acid to the inhibitory neurotransmitter gamma aminobutyric acid, a step requiring both glutamic acid decarboxylase and pyridoxal phosphate. The latter enzyme also is necessary for synthesis of sphingomyelin, interference with which process causes peripheral neuropathy. Pyridoxine in excess is neurotoxic, although the mechanism is debated.

Pantothenic acid

Pantothenic acid combines with ATP and cysteine in the liver to generate coenzyme A (CoA), which serves as a coenzyme in reactions involving transfer of acetyl groups. Such reactions are important in carbohydrate metabolism, gluconeogenesis and synthesis and degradation of fatty acids.

Biotin

Biotin functions in several carboxylation reactions including those involving pyruvate carboxylase and acetyl-CoA. Thus it plays an important role in both carbohydrate and fat metabolism.

Biotin deficiency, producing dermatitis, alopecia, pallor, irritability, lethargy and hypotonia in a 12 month old child receiving parenteral nutrition, has been described, and more recently this clinical picture has been described in some adult patients. It has also been suggested that biotin deficiency may develop in children receiving TPN, particularly if they have malabsorption syndromes or diarrhoea, and in adults on long-term TPN.

Choline

Although not strictly a vitamin, choline has several roles in the body. It affects the mobilisation of fat from the liver, acts as a methyl donor and, together with acetyl-CoA, is synthesised to acetylcholine.

Cyanocobalamin

Cyanocobalamin's two active coenzymes, methylcobalamin and deoxyadenosylcobalamin transfer 1-carbon groups such as methyl groups. They are involved in a number of reactions in fat and carbohydrate metabolism, including the conversion of methylmalonyl-CoA to succinyl-CoA, and also protein synthesis.

Folic acid

Tetrahydrofolic acid (THFA) also functions as a coenzyme to carry 1-carbon groups in nucleoprotein synthesis.

Folic acid deficiency in patients receiving TPN was first described in 1974. Various mechanisms for its occurrence have been proposed, including depletion of body folate stores prior to commencement of TPN, administration of folate-free solutions, interference with folate metabolism by concurrent administration of ethanol in TPN solutions, and the presence of excess methionine or glycine in TPN mixtures.

Most clinicians are in the habit of administering multivitamin preparations parenterally to patients receiving intravenous nutrition. The commonly used solutions in Australia contain thiamine, riboflavine, niacin, pyridoxine, pantothenic acid and ascorbic acid, but none of the other water soluble or fat soluble vitamins. However, with the introduction of MVI–12® and similar products, this practice is changing.

Deficiencies of vitamins B_{12}, A, D and E, are unlikely to occur in short-term parenteral nutrition. However, vitamin A deficiency has been reported in a patient receiving home parenteral nutrition for Crohn's disease. The deficiency, producing a visual defect, occurred after 6 months, while the patient was receiving 900 μg (3000 IU) of retinol per day. Vitamin K deficiency will cause hypoprothrombinaemia, but this is easy to monitor. Vitamin C deficiency has been reported during TPN.

REQUIREMENTS

Current knowledge of vitamin requirements in parenteral nutrition has followed work carried out at Vanderbilt University. Their intravenous recommendations are given in Table 13.2. In their study, all vitamins were

Table 13.2 Daily vitamin recommendations and use (adult intravenous administration and oral administration)

	A.M.A. 1975	Nichoalds 1977	Bradley 1978	R.D.A.* 1980 (oral)
B_1 mg	3.0	21.0	50	1.4/1.0
B_2 mg	3.6	4.2	10	1.6/1.2
Niacin mg	40	42	100	18/13
B_6 mg	4	6.3	15	2.2/2.0
B_{12} μg	5	15	143	3.0
Pantothenate mg	15	10.5	25	4–7†
C mg	100	210	500	60
A (IU) mg	(3300) 1.135	(4200) 1.44	(10000) 3.44	1.0/0.8
D (IU) μg	(200) 5	(420) 10.5	N.R	5.0
E (IU) mg	(10) 10	(2.1) 2.1	(5) 5	10/8
Folate mg	0.4	0.6	2	0.4
K mg	0.5	N.R	1.4	0.07–0.14†
Biotin μg	60	N.R	N.R	100–200†

N.R = No recommendation.
   * Where male and female allowances differ, top figure is daily allowance for male 23–50 years, and bottom figure is daily allowance for female 23–50 years.
   † Estimated safe and adequate daily dietary intake.

added to the infusate and given evenly over 24 hours, and serum concentrations of folic acid, vitamins B_{12}, A, C, E and riboflavine were measured and found to be adequate. Note that if the recommendations are to be followed, none of the commercially available preparations offers a complete solution (Table 13.3 and 13.4). Bradley has reported adequate red cell B vitamins, folate and white cell vitamin C in critically ill patients using a regimen providing approximately two and a half times Nichoalds' recommendations.

In a study in which 39 patients received vitamin doses less than those recommended by the AMA (Table 13.2), plasma concentrations of vitamins A, E, folic acid and vitamin B_6 increased significantly. Three patients developed low concentrations of vitamin A, and 2 patients had evidence of thiamine deficiency. No abnormalities of vitamins B_2, B_6, or B_{12} were observed. The contents of some multivitamin preparations containing water and fat soluble vitamins are given in Tables 13.3 & 13.4.

STABILITY

The addition of vitamins to parenteral nutrition solutions is routine practice. However, there is much debate regarding the stability of some vitamins. Stability and compatibility factors relevant to the preparation of nutrition solutions include:

1. Vitamin A is both absorbed and adsorbed to plastic (PVC) and glass surfaces, the extent of sorption being greater with plastic (up to 75%). Preliminary tests using the recently released multivitamin preparation Berocca PN®, which contains retinyl palmitate to provide vitamin A

Table 13.3   Some vitamin preparations for parenteral use — Water soluble vitamins

Vitamin	Berocca-WS[1] (reconstituted)	Combex[2]	Parentrovite[3] (reconstituted)	Vitamin B group Plus C[4]
B_1 mg/ml	1.5	10	50	5
B_2 mg/ml	1.8	0.33	0.8	2.5
Niacin mg/ml	20	10	32	25
B_6 mg/ml	2	—	10	1.25
B_{12} μg/ml	2.5	10	—	—
Pantothenate mg/ml	7.5	4	1	2.5
Ascorbic acid mg/ml	50	—	100	25
A mg/ml	—	—	—	—
D μg/ml	—	—	—	—
E mg/ml	—	—	—	—
Folate mg/ml	0.2	—	—	—
Biotin μg/ml	30	—	—	—
K μg/ml	—	—	—	—

1. Roche Laboratories
2. Parke Davis & Co.
3. Beecham Research Laboratories
4. Nicholas (Intravite); David Bull Laboratories

Table 13.4 Some vitamin preparations for parenteral use — Water and fat soluble vitamins

	Berocca PN[1] (reconstituted to 2 ml)	Dayamin[2]	M.V.I-12[3]	Soluvit[4] (Solivito) (reconstituted to 10 ml)	Vitalipid[4] Adult[4]
B_1 mg/ml	1.5	10	0.3	0.12	—
B_2 mg/ml	1.8	2.5	0.36	0.18	—
Niacin mg/ml	20.0	37.5	4.0	1.0	—
B_6 mg/ml	2.0	2.5	0.4	0.2	—
B_{12} µg/ml	2.5	2	0.5	0.2	—
Pantothenate mg/ml	7.5	5	1.5	1.0	—
Ascorbic acid mg/ml	50.0	50	10.0	3.0	—
A mg/ml	0.5(a)	—	0.1	—	0.075
D µg/ml	2.5	1.2	0.5	—	0.3
E mg/ml	5.0	12.5	1.0	—	—
Folate mg/ml	0.2	1	0.04	0.02	—
Biotin µg/ml	30.0	—	6.0	30.0	—
K µg/ml	—	—	—	—	15

1. Roche Laboratories
2. Abbott Laboratories
3. USV Laboratories
4. KabiVitrum, AB
(a) as retinyl palmitate

activity, revealed that retinyl palmitate was not absorbed by the PVC infusion system when 5.5 μg/ml was added to glucose 5%. Further studies of the stability of this product in nutrition solutions and delivery systems are required before a conclusion can be drawn regarding the stability of retinyl palmitate. Vitamin A is decomposed quickly in sunlight.

2. Of the B group vitamins, thiamine hydrochloride is reported to be unstable with oxidising and reducing agents (particularly the antioxidant sodium bisulphite present in many amino acid solutions), should be protected from air and light, and is destroyed rapidly by heat:

   a. Riboflavine should be protected from light. Also, it may enhance photo-oxidation of certain amino acids.

   b. Pantothenic acid is stable in a nitrogen atmosphere.

   c. Niacin (nicotinic acid) is incompatible with oxidising agents. Niacin has been reported to be stable in parenteral nutrition solutions under different light conditions.

   d. Pyridoxine has been claimed to be incompatible with iron salts, oxidising agents, and should be protected from sunlight (there is minimal loss only on exposure to fluorescent light).

   e. Folic acid has been claimed by some workers to be incompatible with oxidising and reducing agents and riboflavine, and to decompose rapidly in the presence of light and/or riboflavine solutions. Others have reported that there is minimal to negligible loss of folic acid activity on exposure to fluorescent and ambient light. In a recent report, the degradation of folic acid added in MVI-12 to a TPN solution was described as proceeding by first order kinetics. The half-life of the degradation reaction was 2.7 $\pm$ 0.08 hours when stored at room temperature and exposed to daylight, and 5.36 $\pm$ 0.1 hours when protected from light. If a solution has a pH less than 5.0, folic acid may precipitate from solution.

   f. Cyanocobalamin is stated to be light sensitive. However further studies are required to support these claims.

3. Ascorbic acid is incompatible with many drugs, darkens on exposure to light, and is rapidly oxidised in air (and alkaline media). The degradation reaction for ascorbic acid has been reported to proceed according to first order kinetics with 50% of the initial concentration of 30 mg per litre remaining at 1.13 $\pm$ 0.06 hours when stored at room temperature and exposed to daylight, and 50% remaining at 2.93 $\pm$ 0.09 hours when protected from light. The oxidation rate for ascorbic acid is increased with increasing concentration of dissolved oxygen in the solution. Similarly, trace elements catalyse the oxidation reaction, and the order of effectiveness as catalysts has been reported to be $Cu^{2+} > Fe^{3+} > Zn^{2+} > Mn^{2+}$.

4. Vitamin D should be protected from light and air.

5. Alpha-tocopherol esters are stable in air and light, but alpha-tocopherols

are unstable. One study has suggested that there may be some sorption of alpha-tocopherol acetate (vitamin E) to the plastic of the infusion system. The concentration decreased 34% over 24 hours.

6. Vitamin K is light sensitive and incompatible with a wide range of drugs. However, there is a lack of published data concerning its stability in nutrition solutions and in the presence of ascorbic acid.

The rate of degradation of a number of these vitamins added immediately prior to administration can be reduced by protecting the solution from light with an ultraviolet light protective bag or wrapping.

Until further information is available it is advisable to administer vitamin K, vitamin B_{12} and possibly folic acid, by alternative routes to the parenteral nutrition fluid. Many workers give once weekly intramuscular injections of these vitamins. Those patients receiving long-term TPN should be monitored periodically to assess their status of vitamin A, thiamine and ascorbic acid, which have poor availability from TPN solutions.

It has been recommended that in order to avoid increased excretion of the water soluble vitamins following a rapid intravenous injection, these should be administered over a number of hours. Administration of 1 gram of ascorbic acid intravenously over 3–4 minutes resulted in an average half-life of 3.37 hours.

COMPLICATIONS

Complications of vitamin therapy may be related to excess administration of the fat soluble group, or masking of vitamin B_{12} deficiency by folic acid.

The development of metabolic bone disease in 12 patients receiving long-term parenteral nutrition has been reported. The metabolic and clinical features improved after cessation of vitamin D. Hypervitaminosis A, with alopecia, dermatitis, personality change, and painful bones due to periosteal new bone formation, has been reported recently in a 4 year old child who received 18 mg (60 000 IU) of vitamin A per day. Massive doses of pyridoxine (2–6g/day) have been reported to cause peripheral neuropathy.

REFERENCES AND FURTHER READING

Allwood M C Factors influencing the stability of ascorbic acid in total parenteral nutrition infusions. J Clin Hosp Pharm 1984; 9: 75–85

Bhatia J, Stegink L D, Ziegler E E Riboflavin enhances photo-oxidation of amino acids under simulated clinical conditions. JPEN 1983; 7: 277–279

Bradley J A, King R F J G, Schorah C J, Hill G L Vitamins in intravenous feeding: a study of water-soluble vitamins and folate in critically ill patients receiving intravenous nutrition. Br J Surg 1978; 65: 492–494

Editorial. Further studies of acute folate deficiency developing during total parenteral nutrition. Nutr Rev 1983; 41: 51–53

Food and Nutrition Board. Recommended Dietary Allowances (9th edn). National Academy of Sciences — National Research Council, Washington DC, 1980

Gillis J, Jones G, Pencharz P Delivery of vitamins A, D, and E in total parenteral nutrition solutions. JPEN 1983; 7: 11–14

Gutcher G R, Lax A A, Farrell P M Vitamin A losses to plastic intravenous infusion devices and an improved method of delivery. Am J Clin Nutr 1984; 40: 8–13

Howard L, Bigaouette J, Chu R, Krenzer B E, Smith D, Tenny C Water soluble vitamin requirements in home parenteral nutrition patients. Am J Clin Nutr 1983; 37: 421–428

Levenson J L Biotin-responsive depression during hyperalimentation. JPEN 1983; 7: 181–183

Nichoalds G E, Meng H C, Caldwell M D Vitamin requirements in patients receiving total parenteral nutrition. Arch Surg 1977; 112: 1061–1064

Niemiec P W Jnr, Vanderveen T W Compatibility considerations in parenteral nutrient solutions. Am J Hosp Pharm 1984; 41: 893–911

Nordfjeld K, Pedersen J L, Rasmussen M, Jensen V G Storage of mixtures for total parenteral nutrition. III: Stability of vitamins in TPN mixtures. J Clin Hosp Pharm 1984; 9: 293–301

Nutrition Advisory Group, Department of Foods and Nutrition, American Medical Association. Statement on multivitamin preparations for parenteral use. AMA, Chicago, IL, 1975. Cited in Multivitamin preparations for parenteral use. JPEN 1979; 3: 258–262

Shils M E, Baker H, Frank O Blood vitamin levels of long-term adult home total parenteral nutrition patients: the efficacy of the AMA–FDA parenteral multivitamin formulation. JPEN 1985; 9: 179–188

Velez R J, Myers B, Guber M S Severe acute metabolic acidosis (acute beriberi): an avoidable complication of total parenteral nutrition. JPEN 1985; 9: 216–219

14

Nutritional assessment

In 1975 Butterworth & Blackburn stated that malnourished patients did not tolerate stress well, seemed more prone to infection and tended to remain in hospital longer than well-nourished patients. Thus, they argued that a complex programme of nutritional assessment should be used to identify those patients who were in need of nutritional support. The assessment included a detailed history and physical examination of the patient, together with consideration of a number of indicators of malnutrition. The various indices employed in this study to quantitate initial nutritional status and progress are outlined in Table 14.1.

Table 14.1 Indices of nutritional assessment

Parameter	Indicator
Skeletal muscle protein	Arm-muscle circumference Creatinine-height index Weight/height
Visceral protein	Serum albumin Serum transferrin Total lymphocyte count
Fat stores	Triceps skinfold thickness
Immune status	Lymphocyte count Delayed hypersensitivity skin testing

During the past decade, several studies have reported that malnutrition occurs frequently in hospitalised patients, secondary to their underlying diseases. The proportion of patients cited as being malnourished ranges from 20 to 65%. More recently these proportions have been questioned because of the variable methodology used in such studies, the variable interpretation of results, the wide variability in the judgemental decisions made regarding the decision to operate, and the lack of uniformity as to the number of tests that should be interpreted as 'positive' for 'malnutrition' to be diagnosed.

Of the vast array of anthropometric, biochemical and immunological tests available to define protein-calorie malnutrition, the following have been

135

employed most frequently to assess the patient's nutritional status. A brief definition of each of these indices is provided, together with some of the problems involved in their interpretation.

SKELETAL MUSCLE (SOMATIC) PROTEIN

Anthropometric and biochemical measurements have been used routinely to estimate the skeletal muscle (somatic) protein mass.

Arm-muscle circumference (AMC)

This is a calculated value derived from the triceps skinfold thickness (TSF) and the mid-arm circumference (MAC) using the equation:

$$AMC \text{ (cm)} = MAC \text{ (cm)} - (0.314 \times TSF \text{ (mm)})$$

The upper arm muscle area (AMA) then is derived from the relationship:

$$AMA = \frac{(MAC - 0.314TSF)^2}{4 \times 0.314}$$

The values obtained are compared to existing standards, and the deficit determined.

Errors inherent in these measurements include the false assumption that both the arm and arm muscle are circular and that bone area can be neglected. In addition, there may be considerable variation between observers in the measurements of skinfold thickness and arm muscle circumference. Similarly, the existing 'standards' have changed considerably over the last two decades, just as they change with age and muscularity.

Creatinine-height index

Deficits in lean body mass have been estimated by comparing the actual urinary creatinine excreted over 24 hours with the expected excretion for height.

Several problems associated with the determination of the creatinine-height index have been identified. These include the difficulty in obtaining an accurate 24 hour urine collection, and the inappropriate application of available standards for predicting creatinine excretion from ideal body weight to young and old patients alike. Creatinine excretion may be increased or decreased, depending on the particular disease present. Creatinine excretion is proportional to skeletal muscle mass which relates not only to height, but also to body frame size. Great care must be taken in the application and interpretation of creatinine-height index in the nutritional assessment of hospitalised patients.

Weight (kg) and height (cm)

Although a comparison with ideal weight/height tables may provide a preliminary assessment of skeletal protein status, the patient's disease state may distort the measurement. The patient's body build also is important when considering this index. Changes in body water can easily mask changes in either the fat or muscle compartments of an individual. Weight change is a commonly used parameter and a loss of more than 10% over any period of time is accepted as evidence of malnutrition.

FAT STORES

Fat stores may be assessed by comparing the triceps skinfold measurement with existing standards. The percentage deficit in this measurement is then determined. Technical problems that must be considered when interpreting skinfold thickness include the presence of oedema or subcutaneous emphysema, altered skin pliability with the administration of intravenous fluids, and inter-observer variability. Changes in subcutaneous fat occur slowly with starvation and refeeding, and thus do not reflect acute nutritional changes.

VISCERAL PROTEIN

Visceral protein status reflects the patient's ability to respond clinically to stress, and is measured indirectly by the depression of secretory (transport) proteins synthesised by the liver.

Serum albumin
Albumin is a poor indicator of early protein malnutrition, as serum concentrations fall and recover slowly with changes in the patient's nutritional status. This slow response is due mainly to albumin's relatively long serum half-life (20 days) as well as the relatively large body pool of this visceral protein (4–5 g/kg). Serum thyroxine-binding prealbumin (prealbumin) has been suggested as a more reliable indicator of visceral protein status. It has a serum half-life of approximately 2 days and the body pool is relatively small.

Serum transferrin
Serum transferrin is a circulating glycoprotein that plays a central role in iron metabolism and an approximation of the serum transferrin value can be derived from the total iron binding capacity (TIBC) measurement:

$$\text{Serum transferrin} = (0.8 \times \text{TIBC}) - 43$$

It has a half-life of 8–10 days, and the extracellular pool is smaller than that for albumin, approximately 4 mg. Thus it has been argued that there are several theoretical advantages to using transferrin rather than serum albumin concentration as a measure of the nutritional state.

A recent study has demonstrated that although a highly significant correlation exists between serum transferrin concentration and the nutritional status of a population, there is a large variance of the data about the mean. It was concluded that this measurement lacks sufficient specificity and sensitivity to serve as a measure of an individual patient's nutritional state.

In measuring visceral protein status, the assumption has been made that a decrease in serum concentrations of these proteins is a consequence of decreased liver biosynthesis, which, in turn, is due both to a limited supply of substrate associated with malnutrition and an actual decrease in organ mass. The serum protein concentrations, however, are dependent on a number of factors including rate of metabolic utilisation, excretion, intravascular-extravascular transfer, degree of hydration, and administration of protein products including albumin, fresh frozen plasma and whole blood.

It has been proposed that serum retinol-binding protein (half-life of 10 hours) may be the most specific indicator of acute changes in protein malnutrition. However, retinol binding protein is filtered by the glomeruli and metabolised by the kidney, and high serum concentrations in patients with renal disease may be misleading.

Recently, the usefulness of plasma fibronectin, a glycoprotein which is thought to be of importance for a normal immunoresponse, has been evaluated as an indicator of response to short-term TPN in malnourished patients. The plasma half-life of fibronectin is thought to be about 12 hours.

IMMUNE STATUS

The status of the visceral proteins also mirrors the patient's ability to mount an immune response. The cellular immune status is estimated from the total lymphocyte count. Malnutrition is associated with decreased host resistance and a clear correlation has been established between nutrition and immune competence. There are a variety of approaches to measuring the effect of nutritional depletion and immune competence. Kahan (1981) has summarised the malnutrition-induced defects in specific and non-specific host resistance.

Many reports have been published on the role of delayed hypersensitivity skin testing in identifying those patients who are anergic and at risk of developing sepsis. In some it has been suggested that vigorous nutritional support may reverse the abnormalities of delayed hypersensitivity skin testing, while others have suggested that this testing is an essential component of nutritional assessment.

Twomey et al (1982) undertook an extensive review of the English literature on delayed hypersensitivity skin testing. They concluded that the data did not support the utility of this test in nutritional assessment of hospital patients. The majority of the studies reviewed lacked suitable controls for the non-nutritional variables known to influence skin testing response

Table 14.2 Some non-nutritional variables influencing skin test response

Non-nutritional variables	Examples
Technical	Antigen source and batch
	Storage
	Method of administration
	Site of test
	Criteria of positivity
	Reader variability
Patient	Age
	Race
	Geographical location
	Previous exposure
Diseases	
Benign	Infection
	Uraemia
	Hepatic disease
	Inflammatory disease, e.g. Crohn's, ulcerative colitis
	Immune alterations, e.g. SLE, rheumatoid arthritis
	Trauma, burns, haemorrhage
Malignant	Solid tumours, lymphomas, leukaemias
Iatrogenic	Drugs, e.g.
	immunosuppressants
	most antineoplastics
	antiinflammatory
	anticoagulants
	H_2-receptor antagonists
	X-ray therapy
	General anaesthesia
	Surgery

(Table 14.2), and did not provide evidence that patients with other than obvious malnutrition were detected.

Miller (1978), in a review of immunological assays as measurements of nutritional status, concluded that delayed hypersensitivity skin testing as a means of assessing the effect of malnutrition on immunocompetence was not without certain drawbacks.

PROGNOSTIC NUTRITIONAL INDEX

Mullen et al (1979) studied the value of 16 nutritional and immunological parameters in predicting subsequent morbidity and mortality in surgical patients. They concluded that the visceral protein compartment (serum albumin and serum transferrin concentrations with delayed hypersensitivity reactions) had a significant predictive value and developed an equation, the prognostic nutritional index (PNI), to relate the risk of post-operative complications to these three nutritional parameters and also the triceps skinfold:

$$PNI \% = 158 - 16.6 \text{ (Alb)} - 0.78 \text{ (TSF)} - 0.20 \text{ (TFN)} - 5.8 \text{ (DH)}$$

Because these indices may be affected by factors other than those related to the nutritional status, the utility of the PNI and its advantage over clinical assessment have been questioned.

CLASSIFICATION OF PROTEIN CALORIE MALNUTRITION

On the basis of the above measurements, three basic types of protein calorie malnutrition have been recognised:

Adult kwashiorkor-like state
Well or over-nourished individuals in whom the combination of severe stress and inadequate nutrition has resulted in visceral protein loss and impairment of immunologic competence. Anthropometric measurements such as weight/height, triceps skinfold thickness and arm circumference are maintained, while serum proteins are decreased and cell-mediated immunity depressed.

Adult marasmus
Chronic malnutrition with loss of weight, decreased skinfold thickness and decreased arm circumference but with preservation of normal visceral proteins.

Marasmus-kwashiorkor-like
Patients with a combination of the first and second types.

Nitrogen balance is useful in documenting the effectiveness of nutritional therapy and is determined by measurement of the 24-hour urine urea nitrogen excretion, from which an approximation of nitrogen balance and protein utilisation can be made. However, urinary urea excretion decreases in all forms of protein calorie malnutrition due to the body's attempts to conserve nitrogen. Nitrogen balance measurements, although widely employed to determine the efficacy of total parenteral nutrition, may be misleading due to the large experimental errors associated with nitrogen balance. Body composition measurements are being employed by some workers to monitor body cell mass and thus the efficacy of TPN.

There is no simple single method available for the accurate and clinically meaningful determination of nutritional status. Thus, emphasis must be placed on obtaining as much data as possible from the patient's dietary and clinical history, physical examination, and laboratory and anthropometric measurements, with considerable reliance being placed on the physician's clinical impression and judgement.

A simple programme of nutritional assessment can be established in any hospital with some effort and no expense. Such a programme:

— assists in diagnosing the type and degree of malnutrition
— aids the selection of the most appropriate form of nutritional treatment
— provides data to evaluate the effectiveness of treatment.

ANERGIC METABOLIC PROFILE					
PATIENT		ROOM			
DATE		DEFICIT			
Parameters	Value	Severe	Mod	Mild	Adequate
SOMATIC PROTEINS					
WEIGHT/HEIGHT					
TRICEPS SKINFOLD mm					
ARM MUSCLE CIRCUMFERENCE cm					
CREATININE/HEIGHT INDEX					
VISCERAL PROTEINS					
ALBUMIN					
TRANSFERRIN					
TOTAL LYMPHOCYTE COUNT					
CELL MEDIATED IMMUNITY					

(Left margin labels: MARASMUS spanning WEIGHT/HEIGHT through CREATININE/HEIGHT INDEX; KWASHIORKOR spanning VISCERAL PROTEINS through TOTAL LYMPHOCYTE COUNT)

NITROGEN IN gm/day ___
NITROGEN OUT gm/day ___
NITROGEN BALANCE gm/day [ ]

NUTRITIONAL STATUS   DEGREE
☐ ADEQUATE   ☐ NONE
☐ MARASMUS   ☐ MILD
☐ KWASHIORKOR   ☐ MODERATE
☐ MARASMUS–   ☐ SEVERE
   KWASHIORKOR MIX

Standards	Severe	Moderate	Mild
SOMATIC PROTEINS			
– % DEFICIT	> 30%	>15-30%	> 5-15%
ALBUMIN (gm%)	< 2.5	<3.0-2.5	< 3.5-3.0
TRANSFERRIN (mg%)	< 160	<180-160	< 200-180
LYMPHOCYTE COUNT	< 900	<1500-900	< 1800-1500
CELL MEDIATED IMMUNITY			
– mm	< 5·0	<10·5	< 15-10

Fig. 14.1 Sample nutritional assessment data sheet. (Reproduced with permission from Kaminski & Winborn, 1978)

A record sheet such as that shown in Figure 14.1 has been used to aid documentation.

REFERENCES AND FURTHER READING

Baker J P, Detsky A S, Whitwell J, Langer B, Jeejeebhoy K N A comparison of the predictive value of nutritional assessment techniques. Human Nutr: Clin Nutr 1982; 36C: 233–241

Bistrian B R, Blackburn G L, Hallowell E, Heddle R Protein status of general surgical patients. JAMA 1974; 230: 858–860

Blackburn G L, Bistrian B R, Maini B S, Schlamm H T, Smith M F Nutritional and metabolic assessment of the hospitalized patient. JPEN 1977; 1: 11–22

Grant J P, Custer P B, Thurlow J Current techniques of nutritional assessment. Surg Clin N Am 1981; 61: 437–463

Hill G L, Blackett R L, Pickford I, Burkinshaw L, Young G A, Warren J V, Schorah C J, Morgan D B Malnutrition in surgical patients: an unrecognised problem. Lancet 1977; i: 689–692

Kahan B D Nutrition and host defense mechanisms. Surg Clin N Am 1981; 61: 557–570

Kaminski M V Jnr, Winborn A L Nutritional assessment guide. Midwest Nutrition, Education and Research Foundation, Chicago, 1978

McLaren D S, Meguid M M Nutritional assessment at the cross roads. JPEN 1983; 7: 575–579

Meakins J L, Pietsch J B, Bubenick O, Kelly R, Rode H, Gordon J, MacLean L D Delayed hypersensitivity: indicator of acquired failure of host defenses in sepsis and trauma. Ann Surg 1977; 186: 241–250

Miller C L Immunological assays as measurements of nutritional status: a review. JPEN 1978; 2: 554–566

Mullen J L, Gertner M H, Buzby G P, Goodhart G L, Rosato E F Implications of malnutrition in the surgical patient. Arch Surg 1979; 114: 121–125

Roza A M, Tuitt D, Shizgal H M Transferrin — a poor measure of nutritional status. JPEN 1984; 8: 523–528

Sandstedt S, Cederblad G, Larsson J, Schildt B, Symreng T Influence of total parenteral nutrition on plasma fibronectin in malnourished subjects with or without inflammatory response. JPEN 1984; 8: 493–496

Seltzer M H, Fletcher H S, Slocum B A, Engler P E Instant nutritional assessment in the intensive care unit. JPEN 1981; 5: 70–72

Shizgal H M The use of body composition measurements to assess the efficacy of parenteral nutrition. In: Johnston IDA (ed) Advances in Parenteral Nutrition. MTP Press, Lancaster, 1978; 535–555

Twomey P, Ziegler D, Rombeau J Utility of skin testing in nutritional assessment: a critical review. JPEN 1982; 6: 50–58

15

Monitoring

Almost all of the metabolic complications of total parenteral nutrition can be prevented by adequate monitoring. The extent of monitoring in enteral nutrition is usually dictated by the patient's disease state, rather than by use of EN itself.

1. Clinical monitoring consists of at least daily assessment of the patient's clinical condition, supplemented by routine nursing observations of pulse, temperature, respiratory rate and ward urinalysis. Patients should be on an accurate fluid balance chart and a diabetic urinalysis chart. Body weight should be measured prior to commencement of TPN and at regular intervals. Weight gain may be due to fluid retention rather than anabolism, and will certainly not be due to increased muscle bulk unless the patient actively exercises.

2. Routine biochemical monitoring in the early stages should include:

— daily blood urea, serum creatinine, serum sodium, potassium, chloride, bicarbonate, and blood glucose concentrations
— twice weekly liver function tests including total plasma proteins and albumin, bilirubin and liver enzymes, serum calcium, phosphate and magnesium concentrations, full blood count and a prothrombin estimation. The frequency of both groups of tests may be varied, depending on how the patient progresses. For example, serum potassium concentration may be required several times in 24 hours in a depleted patient with excessive gastrointestinal fluid loss; once a week in a patient who is quite stable, or once a month in a patient on home TPN
— other investigations as indicated, such as blood gases, serum and urine osmolalities, 24 hour urine and gastrointestinal fluid electrolytes, and urine urea from which nitrogen loss can be estimated.

3. Additional investigations may be indicated under special circumstances, such as plasma amino acid concentrations, blood ammonia, serum lipids, uric acid, zinc, copper, folic acid, vitamin B12, iron studies, thyroid status, measurement of 3-methylhistidine excretion.

4. In certain centres, formal nitrogen balance studies may be performed,

and sophisticated measurements such as whole body nitrogen and other measurements of body composition may be made.

Total body water may be measured by isotope dilution, using deuterium or tritium, and total body potassium can be measured similarly. Body cell mass, the metabolically active component of the body can be determined and monitored under different conditions.

Gas exchange measurements have become topical in the last few years. Very old, standard physiological techniques, based on measurement of O_2 consumption and CO_2 production, were incorporated into medicine mainly in areas such as measurement of the basal metabolic rate in relation to diagnosis of thyroid disease. Formerly a laboratory measurement, now there are available commercial portable instruments which can measure inspired and expired oxygen concentrations, and expired carbon dioxide concentrations in ventilated patients. Combined with flow rate, both oxygen consumption and carbon dioxide production are calculated, and respiratory quotient derived.

Table 15.1   Parameters employed to monitor response to TPN

4th hourly	Nursing observations
	    temperature
	    blood pressure
	    pulse
	    respirations
	Urinalysis or ward blood glucose

Daily	Blood urea Serum creatinine Serum electrolytes Blood glucose Blood gases (as indicated) Serum/urine osmolalities (as indicated) Nutrient intake Fluid balance
Twice weekly	Liver function tests Serum Ca/PO$_4$/Mg Complete blood count Prothrombin time Weight
As indicated	Serum lipids Serum urate Serum Zn and Cu Serum B$_{12}$/folate Iron studies Nitrogen balance
Special circumstances	Body protein turnover Body composition measurements Gas exchange measurements Trace element balance Vitamin assays

In a similar way, traditional direct calorimetry for measuring heat loss and energy balance, a complicated laboratory technique, has been modified. Partitional calorimetry is a much simpler method of measurement of metabolic heat production and heat loss. Measurement of resting energy expenditure, and calculation of energy requirement is useful in ensuring that the patient receives an adequate caloric input, but not an excess one, which may result in fat deposition and excess CO_2 production.

As better information becomes available from research in these areas it will become clearer how necessary these methods of monitoring are during routine TPN. However, meticulous adherence to a simple safe system of monitoring is of the essence.

REFERENCES AND FURTHER READING

Damask M C, Forse R A, Kinney J M Clinical applications of gas exchange measurements. In: Nutritional Aspects of Anaesthesia. Clin Anaesthesiol 1983; 1: 599–631

Munro H N, Young V R 3-methylhistidine as an index of rate of muscle protein breakdown. Klin Anasth Intens 1977; 13: 35–42

Park G R Rapid calculation of nitrogen losses. Intens Care Med 1980; 6: 243–246

Shizgal H M The use of body composition measurements to assess the efficacy of parenteral nutrition. In: Johnston IDA (ed) Advances in Parenteral Nutrition. MTP Press, Lancaster, 1978; 535–555

16

Complications

General reviews of the complications of total parenteral nutrition are those of Burri & Krischak (1976), Cetrullo et al (1976), Ryan (1976), Dudrick & Long (1977) and Seashore (1980). This chapter summarises these complications. Individual problems are discussed in the relevant chapters. Complications of enteral nutrition are dealt with in Chapter 27.

Complications may be divided into technical, metabolic and septic (Table 16.1). Technical complications and sepsis have been covered in Chapter 4, and this chapter confines itself to metabolic problems.

Metabolic complications are readily prevented or corrected, provided that monitoring is meticulous. The more obvious ones include:

Overhydration or dehydration: clinical examination, accurate fluid balance, and correct interpretation of daily biochemistry results should prevent both these problems.

Table 16.1 Some complications of TPN

Technical	— failure to catheterise
	— malposition of catheter
	— pneumothorax
	— haemothorax
	— hydrothorax
	— haemomediastinum
	— hydromediastinum
	— neural damage
	— venous thrombosis
	— arterial damage
	— thoracic duct damage
Metabolic	— excess or deficiency of Na, K, Mg, PO_4, Cl, HCO_3, H_2O, glucose, trace elements, vitamins
	— acidosis/alkalosis
	— polymyopathy
	— fat overload
	— hypouricaemia
	— bone disease
Septic	— wound infection
	— septicaemia
	— endocarditis

Hypo- or hyper-natraemia: most commonly due to water excess or deficiency rather than deficiency or excess of sodium.

Hypo- or hyper-chloraemia: interrelated with sodium, potassium, and acid-base balance.

Hypo- or hyper-kalaemia: effective parenteral nutrition may result in increased potassium requirements, due to hyperglycaemia-induced increase in insulin secretion, and to anabolism.

Hypo- or hyper-calcaemia: pancreatitis associated with hypercalaemia has been reported.

Hypo- or hyper-phosphataemia: effective parenteral nutrition implies energy utilisation, hence hypophosphataemia may occur, especially when high glucose concentrations are used to achieve a high caloric input. Hypophosphataemia, which causes increased haemoglobin oxygen affinity, haemolysis, myopathy and reduced cardiac contractility, has been shown to be due to phosphaturia in the first 2 days postoperatively, when it cannot be corrected by phosphate administration. Subsequently, phosphate administration will correct the deficiency.

Hypo- or hyper-magnesaemia: low magnesium concentrations are mainly a problem when the patient has excessive gastrointestinal fluid loss.

Hypo- or hyper-osmolality: especially due to changes in serum sodium or blood glucose.

Acid-base imbalance: this may occur with metabolic acidosis or alkalosis. Acidosis may be associated with chloride excess. Alkalosis may be due to chloride loss or inadequate chloride administration, or to excess base administration, for example, acetate.

Trace element deficiencies: these may occur if supplements are not included, especially zinc (see Chapter 12).

Vitamin deficiencies: these will occur if supplementation is neglected. The water soluble B group vitamins and ascorbic acid are usually given daily. Vitamins which may cause problems if not administered are vitamin K and folic acid in the short term, and vitamins B_{12}, A, D and E in the longer term (see Chapter 13).

Hypo- or hyper-glycaemia: hyperglycaemia is unpredictable. It may occur in some patients with a small glucose load, in others not even with 25 000 carbohydrate kJ (6000 kcal) per 24 hours. It is less likely to occur if glucose administration is slowly increased to allow endogenous insulin production to increase as required. If it does occur, it may be controlled by reducing the glucose load, or by giving insulin. Hyperglycaemia is precipitated by stress, as in burns, post-operative and post-trauma patients, infection, and during administration of certain drugs, for example, corticosteroids and glucagon. It is often an early sign of developing sepsis in a previously euglycaemic patient. Hypoglycaemia may occur in patients on glucose infusions if these are suddenly ceased.

Hyper-ammonaemia: this has been reported, especially in infants (see Chapter 9).

Metabolic bone disease: a disease characterised by hypercalciuria, intermittent hypercalcaemia, reduced skeletal calcium, low circulating parathyroid hormone concentration, negative calcium balance, and osteomalacia has been described in patients on long-term parenteral nutrition. Withdrawal of vitamin D corrected the picture. A syndrome with disabling bone pain and osteomalacia, but with normal serum concentrations of calcium and parathyroid hormone, has also been described. It responded to withdrawal of parenteral nutrition.

Hypouricaemia: this has been described in patients receiving parenteral nutrition.

Polymyopathy: this has been reported and is thought to be due to fat deficiency and to be distinct from that due to deficiency of phosphate, vitamin E or selenium.

Table 16.2   Some causes of some serum electrolyte abnormalities (intracellular electrolytes)

↑ PLASMA K	↓ PLASMA K
Excess intake	Decreased intake
Decreased loss — renal failure — some diuretics — ↓ aldosterone	Increased loss — renal failure — diuretics — GIT secretions — ↑ aldosterone — liver failure
Redistribution — tissue damage — acidosis	Redistribution — insulin — alkalosis
Artefact (e.g. haemolysis)	
↑ PLASMA PO₄	↓ PLASMA PO₄
Excess intake	Decreased intake
Decreased loss — renal failure — hypoparathyroidism — vitamin D excess	Increased loss — renal failure — hypoparathyroidism — vitamin D deficiency
Redistribution — tissue damage — acidosis	Redistribution — alkalosis — TPN
↑ PLASMA Mg	↓ PLASMA Mg
Excess intake	Decreased intake
Decreased loss — renal failure — ↓ aldosterone	Increased loss — renal failure — ↑ aldosterone
	Redistribution — acidosis — pancreatitis

For further information see Walmsley & Guerin, 1984

Table 16.3   Some causes of some serum electrolyte abnormalities (extracellular electrolytes)

↑ PLASMA Na	↓ PLASMA Na
Excess intake	Decreased intake
Water depletion — low intake — renal loss — GIT secretion loss — skin loss	Water excess — high intake — renal failure — liver failure
	Diuretics
	Drugs — morphine — barbiturates
	Artefact — hyperlipidaemia — hyperglycaemia
↑ PLASMA Cl	↓ PLASMA Cl
Hypernatraemia	Hyponatramia
Metabolic acidosis	Metabolic alkalosis
Respiratory alkalosis	Respiratory acidosis
↑ PLASMA HCO₃	↓ PLASMA HCO₃
Acid loss — gastrointestinal — renal	Excess acid — production — administered
Excess bicarbonate	Bicarbonate loss — GIT secretions — renal failure

For further information see Walmsley & Guerin, 1984

Sudden death: death due to cardiopulmonary collapse associated with hypophosphataemia has been attributed to aggressive parenteral nutrition in debilitated patients.

Factors influencing some serum electrolyte concentrations in the patient receiving TPN are shown in Tables 16.2 & 16.3.

REFERENCES AND FURTHER READING

Burri C, Krischak G Techniques and complications of the administration of total parenteral nutrition. In: Manni C, Magalini S I, Scrascia E (eds) Total Parenteral Alimentation. Excerpta Medica, Amsterdam, 1976; 306–315

Cetrullo C, Castelli E, Zanello M Complications of total parenteral nutrition. In: Manni C, Magalini S I, Scrascia E (eds) Total Parenteral Alimentation. Excerpta Medica, Amsterdam, 1976; 316–330

Dudrick S J, Long J M III Applications and hazards of intravenous hyperalimentation. Ann Rev Med 1977; 28: 517–528

Klein G L, Rivera D Adverse metabolic consequences of total parenteral nutrition. Cancer 1985; 55: 305–308

Rudman D, Williams P J Nutrient deficiencies during total parenteral nutrition. Nutr Rev 1985; 43: 1–13

Ryan J A Jnr Complications of total parenteral nutrition. In: Fischer J E (ed) Total Parenteral Nutrition. Little Brown and Company, Boston, 1976; 55–100

Seashore J H Metabolic complications of parenteral nutrition in infants and children. Surg Clin N Am 1980; 60: 1239–1252

Walmsley R N, Guerin M D Disorders of fluid and electrolyte balance. John Wright & Sons, Bristol, 1984

17

Role of the nurse

Nursing staff are responsible for all aspects of patient care. In parenteral nutrition the physician assesses, diagnoses and prescribes, the pharmacist formulates, but it is the nurse who ensures that the regimen is followed. In enteral nutrition, the dietitian replaces the pharmacist in many hospitals, but the final common pathway remains the nurse.

Prime responsibilities of the nurse in relation to TPN may be summarised as follows:

1. Prepare the patient for central venous line insertion. This includes explanation of the procedure, the reasons for it, and its implications, as well as having the patient in the procedure room with site shaved, if indicated, at the agreed time.

2. Assist the physician with line insertion. Equipment should be available, including gown, gloves and mask for the operator, sterile tray with swabs, povidone iodine (Betadine®) solution, forceps, needle holder, scissors, suture material, drapes, syringe, needles, local anaesthetic, and chosen central venous catheter. She lies the patient flat, tips the bed head down, and exposes the site for catheter insertion. She also ensures that the drip set, starting fluid and adhesive tape are ready.

3. Advise the physician of any relevant facts about the patient which may influence management — bleeding disorder or low platelet count, contra-indicating central venous puncture, diabetes, medication such as cortico-steroids and glucagon, which influence tolerance to glucose.

4. Check that a post-insertion chest X-ray is done.

5. Monitor fluid administration according to orders. As well as notifying the physician of problems with fluid administration, she should also know the implications of errors, and their management.

6. Check the monitoring routine required, especially clinical observations, urinalysis, frequency and nature of biochemical investigations. She should ensure that blood is taken and delivered to the laboratory on time, and that results are reported to the physician, especially abnormal values.

7. Ensure that the feeding system is kept sterile, particularly with regard to bag or bottle changes, avoidance of contamination of the line, and maintenance of an intact, sterile dressing.

8. Check the routine for dressing care, and ensure it is followed.

9. Liaise with other members of the nutrition team, and ensure the input of the various members is coordinated, from the patient's point of view.

In relation to EN, similar principles apply. In some hospitals, the nurse inserts the nasogastric tube, as well as managing the feeding, and liaising with the dietitian. In both home TPN and EN, the nurse often is a key figure in patient education prior to discharge from hospital, and as a contact person when problems arise following discharge.

In previous editions of this book, some nurses criticised this chapter because it smacked of an old-fashioned 'doctor orders, nurses obey' attitude. This was never intended. As has been stated by Zena Leider: 'In order to see that the best medical care is obtained for the patient, the nurse must keep current, be aggressive (in a tactful manner), and try to educate physicians regarding the need for specific care for their patients in deficient areas'. The nurse may, in fact, be the person who first draws the doctor's attention to the patient's nutritional state. Because nurses are closer to patients than any other health worker, their role in TPN and EN is a key one.

REFERENCES AND FURTHER READING

Ivey M F The status of parenteral nutrition. Nurs Clin N Am 1979; 14: 285–304
Kennedy G Total parenteral nutrition: down to the basics. Canad Nurse 1981; 77(3): 32–35
Leider Z L The floor nurse's role in nutritional support: a physician's viewpoint. Nutr Supp Serv 1984; 4(4): 18–23

18

Nutrition in the presence of respiratory, cardiac, renal and liver failure

Total parenteral nutrition is usually straightforward in the presence of normal respiratory, cardiac, liver and renal function, but can become quite complicated if these systems are diseased. Such disease, however, is no contraindication to feeding, but often a more urgent indication.

CARDIORESPIRATORY FAILURE

Cardiac failure may limit the amount of fluid and sodium which can be given safely, and use of drugs such as diuretics and digoxin may increase the need for care with potassium balance. Respiratory failure, especially adult respiratory distress syndrome, likewise may be an indication for fluid and sodium restriction. In both situations, and within volume limits, parenteral feeding can be given.

Of considerable interest is the report that high carbohydrate loads may precipitate respiratory distress in the critically ill patient. Kinney's group has studied patients with chronic nutritional depletion, and those acutely ill secondary to injury or infection. Resting energy expenditure (REE) was calculated from oxygen consumption, carbon dioxide production and nitrogen excretion, while the patients were maintained on 5% glucose for 1 day, then on TPN providing approximately 6270–8360 kJ/24 hours (1500–2000 kcal/24 hours) from glucose, or half this intake from glucose and half from lipid. In the chronic nutritionally depleted patients, shifting from the lipid to the glucose system resulted in a 20% increase in CO_2 production with an insignificant increase in oxygen consumption. In the critically ill group, shifting from the lipid to the glucose system resulted in a significant increase in CO_2 production, while O_2 consumption also increased.

There have been reports of the onset of acute respiratory failure in patients with relatively fixed ventilatory response within 12–24 hours of commencing TPN with a high carbohydrate load.

LIVER FAILURE

The liver plays a key role in metabolic functions, and disturbances of its role produce many far-reaching effects (Table 18.1).

153

Table 18.1 Liver failure

Some functions of the liver	
Metabolic	— carbohydrate
	— protein
	— lipid
Storage	— carbohydrate, lipid, vitamins
Synthesis	— bile salts, ketones, plasma proteins, coagulation factors
	— urea, lipoproteins, cholesterol
Detoxification	— steroid hormones, drugs
	— polypeptide hormones
Excretion	— bilirubin
Phagocytosis	

Some results of liver failure:
Hypoalbuminaemia
Sodium retention
Fluid overload
Hyperammonaemia
Jaundice
Hyponatraemia
Hypokalaemia
Renal failure
Coagulopathy
Prolonged drug effect
Hypoglycaemia

There is an association between parenteral nutrition and cholestatic jaundice, and typical biochemical and histological features have been reported in some patients receiving nutrition with a high lipid:glucose ratio (3:2), and a high amino acid intake (2 g/kg per 24 hours). The abnormalities disappear when parenteral nutrition is ceased. Abnormalities of liver function tests due to parenteral nutrition, have been reported. However, these may be due to liver disease, to poor liver perfusion, to disturbed hepatocellular metabolism, or to TPN with excess glucose or excess fat.

In patients with liver failure, as distinct from cholestatic jaundice, intravenous fats should not be given, and amino acids given with care. Fischer observed that in patients with liver disease receiving intravenous amino acids, plasma phenylalanine and methionine concentrations were raised, and there were decreased concentrations of the branched chain amino acids isoleucine, leucine and valine. In a series of studies in dogs, he showed that it was possible to give high protein intakes without adverse effects if the amino acid pattern was manipulated to normalise the plasma amino acid pattern.

In fulminant hepatic failure, it is important to give glucose, with careful monitoring of blood sugar, to avoid hypokalaemia, and to administer large amounts of vitamins. Aggressive parenteral nutrition is indicated in liver failure, but much work is still to be done to determine the optimal ingredients.

RENAL FAILURE

Like the liver, the kidney is a key organ in maintenance of the internal milieu — failure has severe consequences (Table 18.2).

Table 18.2   Renal failure

Some functions of the kidney:	
Homeostasis	— water
	— Na, K, Cl, HCO_3, P, Ca, Mg, Zn, H^+
Synthesis	— erythropoietin
	— prostaglandins
Excretion	— urea, drugs

Some results of renal failure:
Dehydration/overhydration
Hyperkalaemia/hypokalaemia
Hypernatraemia/hyponatraemia
Hypermagnesaemia/hypomagnesaemia
Hypercalcaemia/hypocalcaemia
Hyperphosphataemia/hypophosphataemia
Hyperchloraemia/hypochloraemia
Metabolic acidosis
Anaemia
Uraemia

Fluid requirements may vary from 500 ml to several litres per day. In anuric patients, fluid restriction may be essential, thus limiting caloric input. With the tendency towards early dialysis, this situation is not as common as it used to be. Metabolic disturbances, common in renal failure, may be compounded by TPN. Thus, hyperglycaemia is common during peritoneal dialysis, because of the extra glucose load it provides. Increased serum concentrations of potassium, magnesium, calcium, phosphate and zinc may all occur, unless there is loss from gastrointestinal secretions.

The aim of nutrition in renal failure has been to provide a high calorie, low protein diet. Giovannetti described a low nitrogen diet with addition of essential amino acids and this concept was pursued in the parenteral nutrition field.

Dudrick reported ten patients with acute on chronic renal failure fed intravenously with a specially formulated mixture containing eight essential amino acids, resulting in wound healing, weight gain and positive nitrogen balance. In another, prospective, double-blind study a significant reduction in mortality in patients with acute renal failure treated with intravenous essential L-amino acids (Freamine E®) and glucose was demonstrated. Freund showed a marked increase in mortality in a group of patients parenterally fed with a solution containing both essential and non-essential amino acids, compared with patients previously treated with essential amino acids. However, in a prospective double blind study of 30 patients with acute renal failure fed glucose alone, glucose and 21 g essential amino acids per day or glucose and 21 g essential amino acids + 21 g non-essential amino acids per day, it was concluded that both essential and non-essential amino acids may be beneficial. In a study of 216 patients with end-stage renal disease undergoing major surgery, 40 patients requiring surgery for sepsis were given parenteral or enteral nutrition. The mortality in this group was 22.5%, compared with 71.4% in a smaller group managed without hyperalimentation. The amount of protein recommended tradition-ally has been 0.3–0.5 g/kg per 24 hours, although 1 g/kg per 24 hours is commonly given, and up to 50% more than this in the patient receiving peritoneal dialysis. Another development in the treatment of renal failure has been investigation of the use of keto-analogues of essential amino acids to allow better urea nitrogen utilisation — this has not been found to be useful.

For practical purposes, in the absence of the availability of special solutions, patients with renal failure should receive a high calorie, low protein intake. The latter may be increased depending on blood urea changes and on dialysis. In the critically ill patient in whom renal failure is one of many problems, especially if there is infection and catabolism, aggressive dialysis will allow aggressive nutrition.

A range of special products for use in both TPN and EN in the presence of hepatic and renal failure is now becoming available (see Table 9.6). Their real role has yet to be established.

REFERENCES AND FURTHER READING

Abel R M, Beck C H Jnr, Abbott W M, Ryan J A Jnr, Barnett G O, Fischer J E Improved survival from acute renal failure after treatment with intravenous essential L-amino acids and glucose. Results of a prospective, double-blind study. New Engl J Med 1973; 288: 695–699

Allardyce D B, Salvian A J, Quenville N F Cholestatic jaundice during total parenteral nutrition. Canad J Surg 1978; 21: 332–339

Askanazi J, Nordenstrom J, Rosenbaum S H, Elwyn D H, Hyman A I, Carpentier Y A, Kinney J M Nutrition for the patient with respiratory failure: glucose vs fat. Anesthesiol 1981; 54: 373–377

Barber J R, Teasley K M Nutritional support of patients with severe hepatic failure. Clin Pharm 1984; 3: 245–253

Bower R H Hepatic complications of parenteral nutrition. Sem Liver Dis 1983; 3: 216–224

Cerra F B, Cheung N K, Fischer J E, Kaplowitz N, Schiff E R, Dienstag J L et al. Disease — specific amino acid infusion (F080) in hepatic encephalopathy: a prospective, randomized, double-blind, controlled trial. JPEN 1985; 9: 288–295

Covelli H D, Black J W, Olsen M S, Beekman J F Respiratory failure precipitated by high carbohydrate loads. Ann Int Med 1981; 95: 579–581

Dudrick S J, Steiger E, Long J M Renal failure in surgical patients. Treatment with intravenous essential amino acids and hypertonic glucose. Surgery 1970; 68: 180–186

Feinstein E I, Blumenkrantz M J, Healy M, Koffler A, Silberman H, Massry S G, Kopple J D Clinical and metabolic responses to parenteral nutrition in acute renal failure: a controlled double-blind study. Medicine 1981; 60: 124–137

Fischer J E Nutritional support in hepatic failure. In: Richards J R, Kinney J M (eds) Nutritional Aspects of Care in the Critically Ill. Churchill Livingstone, Edinburgh, 1977; 471–486

Freund H, Atamian S, Fischer J E Comparative study of parenteral nutrition in renal
failure using essential and nonessential amino acid containing solutions. Surg Gynecol
Obstet 1980; 151: 652–656

Giacchino J L, Geis W P, Wittenstein B H, Bansal V K, Gandhi V C, Vertuno L L
Surgery, nutritional support, and survival in patients with end-stage renal disease. Arch
Surg 1981; 116: 634–640

Giovannetti S, Maggiore Q A low-nitrogen diet with proteins of high biological value for
severe chronic uraemia. Lancet 1964; i: 1000–1003

Mirtallo J M, Kudsk K A, Ebbert M L Nutritional support of patients with renal disease.
Clin Pharm 1984; 3: 253–263

Panel Report. Nutritional support of patients with liver, renal and cardiopulmonary
diseases. Am J Clin Nutr 1981; 34: 1235–1245

Wagner W H, Lowry A C, Silberman H Similar liver function abnormalities occur in
patients receiving glucose-based and lipid-based parenteral nutrition. Am J Gastroenterol
1983; 78: 199–202

19

Nutrition in malignant disease

Just as many believed that negative nitrogen balance and wasting were unavoidable post-operatively, so many believed that wasting was an inevitable feature of malignant disease. With more aggressive approaches to therapy in various forms of malignancy, attempts were made to improve patients' nutritional status, especially at the time of chemotherapy, operation or radiotherapy. Cancer has a number of effects on nutritional status, as shown in Table 19.1

Table 19.1 Effects of cancer on nutritional status

Inadequate nutrient intake
Impaired digestion or absorption of nutrients
Fistulous losses
Increased energy expenditure by neoplasm
Increased glucose turnover
Increased lipolysis
Increased proteolysis
Anorexia

Cancer therapy — surgical, chemotherapeutic, and radiotherapeutic — compounds the situation. Surgery and radiotherapy may impair ingestion of nutrients, their digestion and absorption. Chemotherapy often makes it difficult for the patient to swallow and there may be anorexia, nausea, vomiting and diarrhoea.

Changes in intermediary metabolism in cancer are the subject of considerable research effort. There is increased metabolic rate, and a high rate of anaerobic glucose metabolism, with production of lactate. Recycling of this lactate via the Cori cycle requires excessive amounts of energy.

There is increased lipolysis, the stimulus for which is not understood. Protein turnover is increased, and the plasma amino acid profile is altered, with a reduction in concentration of the gluconeogenic amino acids alanine, glucine and threonine, in the presence of normal concentrations of branched chain amino acids.

Copeland has described the nutritional management of 1000 adults with malignant disease of various types. Candidates were chosen because of nutritional depletion, defined as recent weight loss of 4.5 kg (10 lb) or more, low serum albumin, and/or a negative reaction to a battery of recall skin test antigens. Criteria also included a reasonable likelihood of responding to appropriate therapy. In the group who received chemotherapy, an overall tumour response (50% or greater reduction in measurable malignant tissue mass) was obtained in 27.8% of patients. Such patients survived an average of 8.2 months, as opposed to nonresponders (1.9 months). In a series of patients with non-oat cell carcinoma of the lung, 75% of patients with good nutritional status responded to chemotherapy, whereas no nutritionally depleted patients responded. When nutritionally depleted patients were restored to an adequate nutritional state, 47% responded to chemotherapy. As a result of studies in a series of patients having major surgery for malignant disease, he recommended that preoperative nutrition be instituted rather than waiting until a catastrophic postoperative complication occurred. Conclusions from a study of 39 patients were that parenteral nutrition allowed a planned course of radiation therapy to be delivered to a group of poor-risk, malnourished cancer patients; that there was a correlation between tumour response and nutritional status; and that symptoms of radiation stomatitis and enteritis were reduced or eliminated. Complications in a series of 406 patients included catheter related sepsis (2.3%), fluid overload (1%), and subclavian vein thrombosis (1%). These excellent results were obtained only using a nutritional team approach.

Deitel reported 85 cancer patients managed by the nutrition service of his hospital. In 24 patients in whom the cancer was resectable, and who were given TPN pre- and post-operatively, there were no significant complications or deaths. Initially, when TPN was started after life-threatening complications had occurred, the mortality was 37.5%. It was concluded that TPN should be reserved only for patients who could achieve significant palliation with improvement in quality of life.

In another study, 15 patients with protein-calorie malnutrition and cancer were compared to 10 patients with protein-calorie malnutrition alone. 9 of the cancer group and 5 of the non-cancer group received intravenous TPN, while 6 of the cancer group and 5 of the non-cancer group received enteral nutrition. Both groups were monitored clinically, using anthropometric techniques and metabolic balance studies for 17–26 days. The cancer group were studied before, during and after chemotherapy. The study showed that the non-cancer patients increased their lean body mass and visceral protein status. These changes occurred to a minor degree in the cancer patients, while fat synthesis appeared to be unimpaired.

Studies from the National Cancer Institute, Bethesda, have continued to advance knowledge in the area of the effect of TPN in malignant disease. In one such study, 18 patients with localised, squamous cell carcinoma of the distal oesophagus were divided into 4 groups. Groups 1 and 2 had a body weight loss less than 20% of pre-illness weight, and groups 3 and 4 had greater than 20% weight loss, and/or could not swallow. Group 1 continued eating, group 2 received TPN, group 3 received jejunostomy feeding, and group 4 received TPN.

Whole body protein turnover, synthesis and catabolism were determined using ^{15}N glycine, skeletal muscle catabolism was determined by measuring urinary excretion of 3-methylhistidine, and lean tissue mass was evaluated using total body potassium measurements by ^{40}K whole body scanning. TPN was found to be slightly more efficacious than jejunostomy feeding in increasing lean tissue mass and decreasing whole body protein catabolism.

A total of 32 patients with metastatic or locally recurrent sarcomas were studied from initiation of chemotherapy to recovery from myelosuppression. Of this group, 14 were given TPN and 18 were given oral nutrition. No survival or therapeutic advantage was demonstrated for the TPN group.

An excellent review by Brennan has made the following points in relation to TPN in the patient with cancer:

1. The metabolic changes in cancer are related partly to those in starvation, partly to those in the traumatised or catabolic patient, and are partly peculiar to the cancer itself.
2. Administration of TPN can result in weight gain and positive nitrogen balance in some patients.
3. There is no evidence that TPN given to patients with cancer who are receiving anti-tumour therapy promotes tumour growth.
4. While TPN can restore nutritional indices, function and well-being in cachectic cancer patients, some authors have found no change in operative mortality or morbidity, others have shown improvement. Tumour response rates to chemotherapy, radiotherapy or surgery were not shown to improve with TPN in several studies.
5. It is clear that when the tumour is likely to be responsive to therapy, nutritional support is effective and should be employed to maintain the patient through the therapy.
6. When the tumour is likely to be unresponsive to therapy, TPN is not indicated.
7. Investigations currently under way may allow manipulation of the TPN regimen to the advantage of the host, and the disadvantage of the tumour.

There is little evidence that TPN is associated with an unacceptable increase in the risk of infection, or in the promotion of tumour growth. As Valerio & Blackburn have pointed out, cancer is the primary cause of malnutrition in hospital, and the latter requires immediate vigorous nutritional support during therapy. This statement remains valid, even though a controversy exists over which patients can benefit most. TPN can reverse the effect of nutrient loss via fistulae, the effect of impaired ingestion and absorption of nutrients, and the effect of anorexia.

REFERENCES AND FURTHER READING

Brennan M F Total parenteral nutrition in the cancer patient. New Engl J Med 1981;
305: 375–382

Burt M E, Stein T P, Brennan M F. A controlled, randomized trial evaluating the effects
of enteral and parenteral nutrition on protein metabolism in cancer-bearing man. J Surg
Res 1983; 34: 303–314

Copeland E M III Intravenous hyperalimentation and chemotherapy: an update. JPEN
1982; 6: 236–239

Deitel M, Vasic V, Alexander M A Specialized nutritional support in the cancer patient: is
it worthwhile? Cancer 1978; 41: 2359–2363

Donaldson SS Nutritional support as an adjunct to radiation therapy. JPEN 1984;
8: 302–310

Heber D, Byerly L O, Chlebowski R T Metabolic abnormalities in the cancer patient. Cancer
1985; 55: 225–229

Landel A M, Hammond W G, Meguid M M Aspects of amino acid and protein metabolism in
cancer-bearing states. Cancer 1985; 55: 230–237

Nixon D W, Lawson D H, Kutner M, Ansley J, Schwarz M, Heymsfield S et al
Hyperalimentation of the cancer patient with protein-calorie undernutrition. Cancer Res
1981; 41: 2038–2045

Rivlin R S, Shils M E, Sherlock P Nutrition and cancer. Am J Med 1983; 75: 843–854

Shamberger R C, Brennan M F, Goodgame J T Jnr, Lowry S F, Maher M M, Wesley R A,
Pizzo P A A prospective, randomized study of adjuvant parenteral nutrition in the treatment
of sarcomas: results of metabolic and survival studies. Surgery 1984; 96: 1–12

Thomas R J S Nutritional support and the cancer patient: 1982. Aust N Z J Surg 1982;
52: 347–349

Valerio D, Blackburn G L Parenteral feeding and cancer. Lancet 1978; i:883

Wesdorp RIC, Krause R, Von Meyenfeldt M F Cancer cachexia and its nutritional
implications. Br J Surg 1983; 70: 352–355

20

Special techniques — protein sparing, cyclic nutrition

PROTEIN SPARING NUTRITION

It is common practice in many countries to infuse hypocaloric solutions of glucose to provide nutritional support in the post-operative period. However, as a key component of the metabolic response to injury is the translocation of amino acids from muscle to plasma, this form of nutrition has been criticised.

Because of the complexities of TPN, Blackburn et al (1973) proposed that the simpler technique of administration of isotonic amino acid solutions via peripheral veins would spare protein breakdown. By not giving glucose, it was proposed that there would be low circulating glucose and insulin concentrations, elevated concentrations of free fatty acids and ketones, resulting in reduced consumption of glucose and hence reduced gluconeogenesis from protein, mimicking the starvation response. A study of 10 patients showed that nitrogen balance was better maintained in patients when they received 3% amino acid solutions alone, than when they received either glucose alone or glucose plus amino acids. Results of some studies have confirmed that the nitrogen balance obtained using peripherally administered amino acids either alone or in combination with glucose, is superior to the infusion of glucose as the sole nutritional source, while other studies have failed to demonstrate positive nitrogen balance, although they usually showed reduced negative nitrogen balance.

Other evidence of the value of protein sparing therapy includes improved albumin synthesis, and the finding that loss of body weight in post-operative patients receiving protein alone is due to loss of body fat, while in patients receiving glucose alone, it is due to loss of fat and lean body mass. It was proposed that the role of protein sparing therapy was in short-term nutritional support when the potential risks of TPN were not justified. However, the routine use of amino acids post-operatively was not supported.

Rowlands & Clark (1978), while demonstrating the protein sparing effect of amino acids, could not correlate this with elevated plasma nonesterified fatty acids, hyperketonaemia or hypoinsulinaemia. They supported previous workers in their opposition to the routine use of amino acid solutions in post-operative patients who make an uneventful recovery. A further criticism of Blackburn's conclusions was that valid conclusions from nitrogen balance data can only be drawn if the patients are on isonitrogenous regimens, which was not the case in these studies. Two recent studies have pointed out the ineffectiveness of this form of therapy in different groups of surgical patients. It has been observed that the 'pattern of trauma' was maintained irrespective of which of three hypocaloric nutritional regimens was used in patients undergoing total hip replacement.

A list of indications and contraindications for protein sparing nutrition has been submitted, and is summarised in Table 20.1.

Table 20.1 Indications and contraindications for peripheral nutrition (adapted from Watters and Freeman, 1981)

Indications	Contraindications
Inadequate oral intake	Enteral route available
Marginal nutritional status	Peripheral veins not available
Brief period of starvation anticipated	Prolonged period of feeding (> 5–8 days)
Indications for TPN not absolute	Total nutritional support required

The metabolic actions of amino acids and glucose, with or without insulin addition, on nitrogen balance have been evaluated in post-operative patients. The following observations were reported — improved nitrogen balance, lowered ketone body concentration and an increase in glucagon-activated hepatic extraction of amino acids with amino acid infusions. Protein catabolism determined from 3-methylhistidine excretion was not different between the groups. Plasma albumin concentration fell significantly during infusions of glucose and glucose with insulin, but not during amino acid infusions. Insulin secretion was stimulated by amino acid infusions. Further it was suggested that 'protein sparing' by amino acid infusion is probably due to increased protein synthesis rather than decreased breakdown. It was concluded that there is presently little justification for the routine use of isotonic amino acid infusions in maintaining nitrogen balance after operation.

Protein sparing infusions may be prepared by adding 500 ml of 8.5% amino acid solution to 500 ml of sterile water or glucose 10%. The approximate osmolarities of these solutions are 425 mOsm/l and 680 mOsm/l, respectively. The addition of electrolytes further increases the osmolarity. It should be noted that there is a universal incidence of chemical phlebitis in peripheral veins when the osmolarity exceeds 600 mOsm/l, thus the daily nutritional input that can be provided by this route is limited.

Some companies now are marketing solutions specifically for peripheral infusion. Examples include ProcalAmine® (American McGaw) containing amino acids 3%, glycerol 3% and electrolytes (see Table 11.1); Periplasmal®

(B Braun) containing amino acids 3%, xylitol 3% and sorbitol 3% (or glucose 6.6% in place of these polyols) and electrolytes; PE 900® (J Pfrimmer) containing amino acids 2.5%, xylitol 2.5% and sorbitol 2.5%, and electrolytes. Before such solutions can be included in protocols for post-operative nutritional management, a clear and consistent clinical advantage must be demonstrated. We believe the place of protein sparing therapy is not firmly established. Several litres of isotonic amino acid solution per day is expensive therapy. While it may be indicated in some patients, it should not become routine therapy at present, nor should it be used as an alternative to TPN in those patients who need the latter.

CYCLIC NUTRITION

The standard protocol for the provision of total parenteral nutrition to the hospitalised patient provides for the continuous administration of carbohydrates, lipid and amino acids. This practice evolved following the classical studies of Dudrick et al (1968), who demonstrated that optimum growth and nitrogen balance could be achieved with the continuous infusion of glucose and amino acids. This is in contrast to the intermittent, or cyclic, protocol adopted for ambulatory (home) patients.

Continuous administration of hypertonic glucose and amino acid solutions alters the hormonal milieu in which man normally maintains life, body composition and physiological function. Serum insulin concentrations are elevated, glucagon concentrations are suppressed, lipolysis is blocked and lipogenesis is stimulated, particularly in the liver. The release of free fatty acids from the tissues largely is prevented, due to the high prevailing insulin concentrations. Alterations of hepatic function also are characteristic of continuous parenteral nutrition with abnormal deposits of fat and glycogen within the hepatocytes. Hepatic formation of secretory proteins such as albumin also may be inhibited due to the decreased availability of amino acids.

In normal meal-eating man, the fed state is replaced by the post-absorptive state when the serum insulin concentration falls, glucagon concentration rises, and there is mobilisation and redistribution of glycogen, fat and amino acids. These relationships are disturbed by the continuous administration of hypertonic glucose and amino acids.

Maini et al (1976) undertook a study to evaluate the ability of cyclic parenteral nutrition, in which the infusion of glucose was withheld for 8–10 hours each day, to alleviate the effects of the continuous infusion of glucose on the liver. Preliminary results from this and other studies suggest that cyclic nutrition may be beneficial in some patients.

In a further study, the metabolic, hormonal and insulin receptor responses with cyclic parenteral nutrition were assessed in five adult patients with gastrointestinal disorders. It was found in this group of patients, being prepared for home nutrition, that adaptation to the initiation, infusion and cessation of the nutrient infusion is characterised by abrupt alterations in insulin secretion without apparent changes in counterregulatory hormones. It was postulated that the responses to insulin may be modulated by regulatory changes in insulin receptors which could predispose some patients to carbohydrate intolerance, while protecting others from post-infusion hypoglycaemia.

A study of the calciuretic effect of cyclic versus continuous TPN in a group of five patients beginning a program of long-term home parenteral nutrition revealed that daily urinary calcium excretion was increased significantly with cyclic TPN. Three patients developed frank negative calcium balance. The significance of this outcome with the maintenance of negative calcium balance and development of metabolic bone disease in long-term cyclic HPN has yet to be established.

Other workers have evaluated the use of nocturnal cyclic parenteral nutrition in hospitalised malnourished acute patients with various gastrointestinal disorders. A significant improvement in a number of nutritional indices, including weight gain, serum albumin, nitrogen balance, creatinine-height index, and anthropometric measurements was reported, together with good patient tolerance and acceptance, and a low incidence of catheter infection. The successful use of cyclic parenteral nutrition during bone marrow transplantation in children, has also been reported. The infusion free period in this group of patients permitted use of the central venous catheter for administration of blood components and drugs without compromising nutritional management.

Page & Clibon (1980) have summarised the group of patients for whom cyclic nutrition may be preferable to continuous parenteral nutrition (Table 20.2).

Table 20.2   Cyclic parenteral nutrition — patient selection (Page & Clibon, 1980)

Stable patient
  Haemodynamic parameters
  Fluid and electrolyte balance
  Glucose metabolism

Adaptive phase
  Non-stressed
  Non-septic

Requires long-term TPN
  > 3 weeks
  Cannot use gut

No exogenous insulin ($\pm$)

Adequate cardiovascular and renal reserves

Adequate fat stores ($\pm$)

REFERENCES AND FURTHER READING

Askanazi J, Furst P, Michelsen C B, Elwyn D H, Vinnars E, Gump F E et al Muscle and plasma amino acids after injury. Hypocaloric glucose vs amino acid infusion. Ann Surg 1980; 191: 465–472

Benotti P N, Bothe A Jnr, Miller J D, Blackburn G L Cyclic hyperalimentation. Compr Ther (Chicago) 1976; 2: 27–36

Blackburn G L, Flatt J P, Clowes G H A, O'Donnell T E Peripheral intravenous feeding with isotonic amino acid solutions. Am J Surg 1973; 125: 447–454

Byrne W J, Lippe B M, Strobel C T, Levin S R, Ament M E, Kaplan S A Adaptation to increasing loads of total parenteral nutrition: metabolic, endocrine and insulin receptor responses. Gastroenterol 1981; 80: 947–956

Dudrick S J, Wilmore D W, Vars H M, Rhoads J E Long-term total parenteral nutrition with growth, development, and positive nitrogen balance. Surgery 1968; 64: 134–142

Foster K J, Alberti K G M M, Binder C, Hinks L, Karran S, Smythe P et al Metabolic effects of the use of protein-sparing infusions in postoperative patients. Clin Sci 1980; 58: 507–515

Freeman J B, Fairfull-Smith R, Rodman G H Jnr, Bernstein D M, Gazzaniga A B, Gersovitz M Safety and efficacy of a new peripheral intravenously administered amino acid solution containing glycerol and electrolytes. Surg Gynecol Obstet 1983; 156: 625–631

Garden O J, Smith A, Harris N W S, Shenkin A, Sim A J W, Carter D C The effect of isotonic amino acid infusions on serum proteins and muscle breakdown following surgery. Br J Surg 1983; 70: 79–82

Gazitua R, Wilson K, Bistrian B R, Blackburn G L Factors determining peripheral vein tolerance to amino acid infusions. Arch Surg 1979; 114: 897–900

Long J M III, Dudrick S J, Duke J H Jnr A rationale for glucose as primary calorie source. In: Richard J R, Kinney J M (eds) Nutritional Aspects of Care in the Critically Ill. Churchill Livingstone, Edinburgh, 1977; 331–344

Maini B, Blackburn G L, Bistrian B R, Flatt J P, Page J G, Bothe A et al Cyclic hyperalimentation: an optimal technique for preservation of visceral protein. J Surg Res 1976; 20: 515–525

Mascioli E A, Smith M F, Trerice M S, Meng H C, Blackburn G L. Effect of total parenteral nutrition with cycling on essential fatty acid deficiency. JPEN 1979; 3: 171–173

Matuchansky C, Morichau-Beauchant M, Druart F, Tapin J Cyclic (nocturnal) total parenteral nutrition in hospitalized adult patients with severe digestive diseases. Report of a prospective study. Gastroenterol 1981; 81: 433–437

Page C P, Clibon U Man the meal-eater and his interaction with parenteral nutrition . JAMA 1980; 244: 1950–1953

Reed M D, Lazarus H M, Herzig R H, Halpin T C Jnr, Gross S, Husak M P, Blumer J L Cyclic parenteral nutrition during bone marrow transplantation in children. Cancer 1983; 51: 1563–1570

Rowlands B J, Clark R G Postoperative amino acid infusions: an appraisal. Br J Surg 1978; 65: 384–389

Shizgal H M, Milne C A, Spanier A H The effect of nitrogen-sparing, intravenously administered fluids on postoperative body composition. Surgery 1979; 85: 496–503

Watters J M, Freeman J B Parenteral nutrition by peripheral vein. Surg Clin N Am 1981; 61: 593–604

Wood R J, Bengoa J M, Sitrin M D, Rosenberg I H Calciuretic effect of cyclic versus continuous total parenteral nutrition. Am J Clin Nutr 1985; 41: 614–619

Young G A, Hill G L A controlled study of protein-sparing therapy after excision of the rectum. Effects of intravenous amino acids and hyperalimentation on body composition and plasma amino acids. Ann Surg 1980; 192: 183–191

21

Foetus, neonate and child

While many of the principles of parenteral and enteral nutrition described in previous chapters are applicable to children, almost every detail of management is different, especially in infants, in whom parenteral nutrition is a specialised and demanding form of therapy. Because of this, the following chapter only attempts to highlight major differences in the approach to TPN in infants and children. The subject of enteral nutrition in this age group is not addressed, even though extensive knowledge in this area is essential for anyone contemplating TPN. The chapter concludes with some information about maternal TPN, and its effect on the foetus.

INDICATIONS

Parenteral nutrition may be indicated in children following gastrointestinal surgery, prolonged ileus or intestinal fistulae. It has a place in infant malabsorption syndromes, necrotising enterocolitis, and more recently has been used in the management of the low birth weight infant and infants with the respiratory distress syndrome.

As in adult TPN, the value of TPN in infants and children has often not been documented by properly designed studies in many conditions. In a recent review from Columbia University, Winters made the observation that whereas TPN has significantly improved outcome in infants with surgically treatable anomalies of the gastrointestinal tract, and infants with intractable diarrhoea, it has been much more difficult to demonstrate that application of similar regimens to premature infants was of the same value.

Low birth weight infants are at significant nutritional risk due to limited caloric and lean body mass reserves, inability to absorb sufficient nutrients for adequate growth due to immaturity of the gastrointestinal tract, and the need to provide appropriate nutrients to ensure complete neurological development and brain growth. In a study of 34 preterm infants with birth weights < 1200 g assigned to TPN or oral feeding regimens, it was shown that the TPN group had improved weight gain although there was no difference in mortality in the two groups.

VENOUS ACCESS

Venous access may be by means of cannulae inserted into peripheral veins, silastic central venous catheters inserted percutaneously via needle or cannula. Central venous catheters have been inserted following venous cutdown (especially for long-term nutrition), or via percutaneous subclavian puncture. Umbilical artery and vein catheters have been used, but are not recommended. After reviewing 385 children fed by peripheral vein infusion, and 200 by central vein infusion, Ziegler et al concluded that the central venous route was preferable when a high caloric intake was required. The per diem complication rate was not significantly different in the two groups. In a review of 117 Broviac TPN catheters introduced to the superior vena cava via the common facial vein in children aged less than 1 year, eight infants developed superior vena caval thrombosis. Of these, five resolved, two developed intracardiac extension of thrombus, and one developed bilateral chylothoraces. Skin necrosis from extravasation of fluid from peripheral venous cannulae must be avoided. Management and prevention of this problem has been reviewed by Lynch et al (1979).

In line bacterial filters are commonly used, and in infants, constant infusion pumps are required to ensure accuracy at low flow rates.

COMPOSITION OF TPN

There are marked differences in the requirements of the neonate for water, protein, carbohydrate and calories compared with the adult. Fluid requirements are generally of the order of 150 ml/kg per 24 hours in the premature neonate by day 5, compared with 120 ml/kg per 24 hours in the term infant. As in the adult, this volume will be influenced by cardio-respiratory, renal and liver failure and increased losses. As in adults, glucose is the carbohydrate of choice, and amounts up to 15 mg/kg per min have been administered. While it is likely that infusion at rates of greater than 7 mg/kg per min will result in lipogenesis, the work carried out in this area in adults has not been repeated in infants. A minimum energy input of 440 kJ (105 kcal)/kg per 24 hours is necessary to maintain growth of 10 g per day, and it has been proposed that the enteral requirement of 494 kJ (120 kcal)/kg per 24 hours can be met by administration of 376 kJ (90 kcal)/kg per 24 hours because of reduced stool loss and reduced specific dynamic action of enteral feeding. Electrolyte input should be closely monitored to ensure that maintenance daily requirements are met and metabolic complications avoided. Vitamins, both water-soluble and fat-soluble, and trace elements, are integral components of any parenteral nutrition regimen. Although the neonate's precise requirements require further elucidation, recommended daily vitamin and trace element inputs have been published.

Amino acid requirements are different in infants than in adults. Cysteine and tyrosine have been accepted as essential amino acids for the small premature infant because they cannot be synthesised. Histidine and taurine are also considered essential amino acids for neonates and infants. A higher proportion of essential amino acids is required to be administered parenterally than for adults. Increased amounts of arginine, decreased amounts of glycine, and increased amounts of acetate have reduced the incidence of hyperammonaemia and metabolic acidosis, which were a problem with some of the earlier solutions. The appropriate basis for the formulation of an amino acid solution for neonates has yet to be resolved. Initially formulations were based on the amino acid composition of first-class protein such as hydrolysates of casein and fibrin, and then the amino acid composition of egg protein. The composition of mother's breast milk has been considered as an alternative basis (see Table 9.6). Some workers have suggested that the aminogram of plasma should be the basis, while others have suggested that the urinary output of amino acids, as well as the serum concentrations, should be taken into account in determining the ideal amino acid input.

The ideal amino acid solution composition for infants is not yet established. However, it is known that different amino acid solutions influence nitrogen retention to greater or lesser degrees. The maximum amount of amino acid administered per 24 hours is generally regarded as 2.5 g/kg.

Lipid infusions are very commonly used in infant feeding. Intralipid® has been used extensively and, more recently, Liposyn®. As in adults, lipid should not be used in the presence of severe liver disease or bleeding disorders. Plasma clearance must be monitored carefully. Concern has been expressed at the use of intravenous lipid infusion in the preterm infant and in the infant with pulmonary hypertension. Total amounts infused should not exceed 3 g/kg per 24 hours.

Trace element requirements have been separately recommended for infants. Zinc and copper deficiencies have been reported. Vitamins are required in recommended amounts. Recommendations for minerals, trace elements and vitamins are shown in Table 21.1.

MONITORING

Monitoring must be precise, even though blood sampling is a problem. Some investigations, such as serum electrolytes, blood urea and blood glucose, are initially required daily, while others, such as liver function tests, serum calcium, phosphate and magnesium and a full blood count, are normally performed twice a week. Specific investigations are ordered as required, e.g. serum lipids to establish lipid clearance, blood gas estimation, urine amino acids. Clinical monitoring, and plotting of weight, length and head circumference are routine.

Table 21.1   Sample term infant TPN requirements per kg per 24 hours

Water (ml)	70–120
kJ (kcal)	376 (90)
Glucose (g)	10–15
Protein (g)	2.5
Lipid (g)	2
Na (mmol)	2–3
K (mmol)	2–3
Cl (mmol)	3–5
Ca (mmol)	1–1.5
P (mmol)	1–1.5
Mg (mmol)	0.3
Zn (μmol)	1.5–5
Cu (μmol)	0.3
*Vitamin A (μg)	400
*Vitamin D (μg)	10
*Vitamin E (mg)	3
*Vitamin K (μg)	15
*Ascorbic acid (C) (mg)	35
*Thiamine (B_1) (mg)	0.4
*Pyridoxine (B_6) (mg)	0.4
*Cyanocobalamin (μg)	1
Niacin (mg)	7
Riboflavine (B_2) (mg)	0.4
Folic Acid (μg)	40
Biotin (μg)	40
Pantothenate (mg)	2.5

* per 24 hours, not per kg per 24 hours. Refer to references for detailed discussion

COMPLICATIONS

Complications reported during parenteral nutrition in children have included metabolic acidosis, hyperammonaemia, hypophosphataemia, zinc deficiency and sepsis. Good reviews have been provided by Heird & Winters and by Seashore.

Any of the metabolic septic and technical complications which occur in adults can occur in children. In a survey of catheter complications in 60 children between the ages of 1 day and 12 months, complications associated with clinical features included hydrothorax, mediastinal effusion, thrombosis, venous perforation and sepsis. Clinically silent complications included venous thrombosis and endocardial thrombosis.

Disturbances of liver function may occur in children as well as in adults, but the pathophysiology appears to differ. Factors associated with cholestasis include prematurity, sepsis, and prolonged TPN. Amino acid composition of solutions may be relevant, deficiency of glycine or taurine resulting in impaired conjugation of bile acids. There is elevation of serum bilirubin and alkaline phosphatase and cholestasis is evident histologically. Interpretation of results may be difficult in the neonate, and there is no specific treatment except resumption of enteral nutrition. Recovery is usual when TPN is ceased, but it has been proposed that prolonged cholestasis may lead to cirrhosis.

In a prospective study of 21 children receiving long-term TPN, nine were found to have cholelithiasis, and five had undergone cholecystectomy. Length of TPN, aberrant eating patterns, and prior ileal resection were associated with a significantly increased risk of gallstones.

Reviews of many aspects of parenteral feeding in children have been those of Candy (1980), Reimer et al (1980), Coran (1981), Easton et al (1982), Seashore (1984) and Zlotkin et al (1985). It was the view of the last author that parenteral nutrition of neonates should only be undertaken in specialised centres. Home parenteral nutrition is being used in children, and has been reported from the age of 1.5 months. Formulation of the exact requirements of the neonate has been simplified by the application of computers.

A panel report on nutritional support in paediatric patients made the following comments regarding TPN:

1. TPN in children must cope with ordinary nutritional requirements as well as requirements for growth and development of organ systems, in the presence of limited endogenous nutrient stores.
2. TPN is of proven value in the management of congenital gastrointestinal anomalies, intractable diarrhoea and inflammatory bowel disease, but data supporting its value in other conditions are unproven.
3. There is a lack of solid data about many aspects of paediatric TPN, including the ideal amino acid composition of solutions, the metabolic handling of lipids, the pathophysiology of the hepatic dysfunction often seen in infants receiving TPN, the requirements of individual nutrients under different circumstances, and the effects of TPN on immunological function.
4. Desired growth rate of low birth weight infants is controversial. Some believe that intrauterine growth rates should be maintained, others that a lesser growth rate is acceptable.
5. The relative merits of peripheral versus central venous nutrition remain controversial.

TPN FOR MATERNAL DISEASE

Pregnant women may suffer from any of the diseases suffered by nonpregnant women for which TPN is indicated, as well as from diseases peculiar to pregnancy, such as hyperemesis gravidarum. In situations in which oral or enteral nutrition are not possible, TPN may be indicated to preserve the mother's nutritional status, as well as to permit continued foetal growth.

The need to feed a pregnant woman by TPN seldom occurs. In the early days of TPN there was considerable concern over its effects on the foetus. A number of reports in recent years have altered this situation.

There have been several case reports of administration of TPN during the last few weeks of pregnancy, because of Crohn's disease, or some other gastrointestinal problem. In some of these, lipid emulsions have been avoided because of supposed risks, while in others, lipid has been given.

One case report is worth quoting in some detail. It is of a 31 year old married woman with Crohn's disease maintained on TPN with 6700 kJ (1600 kcal)/24 hours, 82% as glucose and 18% as lipid, 12 g nitrogen/24 hours plus all other necessary ingredients. Because of an increase in weight from 41.8 kg to 57 kg, her caloric intake was reduced to 3350 kJ (800 kcal)/24 hours. Nine months after commencement of TPN it was discovered that she was 26 weeks pregnant. Indirect calorimetry gave a resting energy expenditure of 6000 kJ (1450 kcal)/24 hours, and her intravenous intake was increased to 10 000 kJ (2400 kcal)/24 hours. By 36 weeks, maternal plasma oestriol, human placental lactogen and urate concentrations were stable. Delivery occurred spontaneously at 37 weeks, and the infant was 2.62 kg and healthy. The baby's head circumference and length were on the 50th percentile for 37 weeks, and 90th percentile for 40 weeks. Weight was at the 20th percentile for 37 weeks, and below the 10th percentile for 40 weeks. The placenta was normal, with no evidence of lipid thrombi.

TPN has also been used to support foetal growth in twin pregnancy, maternal jejunoileal bypass, pancreatitis, hyperemesis gravidarum and anorexia nervosa.

TPN AND THE FOETUS

It was proposed by Beischer in the early 1970s that pregnant women with low urine oestriol excretion would respond to energy supplementation with intravenous hypertonic glucose infusion. There has not been a lot published on this topic, but two papers from Christchurch are informative. In one study, six patients with very low urine oestriol excretion were infused with hypertonic glucose and amino acids for 48 hours prior to delivery. Amniotic fluid samples were taken pre- and post-infusion.

Lecithin sphingomyelin ratios and insulin concentrations were increased following infusion in all patients. There was usually a fall in amniotic fluid glucose and an increase in ammonia, amino acid, nitrogen and osmolality following infusions, while maternal plasma oestriol and urine oestriol excretion were unchanged. Lactate concentrations in amniotic fluid fell slightly, while pyruvate concentrations rose.

In a follow-up study, ten women with low oestriol excretion and probable intrauterine growth retardation were given either glucose 25% and amino acids 5%, 1.5 litres per 24 hours each, for 2 days (six patients), while two patients received glucose only, and two received amino acids only. All received a normal diet. Amniocentesis was performed prior to and at completion of the infusion. In the amino acid-glucose infusion group, amniotic fluid palmitic acid concentration (an index of foetal lung maturity) increased significantly post-infusion, as did reverse triiodothyronine concentration (rT3). There was no change in growth hormone, prolactin, or ACTH. There were significant increases in insulin, cortisol, and cAMP. The amino acid and glucose only groups gave similar results, except for the change in rT3. There was no significant change in T3 or T4 in any group, and no TSH was detected in any sample. Interpretation of these results was that there had been a significant foetal response to the infusions, with an increase in glucose utilisation and in amniotic fluid surfactant, palmitic acid.

Enteral nutrition also has been used in pregnancy in a number of circumstances. Two patients with insulin-dependent diabetes and hyperemesis gravidarum were managed in the second and third trimesters with enteral nutrition. Both were delivered of infants weighing 2600 g, with no complications.

In summary, it would seem that TPN is useful in maintaining both maternal and foetal nutrition in circumstances in which there is no alternative.

REFERENCES AND FURTHER READING

American Academy of Pediatrics. Commentary on parenteral nutrition. Pediatr 1983; 71: 547–552

Bellini F, Beluffi G, Principi N Total intravenous hyperalimentation (TIH) complications in childhood: a radiological survey. Pediatr Radiol 1984; 14: 6–10

Benny P S, Legge M, Aickin D R The biochemical effects of maternal hyperalimentation during pregnancy. NZ Med J 1978; 88: 283–285

Bower R H Hepatic complications of parenteral nutrition. Sem Liver Dis 1983; 3: 216–224

Candy D C A Parenteral nutrition in paediatric practice: a review. J Hum Nutr 1980; 34: 287–296

Cohen I T Special considerations in the paediatric patient. In: Nutritional Aspects of Anaesthesia. Clin Anaesthesiol 1983; 1: 669–705

Coran A G Parenteral nutrition in infants and children. Surg Clin N Am 1981; 61: 1089–1100

Costanzo J Di, Martin J, Cano N, Mas J C, Noirclerc M Total parenteral nutrition with fat emulsions during pregnancy — nutritional requirements. A case report. JPEN 1982; 6: 534–538

Duffy B, Gunn T, Collinge J, Pencharz P The effect of varying protein quality and energy intake on the nitrogen metabolism of parenterally fed very low birthweight (<1600 g) infants. Pediatr Res 1981; 15: 1040–1044

Easton L B, Halata M S, Dweck H S Parenteral nutrition in the newborn: a practical guide. Ped Clin N Am 1982; 29: 1171–1190

Expert Panel A M A, Department of Foods and Nutrition Guidelines for essential trace element preparations for parenteral use. JAMA 1979; 241: 2051–2054

Filston H C, Grant J P A safer system for percutaneous subclavian venous catheterization in newborn infants. J Pediatr Surg 1979; 14: 564–570

Heird W C, Winters R W Total parenteral nutrition. The state of the art. J Pediatr 1975; 86: 2–16

Hew L R, Deitel M Total parenteral nutrition in gynecology and obstetrics. Obstet Gynecol 1980; 55: 464–468

Legge M, Benny P S, Parker A J, Aickin D R Amniotic fluid endocrine changes during maternal hyperalimentation. JPEN 1984; 8: 433–437

Levene M I, Batisti O, Wigglesworth J S, Desai R, Meek J H, Bulusu S, Hughes E A prospective study of intrapulmonary fat accumulation in the newborn lung following Intralipid infusion. Acta Paediatr Scand 1984; 73: 454–460

Lynch D J, Key J C, White R R IV Management and prevention of infiltration and extravasation injury. Surg Clin N Am 1979; 59: 939–949

MacMahon R A, James B, Shaw P, Hendry P, Yu V, Bornstein J Intravenous solutions in parenteral nutrition. Acta Chir Scand 1981; Suppl 507: 248–257

Martin L F, Voyles C R, Groff D B A method of assuring stabilization of the central venous line in newborn infants. Surg Gynecol Obstet 1981; 153: 93–94

Martin R, Trubow M, Bistrian B R, Benotti P, Blackburn G L Hyperalimentation during pregnancy: a case report. JPEN 1985; 9: 212–215

Mollitt D L, Golladay E S Complications of TPN catheter-induced vena caval thrombosis in children less than one year of age. J Pediatr Surg 1983; 18: 462–467

Panel Report on nutritional support of pediatric patients. Am J Clin Nutr 1981; 34: 1223–1234

Pereyra R, Andrassy R J, Mahour G H Central venous cannulation in neonates. Surg Gynecol Obstet 1980; 151: 253–254

Reimer S L, Michener W M, Steiger E Nutritional support of the critically ill child. Ped Clin N Am 1980; 27: 647–660

Rivera-Alsina M E, Saldana L R, Stringer C A Fetal growth sustained by parenteral nutrition in pregnancy. Obstet Gynecol 1984; 64: 138–141

Roslyn J J, Berquist W E, Pitt H A, Mann L L, Kangarloo H, DenBesten L, Ament M E Increased risk of gallstones in children receiving total parenteral nutrition. Pediatr 1983; 71: 784–789

Seashore J H Metabolic complications of parenteral nutrition in infants and children. Surg Clin N Am 1980; 60: 1239–1252

Seashore J H Nutritional support of children in the intensive care unit. Yale J Biol Med 1984; 57: 111–134

Seifer D B, Silberman H, Catanzarite V A, Conteas C N, Wood R, Ueland K Total parenteral nutrition in obstetrics. JAMA 1985; 253: 2073–2075

Shaw J C L Parenteral nutrition in the management of sick low birth weight infants. Ped Clin N Am 1973; 20: 333–358

Shaw J C L Trace metal requirements of preterm infants. Acta Paediatr Scand, Suppl 1982; 296: 93–100

Smith C V, Rufleth P, Phelan J P, Nelson K J Long-term enteral hyperalimentation in the pregnant woman with insulin-dependent diabetes. A report of two cases. Am J Obstet Gynecol 1981; 141: 180–183

Strobel C T, Byrne W J, Fonkalsrud E W, Ament M E Home parenteral nutrition: results in 34 pediatric patients. Ann Surg 1978; 188: 394–403

Tresadern J C, Falconer G F, Turnberg L A, Irving M H Maintenance of pregnancy in a home parenteral nutrition patient. JPEN 1984; 8: 199–202

Weinberg R B, Sitrin M D, Adkins G M, Lin C C Treatment of hyperlipidemic pancreatitis in pregnancy with total parenteral nutrition. Gastroenterol 1982; 83: 1300–1305

Wilson F E, Yu V Y H, Hawgood S, Adamson T M, Wilkinson M H Computerised nutritional data management in neonatal intensive care. Arch Dis Child 1983; 58: 732–736

Winters R W, Heird W C, Dell R B History of parenteral nutrition in pediatrics with emphasis on amino acids. Fed Proc 1984; 43: 1407–1411

Yu V Y H, James B, Hendry P, MacMahon R A Total parenteral nutrition in very low birthweight infants: a controlled trial. Arch Dis Child 1979; 54: 653–661

Ziegler M, Jakobowski D, Hoelzer D, Eichelberger M, Koop C E Route of pediatric parenteral nutrition: proposed criteria revision. J Pediatr Surg 1980; 15: 472–476

Zlotkin S H, Stallings V A, Pencharz P B Total parenteral nutrition in children. Ped Clin N Am 1985; 32: 381–400

22

The hypermetabolic patient

Throughout this book, reference has been made to TPN and EN in a variety of disease states, including a particularly difficult group of patients, those who are hypermetabolic or hypercatabolic. Patients with severe trauma fit into this category, as do patients with severe sepsis and those with extensive burns. All these patients share one thing in common — they are more or less immobilised, so tend to waste skeletal muscle, and they have an increased metabolic rate.

Metabolic effects of sepsis and trauma are dealt with in Chapter 6. However, it was considered advisable to put together in this chapter a summary of the implications of these changes for TPN, and, where relevant, EN.

Daily energy expenditure can be estimated from one of several formulae, examples of which are for a male patient:

Long's formula
$$(66.47 + 13.75 \text{ W} + 5.0 \text{ H} - 6.76 \text{ A}) \times af \times if$$
where W = weight, H = height, A = age,
af = activity factor, if = injury factor

Quebbeman's formula
$$(\text{kg} \times 12.3 + 754) \times 1.2$$

Without parenteral nutrition this energy will be derived from the patient's skeletal muscle predominantly, and some from fat. Nomograms for calculation of metabolic requirements, and prediction of resting energy expenditure of patients have been devised. None of them predict accurately what nutrition can usefully be utilised.

Calorimetry also may be used to measure energy expenditure and to quantify the fate of administered fuels.

The composition of TPN solutions given is open to debate. The metabolic problem in sepsis is that there is a progressive inability of the skeletal muscle mass to appropriately use carbohydrate and fat. There is increasing use of amino acids, especially branched chain amino acids derived from skeletal muscle, as a fuel source. This appears to be a mitochondrial metabolic failure problem. Inability of the cell to utilise nutrients, even though they abound, is analogous to the inability of cells to use oxygen in cyanide poisoning, even though oxygen is there to be used.

There is increased secretion of catecholamines, glucagon, glucocorticoids and growth hormone, with resultant gluconeogenesis. Non-branched chain amino acids released from muscle are converted to glucose, which cannot be fully utilised, and to ammonia.

If one adds to this picture the complexities of the metabolic changes which occur in trauma (in relevant patients) and starvation, it is clear that the approach to the composition of TPN solutions for these patients should be either simple, or complex to the point where it is unmanageable.

Calorie source and amount is controversial. Infusion of glucose at rates greater than 6–7 mg/kg per minute may result in increased CO_2 production and oxygen consumption, and increased energy expenditure, lipogenesis and water retention. In practice, administration of this glucose load may not be tolerated without elevation of blood glucose concentration. In the non-diabetic patient, glucose infusion should be limited to an amount tolerated without the need for administration of significant amounts of insulin, since its use stimulates lipogenesis.

Lipid, at high calorie intakes, is just as effective a calorie source as glucose, with the advantage that a lesser volume of fluid is required to deliver the same number of calories. In a study in which traumatised or septic patients were given TPN containing nonprotein energy as glucose alone, or as half glucose, half lipid to a total energy input of 149–158 kJ (36–38 kcal)/kg per 24 hours, with 280–290 mg N/kg per 24 hours, there was no significant difference in nitrogen balance between the two systems. Use of lipid also minimises the increased O_2 consumption and CO_2 production which occur with glucose loads in catabolic patients. Even pancreatitis does not exclude administration of lipid, provided it is being cleared from the blood, as evidenced by recording of normal plasma lipids prior to the next 8-hour infusion of lipid. Septic patients clear lipid well. Septic patients given up to 1.4 g lipid/kg per 24 hours as part of their TPN did not have elevated blood concentrations of total lipids, triglycerides, cholesterol, phospholipids or free fatty acids. Daily administration of lipid prevents development of essential fatty acid deficiency.

Calorie:nitrogen ratio remains controversial. Cerra's group (Konstantinidis, et al 1984) has proposed a range from a calorie:nitrogen ratio of 150:1, with input of 1 g/kg per 24 hours of amino acids, and 105 kJ (25 kcal)/kg per 24 hours (with 60% of total calories derived from carbohydrate), for starved patients, up to a calorie:nitrogen ratio of 80:1 with input of 3 g/kg per 24 hours of amino acids, and 146 kJ (35 kcal)/kg per 24 hours (with 70% of total calories derived from carbohydrate), for septic patients.

In an excellent review of energy and protein requirements of general surgical patients, Hill & Church (1984) categorised patients into four groups — normally nourished without stress (trauma or sepsis), depleted without stress, depleted and stressed, and normally nourished and stressed. They stated that total energy expenditure in the different groups ranged from 151 to 218 kJ (36 to 52 kcal)/kg per 24 hours.

The presence of renal failure limits the amount of protein which should be given, to a maximum of 1 g/kg per 24 hours, or 1 litre of 8% amino acid solution. Many authorities would opt for 33–50% of this amount, and determination of calorie:nitrogen ratio and total caloric input then becomes confusing. It seems unlikely that a patient who is septic and immobilised, requires more than 8368 kJ (2000 kcal)/24 hours. A patient who recovers and mobilises, can, of course, utilise much more energy once in the anabolic phase of recovery.

The composition of the amino acid solution best suited to a particular patient is debated, since it is difficult to relate different progress or outcome to any particular solution. Synthetic L-amino acid mixtures should be used, with an essential:non-essential amino acid ratio approaching 40%, and a branched chain:total amino acid ratio approaching 25%. Branched chain amino acids are believed to be important for several reasons, including reduction of the risk of hepatic encephalopathy, and improved nitrogen utilisation. However, it has been suggested recently that the ratio of individual branched chain amino acids may be more critical than the total amount, and that, of the branched chain amino acids, leucine is the most important.

Plasma protein solutions are often used to maintain serum albumin concentration in patients losing protein containing fluids. They should not be used as an amino acid source.

Administration of sodium, potassium, chloride, calcium, phosphate and magnesium is dictated by serum concentrations of these ions, supplemented when indicated by measurement of loss in urine and gastrointestinal secretions. It is common in the patient without renal failure, to have to administer large amounts of potassium and phosphate, and magnesium, if there is excess gastrointestinal fluid loss. In oliguric renal failure, high serum concentrations of all of these may mean that all are contraindicated. Trace elements should be considered similarly. In the short term critically ill patient, only zinc is required, in amounts based on Wolman's formula:

$$\text{Zinc (mg/day)} = 2 + 17.1a + 12.2b$$

where: a = mass (kg) of stool or ileostomy output in a patient with intact small bowel; b = mass (kg) of small bowel fluid loss via fistula/stoma or duodeno-jejuno-colostomy; and 2 = urinary loss.

Zinc is essential for many enzyme systems involved in intermediary metabolism. Adequate amounts cannot be provided as a contaminant of intravenous fluids, or by administration of blood products, and a clinical deficiency syndrome may develop within 2 weeks of commencing TPN. To await the appearance of mental apathy, depression, irritability, tremor, diarrhoea, alopecia and skin lesions before giving zinc, is analagous to awaiting cyanosis before giving oxygen, or hypotension before treating shock.

In an anuric patient with no gastrointestinal fluid loss, no zinc is required. If TPN is required for more than 2–3 weeks, or if the patient is already in a poor state of nutrition prior to commencement of TPN, other essential trace elements should probably be given although there is no satisfactory way of monitoring whether amounts given are appropriate.

Water soluble vitamins should be given daily. The only real controversy at present is whether folic acid should be given daily intravenously or weekly intramuscularly, and whether it is stable in TPN solutions. Fat soluble vitamins are probably unnecessary, with the exception of vitamin K, in short-term TPN. More expensive and more complete vitamin preparations are available for patients on long-term TPN.

The vitamin deficiencies most commonly overlooked, because higher than recommended amounts may be required, involve thiamine, deficiency of which interferes with carbohydrate metabolism in heart and neural tissue, and folic acid, deficiency of which results in a megaloblastic anaemia.

A basic, simple approach to nutrition should be taken as a starting point, fitting in to the fluid volume acceptable to the patient the appropriate amounts of electrolytes required as determined by biochemical results. Trace elements (at least zinc), and vitamins, should be added. A basic amount of protein is 1–2 g/kg per 24 hours, and of energy, 8400 kJ (2000 kcal)/24 hours, 50% as glucose and 50% lipid. From this basic stand, variations can be made based on logical reasoning, from the arguments presented in the literature.

With regard to burns, maintenance of nutritional state has always been regarded as of great importance. Frequently this can be achieved enterally, but TPN is often the only effective way to deliver nutrients in the early stages of extensive burns. Energy requirements may be reduced by nursing the patient in a warm, dry environment and by early skin grafting.

In one study in which patients with over 30% burns were given TPN containing 6700 kJ (1600 kcal) from glucose, 4184 kJ (1000 kcal) from lipid and 24 g nitrogen/24 hours, nitrogen balance was significantly improved when compared to a group receiving the same caloric input without protein. A calorie:nitrogen ratio of 130:1 was used. In another study, caloric requirements were calculated from the formula:

$$\text{Calories} = 25 \times \text{Wt (kg)} + 40 \times \% \text{ BSA burnt}$$
$$(\text{where BSA} = \text{body surface area})$$

and providing 125% of requirements. A calorie:nitrogen ratio of 100:1 was found to achieve positive nitrogen balance, whereas 150:1 did so only in patients with less than 10% burns.

REFERENCES AND FURTHER READING

Berge Hvd, deJong P C M, Soeters P B, Greep J M Clearance of fat emulsions in severely stressed patients. Nutr Supp Serv 1984; 4(12): 18–26

Bonau R A, Ang S D, Jeevanandam M, Daly J M High-branched chain amino acid solutions: relationship of composition to efficacy. JPEN 1984; 8: 622–627

Bradley J A, King R F J G, Schorah C J, Hill G L Vitamins in intravenous feeding: a study of water-soluble vitamins and folate in critically ill patients receiving intravenous nutrition. Br J Surg 1978; 65: 492–494

Cerra F B, Siegel J H, Coleman B, Border J R, McMenamy R R Septic autocannabalism: a failure of exogenous nutritional support. Ann Surg 1980; 192: 570–580

Editorial. Further studies of acute folate deficiency developing during total parenteral nutrition. Nutr Rev 1983; 41: 51–53

Editorial: Fuel mixtures for critically ill patients given total parenteral nutrition. Nutr Rev 1985; 43: 17–20

Hill G L, Church J Energy and protein requirements of general surgical patients requiring intravenous nutrition. Br J Surg 1984; 71: 1–9

Konstantinidis N N, Teasley K, Lysne J, Shronts E, Olson G, Cerra F B Nutritional requirements of the hypermetabolic patient. Nutr Supp Serv 1984; 4(2): 41–50

Liljedahl S-O, Larsson J, Schildt B, Vinnars E Metabolic studies in severe burns. Acta Chir Scand 1982; 148: 393–400

Long C L, Schaffel N, Geiger J W, Schiller W R, Blakemore W S Metabolic response to injury and illness: estimation of energy and protein needs from indirect calorimetry and nitrogen balance. JPEN 1979; 3: 452–456

MacFie J Energy requirements of surgical patients during intravenous nutrition. Ann Roy Coll Surg Engl 1984; 66: 39–42

Matsuda T, Kagan R J, Hanumadass M, Jonasson O The importance of burn wound size in determining the optimal calorie: nitrogen ratio. Surgery 1983; 94: 562–568

Mirtallo J M, Kudsk K A, Ebbert M L Nutritional support of patients with renal disease. Clin Pharm 1984; 3: 253–263

Nachbauer C A, James J H, Edwards L L, Ghory M J, Fischer J E Infusion of branched chain-enriched amino acid solutions in sepsis. Am J Surg 1984; 147: 743–752

Nanni G, Siegel J H, Coleman B, Fader P, Castiglione R Increased lipid fuel dependence in the critically ill septic patient. J Trauma 1984; 24: 14–29

Nordenstrom J, Askanazi J, Elwyn D H, Martin P, Carpentier Y A, Robin A P, Kinney J M Nitrogen balance during total parenteral nutrition: glucose vs fat. Ann Surg 1983; 197: 27–33

Park G R Rapid calculation of nitrogen losses. Intens Care Med 1980; 6: 243–246

Phillips G D Total parenteral nutrition in acute illness. Anaesth Intens Care 1985; 13: 288–299

Quebbeman E J, Ausman R K Estimating energy requirements in patients receiving parenteral nurition. Arch Surg 1982; 117: 1281–1284

Rainey-Macdonald C G, Holliday R L, Wells G A Nomograms for predicting resting energy expenditure of hospitalized patients. JPEN 1982; 6: 59–60

Shils M E, White P L. Trace element conference report. Bull NY Acad Med 1984; 60: 115–212

Silberman H, Dixon N P, Eisenberg D The safety and efficacy of a lipid-based system of parenteral nutrition in acute pancreatitis. Am J Gastroenterol 1982; 77: 494–497

Smith H S, Kennedy D J, Park G R A nomogram for rapid calculation of metabolic requirements on intubated patients. Intens Care Med 1984; 10: 147–148

Wolfe R R, O'Donnell T F Jnr, Stone M D, Richmand D A, Burke J F Investigation of factors determining the optimal glucose infusion rate in total parenteral nutrition. Metabolism 1980; 29: 892–900

Wolman S L, Anderson G H, Marliss E B, Jeejeebhoy K N Zinc in total parenteral nutrition: requirements and metabolic effects. Gastroenterol 1979; 76: 458–467

23

Home nutrition

In the last 15 years significant progress has been made in the development and application of parenteral and enteral nutrition. Home parenteral and enteral nutrition have become recognised as viable means of supporting patients with severe malnutrition who, otherwise, would require prolonged hospitalisation to avert crippling nutritional deficiency or death, from devastating small bowel disease.

HOME PARENTERAL NUTRITION

Some important work which has contributed to the establishment of home parenteral nutrition as a viable therapeutic option, includes that of Scribner et al (1970), Broviac et al, (1973), Jeejeebhoy et al (1976), Solassol et al (1976), Cannon et al (1980), Jarnum & Ladefoged (1981), and Dudrick et al (1984).

A home parenteral nutrition programme should be considered only after careful attention to the following:

— route of administration
— equipment required
— supply of solutions
— rate of administration
— monitoring
— feasibility of subsequent enteral feeding
— availability of immediate assistance of patient, if required.

The success of the programme depends on many factors, including the knowledge and expertise of the personnel involved in the management and training of the patient and a number of centres have emphasised the need for a multidisciplinary approach. The nucleus of personnel involved in a home parenteral nutrition programme generally includes one or more physicians, nurses, a pharmacist and a dietitian. Each individual has a specific role to play, and the coordination of these roles is of paramount importance to the patient's well-being. Other personnel whose services may be required include a psychiatrist, a social worker and a physiotherapist.

Selection of the patient who may be considered as a suitable candidate for long-term home parenteral nutrition is one of the most important aspects of this home-care approach. Patients who have benefited from this form of nutrition include those whose illness has resulted from inflammatory bowel disease (e.g. Crohn's disease), irradiation enteritis, scleroderma and multiple enteric fistulae causing blind loop problems. Other patients who have undergone extensive bowel resection following a mesenteric vascular accident, or small bowel volvulus, or as a result of Crohn's disease, also may benefit from home parenteral nutrition. Patients with cancer have been entered into home parenteral nutrition programmes in order to improve their quality of life. However, this therapy is of extremely limited benefit in patients with 'untreatable' malignancies, and raises a number of ethical issues.

Factors that should be considered in the patient selection process are summarised in Table 23.1. In assessing the prospective patient against each of these criteria, the quality of life versus the quantity of life should be of paramount importance to the physician.

Table 23.1 Factors to consider in assessing suitability of patient for home parenteral nutrition

Personnel	Factors
Patient	Quality of life vs quantity of life Psychologically stable Clinical condition relatively stable Good eye-hand coordination Intellectually capable of learning various techniques Understands importance of compliance Has good image of self Motivated to avoid 'sick role'
Patient's family	Supportive Prepared to learn various techniques Willing and able to support patient psychologically Able to assist with various techniques
Medical support	Trained nurse available to visit patient in the home Willingness of local medical officer to assume some responsibilities for patient Efficient mechanism for delivering solutions and supplies and monitoring use

One of the major obstacles to long-term parenteral nutrition experienced by workers in the early seventies was the technical one of maintaining access to the circulation. In 1970, the first report was published of initial experiences of maintaining patients at home by constructing arteriovenous shunts with silicone rubber sidearms for the delivery of hypertonic nutrient solutions (Scribner et al, 1970). This method was limited by unsatisfactory veins for shunt construction in these malnourished and chronically ill patients and by the frequency of thrombosis and infection. The same group of workers then developed a teflon silastic catheter (the fore-runner of today's catheters) for insertion via the subclavian vein into the superior vena cava. In 1973 and 1976, further reports were published indicating that a cuffed silastic right atrial catheter, called the Broviac catheter, was safe and easy to use (Broviac et al, 1973, Riella & Scribner, 1976). At this time, Jeejeebhoy et al (1976) also reported a number of successful cases of home parenteral nutrition using a non-cuffed silastic rubber catheter (the Langer catheter) inserted into the superior vena cava.

Both the Broviac catheter and the Hickman catheter, a modified version of the Broviac catheter, now have been used successfully by several groups for long-term home parenteral nutrition. Repair kits are available for these two catheters and thus the life of the catheter can be prolonged even when part of the external segment is damaged.

The route of catheterisation (subclavian, internal or external jugular) is dependent on the patency of the patient's veins, whether or not a venous cut-down has been performed previously at a potential catheterisation site, and on the preference of the surgeon performing the procedure. Irrespective of the route selected, it is imperative that the catheter is tunnelled subcutaneously to exit at a site on the chest wall (Fig. 23.1) where it can be:

— readily observed by the patient
— easily manipulated with the patient's dominant hand
— easily dressed
— concealed by the patient's clothing.

The incidence of complications following catheter insertion is related to the diligence of the patient in caring for the catheter and the catheter exit site. Fleming et al (1980) have reviewed catheter-related complications identified in 27 patients treated with home parenteral nutrition for a total of 662 patient-months. These complications included six episodes of catheter-related sepsis, damage to the external segment of the silastic catheter, intravascular catheter displacement, extravascular catheter displacement, occlusion of the catheter, and use of the catheter to infuse narcotic drugs. Venous thrombosis also may occur, although its incidence is low with the silastic-type catheters. Fleming concluded that a well-educated and motivated patient can manage his catheter with a relatively low incidence of complications.

Recently our home nutrition team has replaced a Hickman catheter with a Port-a-Cath® in a long-term home nutrition patient who had presented on two previous occasions with catheter-related fungaemia. The Port-a-Cath® is a totally implanted system consisting of a stainless steel chamber which is implanted subcutaneously, and which is sealed at the top by a rubber disc, or septum, designed to withstand multiple needle punctures. A silicone catheter is connected to the outlet of the chamber and the other end is located in the superior vena cava. At the time of writing, this system has

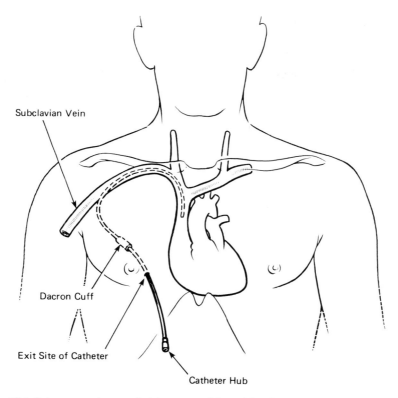

Subclavian Vein

Dacron Cuff

Exit Site of Catheter

Catheter Hub

Fig. 23.1 Subcutaneously tunnelled long-term right atrial catheter.

been in situ for 12 months, and both the patient and her spouse have accepted the system well, finding it easier to use and maintain than the subcutaneously tunnelled Hickman catheter.

Most patients are trained to infuse their solutions on a cyclic basis at a constant rate over an 8–12 hour period. Generally the infusion rate is tapered off over the last half an hour to prevent reactive hypoglycaemia. The catheter is converted to a heparin lock during the 'off' period to maintain its patency. This technique enables the patient to be independent of his nutrition system for a large portion of the day.

Some patients require continuous infusions, in particular those who cannot tolerate the rapid infusion of large volumes of hypertonic solutions over a short period. Dudrick et al (1979) developed an infusion system, based on that designed by Solassol & Joyeux, consisting of a polyester mesh vest, designed to carry two bags of nutrition solution, and a pocket for carrying a miniature battery-powered volumetric pump to control the infusion rate. This system provides these patients with a significant degree of mobility while their nutrients are being infused.

The success of home parenteral nutrition is dependent largely on the

ability of the home parenteral nutrition team members to adequately train
the patient in the following aspects prior to discharge from the hospital —

— the purpose of home parenteral nutrition and the role of the various
   nutrients
— catheter care
— aseptic preparation of solutions
— operation of the infusion pump
— commencing and discontinuing solution infusion
— self-monitoring
— detecting and coping with complications.

Detailed training manuals, which are written for the lay-person, have
been published by some centres, including the Mayo Clinic, Cleveland
Clinic, University of Washington Hospitals, Seattle, Toronto General
Hospital and our own Centre. Typical information included in these illustrated manuals and addressed in patient training programmes is summarised

Table 23.2 Contents of a typical home parenteral nutrition training manual (adapted from
Phillips et al, 1983)

Section	Contents
Introduction	Home parenteral nutrition training personnel Metric system and home parenteral nutrition
Aseptic technique	Principles Hand-washing Disinfectants Syringes, needles — how to use Vials, ampoules — how to withdraw solution Nutrition solution containers — how to use Filters — how to use Aseptic reminders
Catheter care	Care of exit site Potential complications Cleaning hub, heparinising catheter Temporary catheter repair — use of kit Permanent catheter repair
Solution preparation	Premixed TPN solutions Making additions
Pump and solution infusion	Pump connection Pump disconnection Infusing lipid
General information	Glossary of terms
What to do if . . .?	Pump problems Catheter breaks, cracks Air embolism Infusion bag leaks Sterile parts are touched Do's and Dont's Notify your doctor if . . .

in Table 23.2. Those workers planning to establish their own home parenteral nutrition programme and training manual are well advised to review these manuals.

In addition to catheter related problems and sepsis, metabolic complications may result from inadequate or excessive infusion of the various nutrients. These complications may include hyper- or hypoglycaemia, hyper- or hypokalaemia, hyper- or hypocalcaemia, hyper- or hypomagnesaemia, hyper- or hyponatraemia, hyper- or hypophosphataemia, hyper- or hypositaminosis, trace element deficiency and essential fatty acid deficiency. A metabolic bone disease has been reported in some long-term patients, which was corrected by the withdrawal of vitamin D. Other deficiency states that have been reported recently with long-term parenteral nutrition include biotin deficiency, selenium deficiency and carnitine deficiency (see Chapters 11–13). With proper monitoring, accurate record keeping by the patient, and performance of blood tests at regular intervals, most of these metabolic complications can be avoided.

Psychological and social problems have been described in patients on home parenteral nutrition. These are summarised in Table 23.3. Psychosocial problems also may be experienced by the parents of paediatric home parenteral nutrition patients.

Table 23.3 Some psychological and social problems experienced by home parenteral nutrition patients

Problem	Examples
Psychiatric disturbances	Acute brain syndrome Depressive illness Anxiety states Drug abuse Compliance problems Body image disturbance Machine-dependency
Relationship	Family and marital may be stressed — overprotection to rejection
Social activities	Dietary restrictions may prove distressing Unable to fulfill previous life-style

Home parenteral nutrition now has become accepted as a valuable life support system for both paediatric and adult patients. It is an expensive form of therapy. However, it costs substantially less than maintaining a patient in hospital. Home parenteral nutrition can be used to return those patients with gut failure to a near normal life at home and in the community.

HOME ENTERAL NUTRITION

In recent years there has been a significant increase in the number of patients discharged home from hospital on enteral nutrition. Greene et al

(1981) have summarised the criteria used by his group for selecting patients to be maintained on home enteral nutrition. These criteria include:

— moderate to severe malnutrition
— inability to consume calculated nutritional requirements voluntarily
— tolerance of continuously infused formula at the required rate well documented while hospitalised
— continued hospital management of underlying illness no longer warranted
— willingness of patient to continue tube feeding at home
— appropriate family support
— patient is free from complicating neurologic, metabolic, or anatomic disorders, which would be difficult to monitor or control adequately as an outpatient.

Solutions are administered through fine bore silicone or polyurethane nasogastric or nasoduodenal tubes, either continuously or intermittently. Some patients elect to re-insert their tubes each day prior to administration of their enteral diet over a 12 hour period. Other patients prefer to leave their tubes in situ, capping the end of the tube and securing it to the cheek in between infusion cycles. For patients who require jejunostomy feeding, Kaminski (1981) has reported the use of a subcutaneously placed modified feeding jejunostomy tube made of silicon with a proximal Dacron cuff to permit it to become embedded in the subcutaneous tissue — the 'K-tube®'. The feeding solutions are infused over the evening hours by pump control. During the day, the tube is flushed and capped to allow the patient maximum mobility.

The goal of treatment is to provide either complete or supplemental tube feeds sufficient to promote positive nitrogen balance and weight gain.

Gravity infusion has been used to administer feeding solutions. However, unstable infusion rates can be a problem with this infusion method. Pumps are preferred for the continuous delivery of feeding solutions and recently some pumps designed specifically for enteral nutrition have been marketed (see Appendix 3).

Patients who are to receive their nutrition at night should be instructed to sleep with the head of the bed elevated at 30° to avoid regurgitation and to assist gastric drainage. Patients also should be instructed to check the position of their nasogastric tubes daily and for retention of stomach contents by aspirating the stomach. The patients should be instructed to reduce the feeding rate for a period if the residual volume is greater than 100 ml. If the patient experiences anorexia, diarrhoea or abdominal distension, he should decrease the infusion rate. If the symptoms are not controlled by slowing the infusion rate, the patient should contact a member of the enteral nutrition team.

The patient must receive training in the use of his enteral nutrition support system and preparation of his feed. He must receive instruction in the detection of problems and complications and should be monitored regularly by his physician for complications relating to the volume load and the composition of the solution infused.

REFERENCES AND FURTHER READING

Baptista R J, Bistrian B R, Blackburn G L, Miller D G, Champagne C D, Buchanan L Utilizing selenious acid to reverse selenium deficiency in total parenteral nutrition patients. Am J Clin Nutr 1984; 39: 816–820

Baptista R J, Lahey M A, Bistrian B R, Champagne C D, Miller D G, Kelly S E, Blackburn G L Periodic reassessment for improved, cost-effective care in home total parenteral nutrition: a case report. JPEN 1984; 8: 708–710

Blackburn G L, Bothe A Jnr, Lahey M A Organization and administration of a nutrition support service. Surg Clin N Am 1981; 61: 709–719

Bloch A S Special needs of the home enteral patient. Nutr Supp Serv 1983; 3(9): 8–14

Bowyer B A, Fleming C R, Ludwig J, Petz J, McGill D B Does long-term nutrition in adult patients cause chronic liver disease. JPEN 1985; 9: 11–17

Broviac J W, Cole J J, Scribner B H A silicone rubber atrial catheter for prolonged parenteral alimentation. Surg Gynecol Obstet 1973; 136: 602–606

Cannon R A, Byrne W J, Ament M E, Gates B, O'Connor M, Fonkalsrud E W Home parenteral nutrition in infants. J Pediatr 1980; 96: 1098–1104

Dudrick S J, Englert D M, MacFadyen B V Jnr, Souchon E A A vest for ambulatory patients receiving hyperalimentation. Surg Gynecol Obstet 1979; 148: 587–590

Dudrick S J, O'Donnell J J, Englert D M, Matheny R G, Blume E R, Nutt R E et al 100 patient-years of ambulatory home total parenteral nutrition. Ann Surg 1984; 199: 770–781

Dzierba S H, Mirtallo J M, Grauer D W, Schneider P J, Latiolais C J, Fabri P J Fiscal and clinical evaluation of home parenteral nutrition. Am J Hosp Pharm 1984; 41: 285–291

Fleming C R, Witzke D J, Beart R W Jnr Catheter-related complications in patients receiving home parenteral nutrition. Ann Surg 1980; 192: 593–599

Gaffron R E, Fleming C R, Berkner S, McCallum D, Schwartau N, McGill D B Organization and operation of a home parenteral nutrition program with emphasis on the pharmacist's role. Mayo Clin Proc 1980; 55: 94–98

Gilchrist P N, Phillips P J, Odgers C L, Hoogendorp J The psychological aspects of artificial nutritional support. ANZ J Psych 1985; 19: 54–59

Greene H L, Helinek G L, Folk C C, Courtney M, Thompson S, MacDonell R C Jnr, Lukens J N Nasogastric tube feeding at home: a method for adjunctive nutritional support of malnourished patients. Am J Clin Nutr 1981; 34: 1131–1138

Gulledge A D, Gipson W T, Steiger E, Hooley R, Srp F Short bowel syndrome and psychological issues for home parenteral nutrition. Gen Hosp Psychiatry 1980; 2: 271–281

Jarnum S, Ladefoged K Long-term parenteral nutrition. I: Clinical experience in 70 patients from 1967 to 1980. Scand J Gastroent 1981; 16: 903–911

Jeejeebhoy K N, Langer B, Tsallas G, Chu R C, Kuksis A, Anderson G H Total parenteral nutrition at home: studies in patients surviving 4 months to 5 years. Gastroenterol 1976; 71: 943–953

Kaminski M V Jnr Enteral hyperalimentation: prevention and treatment of complications. Nutr Supp Serv 1981; 1(4): 29–35

Kennedy G, Jeejeebhoy K N Home total parenteral nutrition. In: Jeejeebhoy K N (ed) Total Parenteral Nutrition in the Hospital and at Home. CRC Press, Boca Raton, 1983, p 89–122

Khalidi N, Wesley J R, Thoene J G, Whitehouse W M Jnr, Baker W L Biotin deficiency in a patient with short bowel syndrome during home parenteral nutrition. JPEN 1984; 8: 311–314

Ladefoged K Quality of life in patients on permanent home parenteral nutrition. JPEN 1981; 5: 132–137

MacRitchie K J Life without eating or drinking. Total parenteral nutrition outside hospital. Can Psychiatr Assoc J 1978; 23: 373–379

Miller D G, Ivey M F Use of home parenteral nutrition in 4 patients with 'untreatable' malignancies. JPEN 1979; 3: 457–458

Newmark S R, Simpson M S, Beskitt M P, Black J, Sublett D Home tube feeding for long-term nutritional support. JPEN 1981; 5: 76–79

Phillips P J, Hoogendorp J, Odgers C L, Gilchirst P Home parenteral nutrition training manual. Flinders Medical Centre, Bedford Park, South Australia, 1983

Riella M C, Scribner B H Five years' experience with a right atrial catheter for prolonged parenteral nutrition at home. Surg Gynecol Obstet 1976; 143: 205–208

Scribner B H, Cole J J, Christopher T G, Vizzo J E, Atkins R C, Blagg C R Long-term total parenteral nutrition. The concept of an artificial gut. JAMA 1970; 212: 457–463

Shike M, Harrison J E, Sturtridge W C, Tam C S, Bobechko P E, Jones G et al Metabolic bone disease in patients receiving long-term total parenteral nutrition. Ann Int Med 1980; 92: 343–350

Solassol C, Joyeux H, Pujol H, Romieu C Long term parenteral nutrition: an artificial gut. Inter Surg 1976; 61: 266–270

Srp F, Steiger E, Montague N, Grover M, Gulledge A D, Gipson W T et al Patient preparation for cyclic home parenteral nutrition: a team approach. Nutr Supp Serv 1981; 1(1): 30–34

24

Two peculiar problems

Two topics not so far mentioned in this book, but of interest to the authors, are the use of TPN in the management of patients with liver derangement secondary to intestinal bypass for morbid obesity and in the management of anorexia nervosa.

JEJUNO-ILEAL BYPASS

In 1963, Payne et al reported observations on metabolic changes which occurred in ten patients who had jejunocolic shunts for uncontrolled obesity. Following the shunts, the patient's blood pressure was lowered, hypokalaemia and hypocalcaemia occurred, serum cholesterol and carotene concentrations fell, and weight loss was associated with fatty change in the liver. Two patients had to have normal intestinal continuity restored because of serious metabolic problems.

In 1975, Heimburger et al reported the development of fatty infiltration of the liver in four patients who had undergone jejunoileal bypass. One patient had restoration of intestinal continuity, but the other three were treated by infusion of a calorie-free amino acid/electrolyte/vitamin solution, with resolution of the liver infiltrates.

This report was followed by another, in which a patient in the same condition was managed with parenteral nutrition, and improved. Two patients who had progressed to a state of jaundice, encephalopathy, and severe malnutrition following jejunoileal bypass were managed with parenteral and oral nutrition, followed by reversal of the bypass.

In a patient managed recently in our institution, obesity had been refractory to both gastric stapling and jejuno-ileal bypass. Four months after this latter procedure, the patient had suffered the following consequences: persistent vomiting and diarrhoea, hypokalaemia, hypomagnesaemia, hypophosphataemia, fatty infiltration of the liver, and clinical manifestations of zinc deficiency.

TPN was instituted and carefully escalated until all measured parameters were normal. A total of 12 500 kJ (3000 kcal), as 70% carbohydrate and 30% lipid, with 16 g N/24 hours were given for 10 days prior to reversal of the bypass, and for 2 weeks post-operatively because of paralytic ileus.

The following observations have been made about this interesting clinical entity:

— liver biopsies from patients with refractory obesity usually demonstrate fatty infiltration
— histologic findings increase in severity in most patients during the first year after jejunoileal bypass, but clinical features of liver disease do not develop
— 1% of patients develop progressive liver failure and die
— the histologic features resemble those of alcoholic hepatitis and cirrhosis
— the pathogenesis of the lesion is not clear. Contributing factors may be absorption of bacterial toxins from the bypassed bowel and malnutrition
— treatment initially is nutritional repletion, usually via the parenteral route. Reconstitution of normal anatomy may be indicated.

ANOREXIA NERVOSA

Anorexia nervosa is one of the more common causes of malnutrition in young women in developed countries. Mortality is currently said to be less than 2% in major centres, although how many die from starvation is unclear. Nutrition via the gastrointestinal tract is ideal, but there are some circumstances in which TPN is more appropriate. In one recent study, weight gain during hospitalisation was found to be greater in a group receiving TPN and psychotherapy, than in another group receiving psychotherapy alone. The authors suggested two indications for TPN in anorexia nervosa — life-threatening weight loss, and failure to respond to psychotherapy and hospitalisation.

If TPN is given to a patient with anorexia nervosa, it is essential to commence feeding gradually, after correction of fluid and electrolyte balance. As with any nutritionally depleted patient, deficiencies of potassium, phosphate, folic acid and zinc, especially, may become manifest rapidly if high caloric nutrition is introduced.

REFERENCES AND FURTHER READING

Ames F C, Copeland E M, Leeb D C, Moore D L, Dudrick S J Liver dysfunction following small-bowel bypass for obesity: nonoperative treatment of fatty metamorphosis with parenteral hyperalimentation. JAMA 1976; 235: 1249–1252

Baker A L, Monroe P, Glagov S, Sitrin M Management of liver failure in a patient following jejunoileal bypass. Gastroenterol 1980; 78: 1593–1601

Croner S, Larsson J, Schildt B, Symreng T Severe anorexia nervosa treated with total parenteral nutrition. Clinical course and influence on clinical chemical analyses. Acta Paediatr Scand 1985; 74: 230–236

Dempsey D T, Crosby L O, Pertschuk M J, Feurer I D, Buzby G P, Mullen J L Weight gain and nutritional efficacy in anorexia nervosa. Am J Clin Nutr 1984; 39: 236–242

Heimburger S L, Steiger E, Gerfo P L, Biehl A G, Williams M J Reversal of severe hepatic infiltration after intestinal bypass for morbid obesity by calorie-free amino acid infusion. Am J Surg 1975; 129: 229–235

Nakazawa T, Okada Y, Onishi T, Azukizawa M, Kumahara Y Hyperalimentation in treatment of anorexia nervosa. Endocrinol Japan 1982; 29: 99–103

Payne J H, DeWind L T, Commons R R Metabolic observations in patients with jejunocolic shunts. Am J Surg 1963; 106: 273–289

Richard J L, Bringer J, Mirouze J, Monnier L, Bellet M H Interet de l'alimentation enterale a faible debit continu dans le tratement de l'anorexie mentale. Ann Nutr Metab 1983; 27: 19–25

Zsigmond G L, Verrier E, Way L W Sudden reversal of renal failure after take-down of a jejunoileal bypass: report of a case involving hemorrhagic proctocolitis and renal and hepatic failure late after jejunoileal bypass for obesity. Am J Gastroenterol 1982; 77: 216–219

25

Pharmaceutical considerations

The assistance of a pharmacist can minimise a number of complications associated with parenteral nutrition through skills and knowledge of solution formulation and preparation, knowledge of drug-nutrient and/or drug-drug incompatibilities and knowledge of drug-nutrient interactions (see chapter 26)

SOLUTION FORMULATION AND PREPARATION

Optimal utilisation of the various components of nutrition solutions is achieved when they are infused simultaneously. In the early days of parenteral nutrition this goal was achieved by hanging multiple containers of nutrient solutions in parallel — amino acid solution, glucose solution, saline solution (often with added electrolytes and vitamins), and then infusing these simultaneously via the central catheter. Lipid generally was infused via a separate peripheral line. This method was very cumbersome and allowed an unacceptable number of breaks in aseptic technique, thus increasing the risk of infectious complications.

The obvious solution to this problem was for the pharmaceutical industry to prepare and market sterile premixed amino acid-glucose solutions with or without electrolytes, to which additional electrolytes, vitamins and trace elements could be added immediately prior to use. However, most manufacturers who adopted the procedure of terminal heat sterilisation used for amino acid solutions or glucose solutions found that the amino acid-glucose solutions were discoloured (brown) and the free amino acid content lowered as a result of the sterilisation process. They were observing some of the changes and products of the *Maillard reaction* and the *Amadori rearrangement*.

In the Maillard reaction, a reducing sugar (e.g. glucose) and an amine (e.g. amino acid) react to form an aldosylamine (see Fig. 8.2.). The extent to which an amino acid reacts with glucose depends not only on its concentration in the solution and the glucose concentration, but also on the chemical characteristics of the amino acid. For example, isoleucine, leucine and valine, which have bulky hydrophobic side chains, react less readily

192

than other amino acids. Serine and threonine, which have aliphatic hydroxy side chains, react more rapidly.

In the presence of an acidic catalyst, the aldosylamines undergo the Amadori rearrangement to the corresponding ketosamines. These initial products react further, yielding a wide variety of other compounds and the solutions change colour to yellow through reddish-brown to brown and polymeric precipitates develop. The reaction rates for these conversions are temperature dependent. Thus, as a result of heat sterilisation, significant quantities of these products are formed. Other factors that influence the rates of reaction are solution pH, and the presence of electrolytes and trace elements. A number of amino acids bind trace metal ions such as zinc, forming chelates, which react with glucose to form Maillard products at rates greater than the amino acids alone.

For a detailed account of these reactions and products, refer to Ellis (1959) and Stegink et al (1981) for an investigation of their formation in parenteral nutrition solutions.

Further experimental work demonstrated that amino acid-glucose solutions sterilised by membrane filtration and stored at 4°C have the lowest conversion of amino acids to Maillard products, although the quantity of Maillard products present in solution increases with storage time. This fact, together with the increased possibility of microbial or fungal contamination with this method of sterilisation, argued against large batch production and long time storage. Thus it became common practice for hospital pharmacists to prepare amino acid-glucose solutions on a daily basis and to tailor the solution composition to satisfy the patient's specific requirements. This approach is adopted still in a number of centres, including our own, although we use commercially premixed solutions for our home nutrition patients and for some adult inpatient formulations.

Prior to commencing solution preparation, the pharmacist determines the correct solution formulation from the physician's order. This may be accomplished by having a set number of formulations which are ordered by a unique name, or by using a simple calculation sheet, a programmable calculator or a computer to derive the solution formulation. Alternatively, the prescriber may use a computer to assist him order a patient's TPN solution and as a consequence, the formulation is automatically derived for the pharmacist.

Techniques in preparation of solutions

Commercially available solutions of amino acids (with or without electrolytes), glucose solutions, electrolyte solutions, trace element solutions and vitamin preparations are combined, using aseptic technique, to prepare the parenteral nutrition solution. In some countries a range of commercially premixed solutions of different concentrations of amino acids and glucose, with or without electrolytes, is available, and additional electrolytes, vitamins and trace elements are added aseptically on a daily basis by the pharmacist.

Vacuum bottle technique (Fig. 25.1)

One method of combining the various ingredients is to use a partially filled 1 litre bottle containing glucose 50%, 500 ml, and having sufficient vacuum

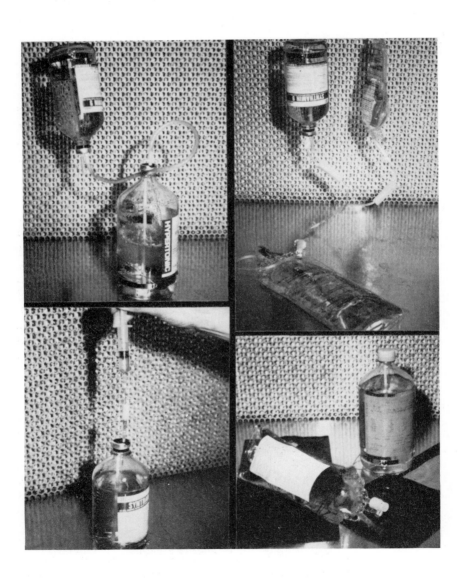

to effect solution transfer. The appropriate electrolytes and vitamins are added to the amino acid solution under laminar air flow conditions using aseptic techniques, through either a membrane filter or a 5 μm depth filter to remove any particles of glass or rubber. The solution is thoroughly mixed after each addition. Once all the additions have been made, the bottle is vented and a sterile transfer set is inserted. The flow adjustment clamp should be closed and then the other spike of the transfer set is inserted into the appropriate site in the rubber closure of the partially filled glucose bottle to effect solution transfer. The spike adaptor is removed, the closure prepped, and a sterile additive cap affixed. The solution is inspected for particulate contamination, labelled and refrigerated until use. If not used within 24 hours of preparation, these solutions should be discarded due to the labile nature of some of the ingredients (vitamins) and as a safeguard against growth of micro-organisms if the solution has been accidentally contaminated during preparation. In some countries, evacuated containers are available in a range of sizes: 1 litre, 500 ml, 250 ml, and these facilitate the combination of different volumes of solutions and also different strengths of glucose.

Empty sterile plastic bag technique (see Fig. 25.1)

Empty sterile plastic bags made of polyvinyl chloride (PVC) or polyolefin or ethylene vinyl acetate (EVA) are available commercially. These are fitted with either a single filling tube, a Y-tube, or up to six filling tubes, spike connectors, flow adjustment clamps and an injection port. They are available in different sizes, ranging from 250 ml to 3 litres. The PVC bags contain the plasticer di-(2-ethylhexyl)phthallate (DEHP). Extraction of DEHP from these bags when they contain parenteral nutrition solutions, has been found to be consistent with the concentrations normally obtained for simple aqueous solutions stored in these containers. However, if a lipid emulsion is added to a PVC bag, then considerable amounts of DEHP may be leached out by the lipid.

Using these bags it is possible to combine any strength or volume of glucose and amino acid solutions. Additives may be added through a membrane filter or depth filter to the ingredient solutions prior to venting the glass containers and inserting the spike connectors from the bag. Or having vented the glucose and amino acid containers, inserted the spike adaptors and inverted the bottles (and bags) in the laminar air flow cabinet to allow the solutions to run (under gravity) into the empty bag, any additions can then be made via a filtration unit into the injection port at the junction of the Y-transfer tubing. A vacuum unit may be used to draw a vacuum around the empty bag and thus speed the transfer of the solutions. Once the appropriate volumes of solutions have been transferred into the sterile bag, the transfer tubing is clamped, the tube sealed adjacent to the bag, and the remaining portion of the transfer tubing cut off. The solution is inspected for particulate matter, labelled and, if not to be used immediately, refrigerated.

A variety of mechanical aids may be used to facilitate solution preparation, including electronic 3-gang pumping devices which facilitate accurate delivery of the base solutions.

Results

These two methods, and various modifications, have been adopted by hospital pharmacists for preparing parenteral nutrition solutions because of their simplicity. However, these methods suffer from certain disadvantages in that they may be more expensive than the bulk preparation method and require more time to formulate and to prepare on a per bottle or bag basis. The nutrient solution generally is used or discarded within 24 hours from the time of preparation and pyrogen, sterility and analytical tests are performed infrequently. Some hospital pharmacy departments perform these tests on unused solutions or on randomly selected samples from the day's workload in order to monitor compounding techniques. Such monitoring should be a routine component of parenteral nutrition services provided by a pharmacy department.

In some hospitals, the pharmacists chose to prepare small batches of amino acid-glucose solutions ($\pm$ electrolytes), to sterilise them by membrane filtration and to give them an 'arbitrary' shelf-life at 4°C of 1 month. Although these solutions were subjected to sterility testing, it was not common practice for the free amino acid concentration, hence formation of Maillard products, to be monitored during the storage period.

Bulk preparation of solutions

When a small fixed range of parenteral nutrition formulae has been approved for use within the hospital, the most economical method of preparing solutions is on a bulk basis. The amino acid solution and concentrated glucose solution or granular anhydrous glucose are combined in appropriate quantities in a sterilised mixing tank. Appropriate volumes or quantities of electrolytes are added and the mixture is made to volume with water for injection. The solution is mixed well, the mixing tank pressurised with nitrogen and the solution filtered through appropriate sterile clarifying and sterilising membrane filters under laminar air flow conditions into the final container. Either sterile glass bottles or sterile empty plastic bags may be used as the final container. If sterile glass bottles are used, it is recommended that the solution be sealed under nitrogen to prevent oxidation of any of the ingredients on storage.

Depending on the batch size, one or more containers are forwarded for pyrogen and sterility testing and one container should be forwarded for analysis of solution content. The remaining containers are inspected for particulate contamination, then placed in quarantine at 4°C, protected from light, until clearance is received. These solutions are generally dated with an expiration period of 30 days from the date of manufacture.

Additives such as insulin, trace elements and vitamin preparations, should be added aseptically under laminar air flow conditions immediately prior to the issue of the solutions, due to the labile nature of some of the additives. Solutions should be given a 24 hour expiry period once any further additions have been made.

The main advantages of bulk preparation of parenteral nutrition solutions are significant savings in cost and time in preparation and also the ability to test for sterility prior to administration. If a number of further additions are required to the basic formulation prior to administration, some of these advantages are lost.

Recent advances in solution preparation

More recently, the pharmaceutical industry has developed techniques whereby a range of pre-sterilised amino acid and glucose solutions can be combined aseptically and the resultant solutions, when stored at 4°C, may, depending on their particular formulations, have a shelf-life of approximately 3 months. These premixed amino acid-glucose solutions are marketed in Australia by Travenol Laboratories and are available from Travenol and other companies in USA, Canada and Europe. The solutions do not contain vitamins, some of which have limited chemical stability, or trace elements. These nutrients should be added aseptically and the electrolyte profiles modified if necessary, just prior to administration.

Abbott Laboratories recently released its Nutrimix® delivery system in USA. This system consists of a dual-chambered plastic intravenous container filled with Aminosyn® in the upper 500 ml chamber and glucose in the lower 1000 ml capacity chamber. It takes approximately 15 seconds to effect transfer of the Aminosyn® to the lower chamber, and hence admixture with the glucose solution.

In most countries the range of commercially available electrolyte additive solutions is extensive and some examples are included in Table 25.1. The ranges of commercially available trace element preparations and vitamin preparations are more limited. Examples of these preparations are included in Chapters 12 and 13, respectively.

The next pharmaceutical challenge regarding solution formulation and preparation followed the acceptance that intravenous lipid should be used to provide a proportion of the patient's daily caloric needs. The obvious request was for the lipid emulsion to be mixed with the TPN solution in a single container. Once again, such a product could not be produced on an industrial scale, this time because of the limited physical stability of lipid emulsions. Studies conducted on the stability of admixtures of lipid with amino acid, glucose and electrolyte solutions allowed to stand at room

Table 25.1 Some electrolyte injection solutions available for addition to parenteral nutrition solutions

Electrolyte	Injection solution	Millimoles per 1 ml solution	
Sodium	Sodium Chloride 2 g/10 ml (20%)	Na^+ Cl^-	3.42 3.42
	Sodium Acetate 1.63 g/10 ml (16.3%)	Na^+ Acetate$^-$	2.0 2.0
Potassium	Potassium Acetate 2.45 g/5 ml (49%)	K^+ Acetate$^-$	5.0 5.0
	Potassium Chloride 2 g/8 ml (25%)	K^+ Cl^-	3.35 3.35
Magnesium	Magnesium Sulphate 2.49 g/5 ml (49.8%) (as heptahydrate)	Mg^{++} $SO_4=$	2.00 2.00
Calcium	Calcium Chloride 1 g/10 ml (10%)	Ca^{++} Cl^-	0.7 1.4
	Calcium Gluconate 1 g/10 ml (10%)	Ca^{++} Gluconate	0.22 0.44
Phosphate	Potassium Acid Phosphate $KH_2 PO_4$ 1.36 g/10 ml (13.6%)	PO_4^{3-} K^+ H^+	1.0 1.0 2.0
	Potassium Phosphates (mixed) $K_2HPO_4:KH_2PO_4$ 1.83 g:0.54 g/10 ml	PO_4^{3-} K^+ H^+	1.45 2.5 1.9
	Phosphate Ions 0.67M® (D.B.L.)	PO_4^{3-} K^+ Na^+ H^+	0.67 0.13 1.07 0.8

temperature, and also at 4–8°C for periods of 24 or more hours, produced variable results ranging from physically stable to creaming, flocculation and coalescence of the emulsion. However, now there is data available which indicates that the lipid emulsion may be stable for a sufficient period of time in various nutrition admixtures, which are within certain defined ranges, to allow practical use within a hospital setting.

Recently, workers at KabiVitrum (Sweden) have published the results of investigations of the physicochemical properties of several TPN admixtures with Intralipid®, which corresponded to commonly used regimens. In particular, they determined the influence of various cations, phosphate, amino acids, glucose concentration and pH on the zeta potential of the lipid particles. In the lipid emulsion (Intralipid®), the lipid particles have a negative zeta potential of c. 35 mV, which contributes to the repulsion of the particles and the stability of the emulsion. (The emulsion also is stabilised by the aqueous layer surrounding the fat globules). Although the results demonstrated that the physical stability of the fat emulsion was reduced in all admixtures and slight creaming was observed after 96 hours at room temperature (20–25°C), it was concluded that the specific admixtures studied (using Intralipid®, Vamin®, glucose and other additives) were stable at room temperature for 96 hours.

However, because several investigators have reported problems when attempting to produce a safe and stable final product, those companies that have tested the stability of defined combinations of their lipid emulsions with defined amino acid, glucose and other nutrient products, have produced specific guidelines for pharmacists regarding admixture, storage and administration. For example, Cutter Laboratories, which markets Intralipid® in the USA, includes specific mixing guidelines and limitations in its product leaflet (Table 25.2). Travenol Laboratories (USA), similarly, includes specific mixing guidelines and limitations for the soybean oil emulsion (Travamulsion®). Both these companies stipulate that the admixtures must be administered within 24 hours of preparation and that polyvinyl chloride (PVC) plastic containers should not be used in combination with lipid emulsions because of the risk of extraction of phthallate plasticisers. Polyolefin or ethylene vinyl acetate polymer (EVA) bags are recommended as these are free of phthallate plasticisers.

Table 25.2 Maximum admixture concentrations studied below which physical stability has been demonstrated (based on data from Anon, Cutter Medical, 1982; Jeppsson & Sjoberg, 1984)

		AMINO ACID SOLUTIONS			
Ingredients	Freamine III® 8.5%*	Travasol® w/out elec 8.5%	10%	Vamin® glucose 7% : 10%	Veinamine® 8%
Intralipid 10% or 20%, ml	250–500	250–500		500–1000	250–500
Amino acids, ml	500	500		1000–2000	500
Glucose, g	50 or 350	50 or 350		100–550	50 or 350
Addamel®, ml	—	—		10†	—
Sodium, mmol/l	107	103	103	70	119
Potassium, mmol/l	84	84	84	55	96
Calcium, mmol/l	4	4	4	2.9	4
Magnesium, mmol/l	5.2	5.2	5.2	3.1	6.4
Acetate, mmol/l	30	21	35	—	20
Chloride, mmol/l	196	209	211	71	223
Phosphorus, mmol/l	10	6	6	9.2	6
Sulphate, mmol/l	5	5	5	1.5	5
Zinc, mmol/l	0.048	0.048	0.048	0.03	0.048
Copper, mmol/l	0.02	0.02	0.02	†	0.02
Chromium, mmol/l	<0.001	<0.001	<0.001	†	<0.001
Manganese, mmol/l	0.012	0.012	0.012	†	0.012
Vitamins — as MVI® Conc, ml	5	5	5	—	5

* Freamine II 8.5% also studied
† Addamel® contains per 10 ml — Ca 5 mmol, Mg 1.5 mmol, Fe 0.05 mmol, Zn 0.02 mmol, Mn 0.04 mmol, Cu 0.005 mmol, F 0.05 mmol, I 0.001 mmol, Cl 13.3 mmol

The specific order for admixing recommended for the KabiVitrum product is to add the required electrolytes, trace elements (and vitamins) to the recommended amino acid and glucose solutions, which are then transferred to a phthallate-free bag. The lipid emulsion is added to this bag containing the combined amino acid-glucose solutions, and the bag gently agitated to ensure complete mixing. Electrolytes should never be added directly to the lipid emulsion. Total quantities of electrolytes, trace elements and vitamins in the admixture must not exceed those evaluated and published to be compatible over the specific study period (Table 25.2). The proportions of specific amino acid to glucose solution to Intralipid® 20% emulsion (V:V:V) recommended are 1:1:1 or 1:1:0.5. The final product must be used within 24 hours of admixing.

It should be noted that not all health administration authorities in western countries have approved the admixture of lipid emulsions with additives other than heparin.

COMPATIBILITY AND STABILITY CONSIDERATIONS

Most hospitalised patients receiving parenteral nutrition are acutely ill, often septic, and require treatment with a range of drugs and anti-infective agents. These drugs, in most instances, are administered parenterally, the intravenous route being the preferred route. Thus, the question is invariably asked: 'Is this drug compatible with TPN and, if not, how should we give it?'

Over the last decade an extensive body of literature has developed pertaining to drug stability and compatibility with parenteral nutrition solutions. Some of this literature is conflicting, some of it is not directly applicable to those products currently in use in specific countries. A useful review and assessment of this literature was published recently by Niemiec & Vanderveen (1984).

CALCIUM AND PHOSPHATE

The addition of electrolyte solutions should be approached with caution and consideration should be given to the compatibility of the electrolytes with other components of the parenteral nutrition solution. One of the more perplexing compatibility issues is that of the amounts of calcium and phosphate salts that can be combined safely in nutrition solutions, particularly those formulated for neonates who have relatively much higher requirements for these nutrients than adults. The compatibility of these salts in nutrition solutions is dependent on a complex set of interrelating factors which influence precipitation of dibasic calcium phosphate. A number of these factors are summarised in Table 25.3.

Phosphate, unlike other electrolytes, exists in aqueous solution as the following species: H_3PO_4, $H_2PO_4^-$, $HPO_4^=$, PO_4^{3-}. Within the range pH

Table 25.3 Some factors influencing dibasic calcium phosphate precipitation

Factor	Influence
Solution pH	As pH increases (e.g. 5.0 to 7.4) amount of $HPO_4^=$ increases favouring calcium phosphate precipitation
Ionic strength of solution	High ionic strength of blood and TPN solutions influence ($\uparrow$) valence of phosphate
Species of salts: *Calcium*	Calcium chloride dissociates more readily than gluconate salt — favouring calcium phosphate precipitation
Phosphate	Phosphate ions 0.67 M (DBL®) and Mixed Potassium Phosphates (DBL®) — pH 7–8, dibasic phosphate species predominates (c. 4:1) Potassium dihydrogen phosphates 13.6% (DBL®) — pH 4–5, $H_2PO_4^-$ predominates
Amino acids: *Titratable acidity of formulation*	Inherent buffering capacity, affects compatibility tolerances of calcium and phosphate salts
Presence of ionised species	At midrange pH, ionised amino acids form soluble complexes with calcium and phosphate
Concentration	<2.5% amino acids limited buffering capacity, less tolerant to calcium and phosphate salts
Albumin	Refer amino acids
Lipid emulsion	Admixture/contact in infusion line may result in pH increase and decreased calcium and phosphate solubility
High molar calcium and phosphate concentrations	Exceed solubility of dibasic calcium phosphate at pH of solution
Order of adding calcium and phosphate salts	Addition of calcium salts before phosphate, or before final formula dilution increases probability of precipitation (concentration effect)
Temperature *Environment* *Catheter* *Body*	Increasing solution temperature decreases calcium phosphate solubility

4 through 10, the principal phosphate species are $H_2PO_4^-$ and $HPO_4^=$, with H_3PO_4 and PO_4^{3-} being present in negligible amounts. At pH 7.4, the ratio of $HPO_4^=:H_2PO_4^-$ is approximately 4:1, and the average valence is 1.8. At pH 5.4, the ratio of $HPO_4^=:H_2PO_4^-$ is approximately 4:100 and the average valence is 1.04.

Calcium phosphate precipitates primarily in the form of dibasic calcium phosphate (Ca HPO_4) which is less soluble than the monobasic form (Ca

[H$_2$PO$_4$]$_2$). Therefore, the solubility of increasing concentrations of calcium and phosphate will be greater in solutions of decreasing pH as the ratio of HPO$_4^=$:H$_2$PO$_4^-$ decreases.

The pH of parenteral nutrition solutions is determined mainly by the composition and titratable acidity of the amino acid solution used, and the concentration of amino acids present. The pH of the nutrition solution decreases with increasing amino acid content, thus increasing the solubility of calcium and phosphate. The addition of albumin to a nutrition solution increases the pH through the buffering capacity of albumin, thus decreasing the solubility of calcium and phosphate. However, amino acids exist in solution as ionic species and can form soluble complexes with calcium and phosphate. Complex formation increases in the midrange pH, thus decreasing the free concentrations of calcium and phosphate available to interact.

Nedich reported on studies conducted to determine the effect of pH on calcium phosphate precipitation and also concentration (ionic ratio) effects associated with phosphate and added calcium ions to Travasol® (Synthamin®) solutions. These results are depicted in the calcium phosphate precipitation curves illustrated in Figures 25.2 & 25.3 respectively. Other workers have produced similar curves for nutrition solutions formulated using other amino acid preparations, including Freamine® II and Freamine® III, and Veinamine®.

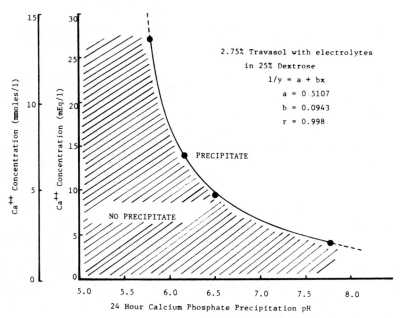

Fig. 25.2 Calcium ion concentration in an extemporaneously prepared parenteral nutrition solution as a function of admixture pH for calcium phosphate precipitation at 24 hours. (Reproduced with the permission of Nedich, 1978 and MTP Press)

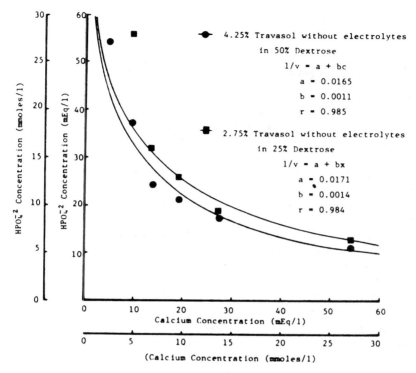

Fig. 25.3 Phosphate concentration as a function of calcium concentration for calcium phosphate precipitation in parenteral nutrition mixtures at 24 hours. (Reproduced with permission of Nedich, 1978, and MTP Press)

As a further measure to avoid the precipitation of calcium phosphate, it is recommended that phosphate salts should be added before the addition of calcium and that the solution should be thoroughly mixed prior to this latter addition. The pH of the parenteral nutrition admixture should not be adjusted to the physiological range if calcium and phosphate ions are present in the solution. With increasing pH, the proportion of the divalent phosphate species in solution increases, facilitating precipitation of calcium phosphate.

An additional factor that should be considered is the effect of temperature on the incompatibility of calcium and phosphate. As the temperature increases, the calcium salt becomes increasingly dissociated, thus providing more free calcium ion available to complex with phosphate. This is a crucial factor influencing calcium phosphate precipitation and has resulted in calcium phosphate occlusion of catheters, particularly in infants placed in incubators. Similarly, body heat may mediate calcium phosphate precipitation in adult patients.

It is important that the pharmacist maintains an acute awareness of those factors which are likely to cause precipitation of calcium phosphate during the infusion of a TPN solution where the compatibility of these salts is considered 'borderline'. Evidence of incompatibility of these 'borderline' solutions — floating, translucent flakes or catheter occlusion — may not occur for 12 or more hours after mixing.

OTHER ELECTROLYTES

Magnesium may influence the interaction between calcium and phosphate competing with the free calcium ions for phosphate.

Sodium bicarbonate added to parenteral nutrition solutions results in the formation of carbon dioxide with loss of the bicarbonate ion. This reaction is facilitated because of the acidic pH of these solutions and also their buffering capacity. Insoluble carbonate salts may be formed with calcium and magnesium ions present in the solution. Since acetate serves as a physiological precursor for bicarbonate, this incompatibility can be avoided.

When supplementing electrolytes, consideration should be given to the total chloride content and also the pH of the final solution. Hyperchloraemic acidosis may occur if cations are all added as the chloride, and not as a buffer. This can be avoided if the acetate:chloride ratio is adjusted to approximately 1:1, using acetate salts instead of chloride salts. Hypochloraemic metabolic alkalosis also may occur if excess acetate is used.

The addition of hydrochloric acid to parenteral nutrition solutions has been considered as an alternative treatment for metabolic alkalosis in patients with acute or chronic renal failure. Hydrochloric acid has been demonstrated to be physiologically available from a Travasol®–glucose solution. However, the pH of the resulting solutions decreased with increasing amounts of hydrochloric acid. The concentrations of the amino acids proline and histidine decreased with time and increasing acid concentration. No other stability effects were reported. The authors concluded that hydrochloric acid in concentrations up to 100 mmol/l may be added to parenteral nutrition solutions and used successfully in the short-term treatment of severe metabolic alkalosis when conventional treatment is contraindicated.

TRACE ELEMENT SOLUTIONS

The stability of combined trace element solutions containing zinc, copper, chromium and manganese has been demonstrated in parenteral nutrition solutions at room temperature and under refrigeration for periods ranging from 24 hours to 4 months (at 2–6°C). Selenium added as sodium selenite to TPN solutions containing a multivitamin preparation, MVI® concentrate and copper (in addition to other trace elements) resulted in the precipitation of selenium. The MVI and copper were considered to be responsible for this effect.

A number of amino acids chelate with trace elements and it is considered that these chelates may react with glucose to form Maillard products at a greater rate than amino acid alone. Thus, until further evidence is available to confirm or dispute this hypothesis, it is recommended that trace elements should be added to nutrition solutions immediately prior to use.

Iron has been added to nutrition solutions as iron dextran and ferrous citrate. Only limited information is available on the stability of these iron salts in TPN solutions over periods of 12–18 hours.

VITAMINS

Vitamin stability in parenteral nutrition solutions may be affected by a number of factors pertaining to the solution and its composition, including the pH, presence of electrolytes, trace elements, or other vitamins; and environmental conditions including storage time, temperature and light exposure. In addition, some vitamins may be lost from the solution through absorption and/or adsorption by the plastic bag used to contain the nutrition solution.

The available information relating to the stability of vitamins often is conflicting and, in some instances, has been based on uncontrolled observations using massive vitamin doses tested over weeks under varying conditions. A summary of recently published data is presented in Table 25.4. For a more detailed discussion of vitamin stability, the reader is referred to Chapter 13.

A number of vitamins are light sensitive, and thus it is recommended that the nutrition solutions should be protected from light to retard the degradation rate of the vitamins. An ultra-violet light protective bag also provides protection against light sensitised photo-oxidation of certain amino acids, and also the light catalysed oxidation of L-tryptophan to indigo carmine.

SOME INTRAVENOUS DRUGS

Patients receiving parenteral nutrition solutions often require treatment with one or more therapeutic agents. In those who have limited venous access, or who are fluid restricted, compatibility information regarding a prescribed intravenous drug with the nutrition solution may be sought. In the past there has been a consensus of opinion that intravenous drugs, particularly antibiotics, should not be added to amino acid containing solutions. However, data is beginning to accumulate regarding the stability — physical, chemical and microbiological — of antibiotics and other anti-infective agents administered by co-infusion with nutrition solutions or as an additive to the solution. Some of this data is summarised in Table 25.5.

Schuetz & King (1978), using physical examination and chemical and microbiological assay methods, found that although ampicillin, kanamycin, cephalothin and gentamicin were physically compatible and microbiologically stable for 12 hours in amino acid-glucose solutions containing specified

Table 25.4 Stability of vitamins in parenteral nutrition solutions (according to recent literature, 1980–1984)

Vitamin	Stability	Comment
Vitamin A		
Retinol/retinyl acetate	Decreased (up to 75% loss)	Loss caused by: — sorption by PVC bag/set — exposure to light (sun, c. 2000 lux)
Vitamin B Group		Degradation caused by:
Thiamine (B1)	Decreased (up to 90% loss)	— greater than 1.5 mmol/l sodium bisulphite (anti-oxidant in AA solutions) — direct sunlight — temperature
Riboflavine (B2)	Decreased	— direct/indirect sunlight
Niacin	Not affected	— different light conditions
Pyridoxine (B6)	Decreased (up to 86% loss)	— direct sunlight only
Folic acid	Decreased (up to 50% in 5.4 h at 24 °C in dark)	Rapid degradation in: — presence of other vitamins — temperature — light
	Not affected (at 8, 48 h)	— in sunlight or fluorescent light — room temperature or at 4 °C
Cyanocobalamin (B12)		Conflicting data
Ascorbic acid (C)	Decreased (variable to >90%)	Rapid degradation in: — presence of other vitamins — oxygen — room temperature — light — copper, other trace elements
Vitamin D	Decreased (up to 20–40%)	— possible sorption to plastic infusion system
Vitamin E	Stable	— at conditions tested
α-tocopherol acetate	Decreased (up to 36%)	— possible sorption to plastic infusion system
Vitamin K	Uncertain	— insufficient data — light may decrease potency

sorption = processes of absorption and adsorption

concentrations of calcium and phosphate. Elevated concentrations of these electrolytes and vitamin preparations were likely to cause precipitation.

Stability studies of cimetidine hydrochloride at concentrations of 120 mg and 500 mg per 100 ml in amino acid solutions, with or without electrolytes, stored at room temperature, revealed this drug to be both physically and chemically compatible in the test solutions. Initial investigations have been undertaken in patients receiving cimetidine added to continuously

Table 25.5   Results of some compatibility studies of anti-infectives in parenteral nutrition solutions

Anti-infective	Concentration	Stability	Comment
Amphotericin	100 mg/l	I–P	Disruption of colloidal suspension
Ampicillin sodium (1)(2)	1 g/l	I/LA	After 24 h at 25–37 °C
	1 g/l	C	After 12 h at 22 °C
Carbenicillin disodium (2)	1–1.5 g/l	C	After 24 h at 4–37 °C
	>1.5 g/l	LA	Visually compatible
Cefamandole	2 g/l	C	After 24 h at 5–25 °C
Cefazolin sodium	1 g/100 ml	C	After 24 h at 22 °C
Cefoxitin	1 g/l	C	After 24 h at 4, 25 °C
Cephalothin sodium	1 g/l	C	After 24 h, 4–25 °C
		LA	With higher temperatures
Chloramphenicol sodium succinate	0.7 g/l	C	After 24 h at 4, 25 °C
Cloxacillin sodium (2)	1 g/100 ml	C	After 24 h at 22 °C
Gentamicin sulphate	80 mg/100 ml	C	After 24 h at 22 °C
	80 mg/l	I–P	After 24 h at 22 °C
Methicillin sodium (2)	1–1.5 g/l	C	After 24 h at 4–25 °C
		LA	With higher temperatures
Metronidazole	2 g/l	I	After 24 h at 30 °C
Penicillin G potassium (2)	1.5 g/100 ml	C	After 24 h at 22 °C
Tobramycin	80 mg/l	C	After 24 h at 4, 25 °C

C   compatible and antimicrobial activity retained
I   incompatible
P   precipitate
LA   loss of antimicrobial activity
(1)   Ampicillin is considered to be unstable in acid solutions
(2)   Addition of penicillins should be discouraged until the immunologic properties of mixtures of crystalline amino acids and penicillins are clarified, since allergenic potential may increase during time admixture stands.

administered parenteral nutrition solutions for the treatment of gastric hypersecretory conditions. There were no apparent adverse consequences detected as a result of mixing cimetidine with the nutrition solutions in this short-term study.

The availability of insulin added to parenteral nutrition solutions is discussed in Chapter 8.

It must be recognised that physical or visual compatibility data are often not a complete indication of a drug additive's effect on the formulation, activity and possible subsequent toxicity of a TPN solution. Until chemical data are made available, the addition of agents to TPN solutions other than those that have been investigated and documented as compatible, should be approached with caution.

LABELLING OF SOLUTIONS

Uniform labelling of parenteral nutrition solutions is essential and should include all relevant information pertaining to the contents of the solution and the patient for whom it has been ordered. The basic format of the label should include:

— patient's name, medical record number, ward/room location
— infusion rate, ml/hour
— content per total volume of solution, namely:
    amount of amino acids and source
    amount of glucose as grams or % w/v in final solution
    content of electrolytes expressed as millimoles/litre
    vitamin source and volume
    grams of nitrogen
    approximate non-protein kilojoules (kilocalories)
    approximate osmolality
    approximate pH
— name and amount of any other ingredients, for example, insulin, trace elements
— bottle/sequence number for specific patient
— space for administering nurse to indicate name and time of administration
— date and time of preparation
— initials of pharmacist preparing solution
— date and time of expiration of solution
— storage information
— name and address of pharmacy department

A number of examples of labels are reproduced in the literature. Some hospital pharmacy departments have designed a 'multiple copies' order form to serve as the order from the physician, the label, and also a record for the patient's medical notes. An example of this type of stationery is illustrated in Figure 25.4.

More detailed information can be produced readily in label format (Fig. 25.5) by utilising a computer program designed to process parenteral nutrition requirements for adult and paediatic patients. Nutritional data sheets can be generated for inclusion in the patient's medical notes (Fig. 25.6). The formula to be used for preparing the nutrition solution also can be produced by the program.

MONITORING OF SOLUTION PREPARATION

Monitoring of the manufacturing process and testing of the final product is essential. Solutions should be monitored for particulate contamination, bacterial and fungal contamination, absence of pyrogens, and should be quantitatively analysed to determine accuracy of formulation.

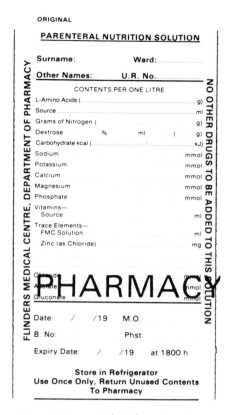

ORIGINAL

PARENTERAL NUTRITION SOLUTION

Surname: Ward:.................

Other Names: U.R. No.................

CONTENTS PER ONE LITRE

| L-Amino Acids (.. g) |
| Source .... ml |
| Grams of Nitrogen (.. g) |
| Dextrose   %   ml   (g) |
| Carbohydrate kcal (.................../............... kJ) |
| Sodium   mmol |
| Potassium   mmol |
| Calcium   mmol |
| Magnesium   mmol |
| Phosphate   mmol |
| Vitamins— |
| Source   ml |
| Trace Elements— |
| FMC Solution   ml |
| Zinc (as Chloride)   mg |

Chloride   mmol
Acetate   mmol
Gluconate   mmol

Date: /   /19   M.O.

B. No: Phst:

Expiry Date: /   /19   at 1800 h

Store in Refrigerator
Use Once Only, Return Unused Contents
To Pharmacy

(left vertical text) FLINDERS MEDICAL CENTRE, DEPARTMENT OF PHARMACY

(right vertical text) NO OTHER DRUGS TO BE ADDED TO THIS SOLUTION

Fig. 25.4 Parenteral nutrition solution order/label/record stationery.

Particulate contamination

Whether solutions are prepared by making additions to commercial premixed amino acid-glucose solutions, as individual units on a daily basis or by bulk technique, all units should be examined visually for particulate contamination prior to distribution. The base solutions and additives should be examined for particulate matter prior to admixture, and the final solution also must be examined as particulate matter may be introduced during compounding. The use of a filter device on the administration set does not relieve the pharmacist of the responsibility of preparing a solution that is low in particulate content.

Bacterial and fungal contamination

Bacterial and fungal septicaemia were reported as major complications of parenteral nutrition from the years 1969 to 1972. The growth of certain bacteria and fungi in patenteral nutrition solutions, particularly *Candida*

H

albicans and *Torulopsis glabrata*, has been demonstrated by numerous investigators within 24–48 hours, when these solutions have been incubated at room temperature. Although a number of studies have reported no growth

```
                    PAEDIATRIC PARENTERAL NUTRITION

    PATIENT NAME: BABY ******                U/R NUMBER: 275498.1
    DATE: 20/03/85          TO RUN AT  6.3 ML/H

       INGREDIENTS        CONTENT PER  150.0 ML   CONTENT PER LITRE
    ------------------ (IE 24 HOUR FLUID) --------------------
    L-AMINO ACIDS  (EX I                       I
    SYNTHAMIN 10% -E)  I   3.50 GRAMS          I   23.33 GRAMS
    GRAMS OF NITROGEN  I   0.59 GRAMS          I    3.90 GRAMS
    DEXTROSE           I  18.75 GRAMS          I  125.00 GRAMS
    CARBOHYDRATE KJ    I  294.94 KJ            I 1966.25 KJ
    TOTAL KILOJOULES   I  353.51 KJ            I 2356.76 KJ
    TOTAL Kcals        I   84.49Kcal           I  563.28Kcal
    CARBOHYDRATE Kcals I   70.49Kcal           I  469.95Kcal
    SODIUM             I    4.20 MMOL          I   28.00 MMOL
    POTASSIUM          I    2.10 MMOL          I   14.00 MMOL
    CALCIUM            I    1.40 MMOL          I    9.33 MMOL
    MAGNESIUM          I    0.39 MMOL          I    2.61 MMOL
    CHLORIDE           I    2.80 MMOL          I   18.67 MMOL
    PHOSPHATE          I    1.12 MMOL          I    7.47 MMOL
    ACETATE            I    6.53 MMOL          I   43.52 MMOL
    GLUCONATE          I    2.80 MMOL          I   18.67 MMOL
    NEONATAL T.E.S.    I    1.40 ML            I    9.33 ML
    B GROUP VITAMINS   I    1.40 ML            I    9.33 ML
    ZINC               I   10.50 MICROMOLES    I   70.00 MICROMOLES
                       I                       I
                       I                       I
    ----------------------------------------------------------
       BATCH NUMBER: SAA200385      EXPIRY:21.3.85    AT 1800H

          FLINDERS MEDICAL CENTRE PHARMACY DEPARTMENT
                      BEDFORD PARK 5042
```

Fig. 25.5 Paediatric parenteral nutrition solution label, generated by a computer program.

```
           PAEDIATRIC PARENTERAL NUTRITION DATA SUMMARY
           -----------------------------------------------
    PATIENT NAME: BABY ******         U/R NUMBER: 275498.1  DATE: 20/03/85

        PATIENT WEIGHT: 1.400           IVN FLUID INPUT:     6.25 ml/h

    -----------------------------------------------------------------
    SOYA OIL EMULSION 20%  10.00 ml/day I TOTAL (IVN & IVL) FLUID INPUT:
    AMINO ACID SOURCE SYNTHAMIN 10% -E  I    160.00 ml/day
    AMINO ACID INPUT    2.50 g/Kg/day   I    114.29 ml/Kg/day
    DEXTROSE           12.50 % w/v       I
    SODIUM              3.00 mmol/Kg/day I IVN RATE:   6.25 ml/h
    POTASSIUM           1.50 mmol/Kg/day I IVL RATE:   0.50 ml/h
    CALCIUM             1.00 mmol/Kg/day I--------------------------------
    MAGNESIUM           0.28 mmol/Kg/day I KILOJOULESI   ex IVN    I   ex IVL
    CHLORIDE            2.00 mmol/Kg/day I per Kg/dayI            I1.43g/Kg/day
    ACETATE             4.66 mmol/Kg/day I--------------------------------
    PHOSPHATE           0.80 mmol/Kg/day I PROTEIN  I  41.84 kJ/Kg I
    BICARBONATE         0.00 mmol/Kg/day I NONPROTEINI 210.67 kJ/Kg I  59.14 kJ/Kg
    B GROUP VITAMINS    1.00 ml/Kg/day   I TOTAL     I 252.51 kJ/Kg I  59.14 kJ/Kg
    DAYAMIN             0.00 ml/Kg/day   I--------------------------------
    NEONATAL T.E.S.     1.00 ml/Kg/day   I TOTAL ENERGY INPUT
    FOLIC ACID          0.00 mcg/Kg/day  I    311.65 kJ/Kg/day
    CYANOCOBALAMIN      0.00 mcg/Kg/day  I    436.31 kJ/day
    ALBUMIN             0.00 g/Kg/day    I 154NON-N Kcal per gram of NITROGEN
    ZINC            7.50 micromoles/Kg/day I 645 NON-N kJ per gram of NITROGEN
    -----------------------------------------------------------------
```

Fig. 25.6 Paediatric parenteral nutrition data sheet, generated by a computer program.

of bacteria and fungi in parenteral nutrition solutions incubated at 4°C for as long as 1 month, rapid proliferation occurred when the contaminated solutions were brought to room temperature. Each addition of an additive or manipulation of a parenteral nutrition solution must be recognised for its potential of introducing microbial contamination to the solution and every effort should be made by the pharmacist to ensure sterility of the final product. Lipid emulsions also support growth of a range of bacteria and *Candida albicans* at room temperature.

Random samples of all bulk prepared solutions should be tested for microbial contamination prior to their release. Although it is not possible to test and receive results on randomly selected solutions prior to administration when parenteral nutrition fluids are prepared daily, it is possible to monitor the operator's technique by:

— testing randomly selected solutions returned unused to the pharmacy for microbial contamination
— randomly selecting a solution from those prepared to meet the requirements of the next 24 hours and testing for microbial contamination. This then necessitates the preparation of another solution to replace the one selected
— obtaining samples of solutions prior to distribution to patients and using the Limulus amoebocyte lysate test to monitor for pyrogens and consequent possible microbial contamination. (This method requires further evaluation)
— using the Addi-chek® quality control system to sample whole containers of nutrition solutions for microbial contamination.

To reduce the potential for extrinsic contamination of parenteral nutrition fluids, it has been recommended that all parenteral nutrition solutions should be prepared by a pharmacist using aseptic technique in a well-maintained laminar air flow cabinet. The nutrient solution should be used immediately after compounding or stored at 4°C until use, and then used within 24 hours of removal from these storage conditions. No further additions should be made to the solution at ward level.

Quantitative analysis

The pharmacist should include quantitative analysis of the various solution components — determination of total nitrogen content, glucose content, the various concentrations of anions and cations present in the solution, pH and osmolality — as part of the routine quality control, quality assurance programme for the parenteral nutrition service. A 5% deviation from theoretical values is acceptable for all values except osmolality, which is not able to be determined with the same degree of accuracy.

Facilities and environment

The facility used for the preparation of nutrition solutions should be inspected regularly to ensure that it complies with the recommendations of the Code of Good Manufacturing Practice. The equipment should be maintained in accordance with these recommendations and those of the manufacturer. Regular tests should be performed to confirm proper functioning and integrity. The environment also should be sampled regularly to ensure that the house-keeping measures adopted to maintain a clean environment are effective.

FILTERS

Membrane filters of pore size 0.45 or 0.2 μm have been advocated for some years for parenteral nutrition fluid therapy. Conflicting reports have been published relating to their efficacy in reducing the incidence of infusion-related septicaemia and infusion phlebitis. A number of authors also have commented that administration sets with attached filters require many more manipulations than do sets without filters, thus increasing the risk of extrinsic contamination. Further evaluation of the potential benefits of 0.45 and 0.2 μm membrane filters is required as new products are marketed before final conclusions can be made regarding the advantages of these devices in reducing the risk of septicaemia. Whether or not inline filters are used, it behoves the pharmacist to monitor the aseptic technique of the operator to ensure sterility of the final product.

REFERENCES AND FURTHER READING

Allwood M C The compatibility of four trace elements in total parenteral nutrition infusions. Int J Pharmaceutics 1983; 16: 57–63
Anon. Intralipid Admixture Manual. Cutter Medical, Berkeley, CA, 1982; H–526
Athanikar N, Boyer B, Deamer R, Harbison H, Henry R S, Jurgens R Jnr et al Visual compatibility of 30 additives with a parenteral nutrient solution. Am J Hosp Pharm 1979; 36: 511–513
Bivins B A, Rapp R P, DeLuca P P, McKean H, Griffen W O Jnr Final inline filtration: a means of decreasing the incidence of infusion phlebitis. Surgery 1979; 85: 388–394
Black C D, Popovich N G A study of intravenous emulsion compatibility: effects of dextrose, amino acids, and selected electrolytes. Drug Intell Clin Pharm 1981; 15: 184–193
Davis M R: A simple method for pharmacy-based microbiological quality control of parenteral products. Aust J Hosp Pharm 1981; 11: S2–S9
Eggert L D, Rusho W J, MacKay M W, Chan G M Calcium and phosphorus compatibility in parenteral nutrition solutions for neonates. Am J Hosp Pharm 1982; 39: 49–53
Ellis G P The Maillard reaction. Adv Carbohyd Chem 1959; 14: 63–134
Farago S Compatibility of antibiotics and other drugs in total parenteral nutrition solutions. Can J Hosp Pharm 1983; 36: 43–52
Giacoia G P, Chopra R The use of a computer in parenteral alimentation of low birth weight infants. JPEN 1981; 5: 328–331
Graham D T The Limulus amoebocyte lysate pyrogen test. Aust J Hosp Pharm 1978; 8: 96–102

Henry R S, Jurgens R W Jnr, Sturgeon R, Athanikar N, Welco A, Van Leuven M Compatibility of calcium chloride and calcium gluconate with sodium phosphate in a mixed TPN solution. Am J Hosp Pharm 1980; 37: 673–674

Jeppsson R I, Sjoberg B Compatibility of parenteral nutrition solutions when mixed in a plastic bag. Clin Nutr 1984; 2: 149–158

Knight P, Heer D, Abdenour G Ca×P and Ca/P in the parenteral feeding of preterm infants. JPEN 1983; 7: 110–114

MacMahon P Prescribing and formulating neonatal intravenous feeding solutions by microcomputer. Arch Dis Child 1984; 59: 548–552

May F, Robbins G A computer program for parenteral nutrition solution preparation, JPEN 1978; 2: 646–651

Miller R C, Grogan J B Efficacy of inline bacterial filters in reducing contamination of intravenous nutritional solutions. Am J Surg 1975; 130: 585–589

Mirtallo J M, Rogers K R, Johnson J A, Fabri P J, Schneider P J Stability of amino acid and the availability of acid in total parenteral nutrition solutions containing hydrochloric acid. Am J Hosp Pharm 1981; 38: 1729–1731

National Coordinating Committee on Large Volume Parenterals. Recommended guidelines for quality assurance in hospital centralized intravenous admixture services. Am J Hosp Pharm 1980; 37: 645–655

Nedich R L The compatibility of extemporaneously added drug additives with Travasol* (amino acid) injection. In: Johnston IDA (ed) Advances in Parenteral Nutrition. MTP Press, Lancaster, 1978; 415–426
*Synthamin

Niemiec P W Jnr, Vanderveen T W Compatibility considerations in parenteral nutrient solutions. Am J Hosp Pharm 1984; 41: 893–911

Robinson L A, Wright B T Central venous catheter occlusion caused by body-heat-mediated calcium phosphate precipitation. Am J Hosp Pharm 1982; 39: 120–121

Sayers M H, Johnson D K, Schumann L A, Ivey M F, Young J H, Finch C A Supplementation of total parenteral nutrition solutions with ferrous citrate. JPEN 1983; 7: 117–120

Schuetz D H, King J C Compatibility and stability of electrolytes, vitamins and antibiotics in combination with 8% amino acids solution. Am J Hosp Pharm 1978; 35: 33–44

Shils M E, Levander O A Selenium stability in TPN solutions. Am J Clin Nutr 1982; 35:829

Smith J L, Canham J E, Wells P A Effect of sodium bisulfite and light on vitamin stability in a TPN admixture. Am J Clin Nutr 1984; 39:674

Solassol C, Joyeux H, Yakoun M, Pujol H, Romieu C Nouvelles techniques pour nutrition parenterale chronique. Ann Chir 1974; 28: 785–794

Stegink L D, Freeman J B, Den Besten L, Filer L J Jnr Maillard reaction products in parenteral nutrition. Prog Fd Nutr Sci 1981; 5: 265–278

United States Pharmacopeial Convention Inc. Bacterial endotoxins test. In: The United States Pharmacopeia, 20th edition. Rockville, 1980; 888–889

Yuhas E M, Lofton F T, Mayron D, Baldinus J G, Rosenberg H A Cimetidine hydrochloride compatibility. II: Room temperature stability in intravenous infusion fluids. Am J Hosp Pharm 1981; 38: 879–881

26

Responsibilities of the pharmacist

The hospital pharmacist is trained in aseptic techniques and the formulation of stable and safe parenteral fluids. It is his responsibility to prepare parenteral nutrition solutions for patients receiving this form of therapy, and to ensure the quality of these solutions.

When a parenteral nutrition programme is to be established in a hospital, the pharmacist should work together with the physician responsible for the programme to:

— design a logical and meaningful order form
— evaluate the range of amino acid solutions, glucose solutions, combined amino acid-glucose solutions, electrolyte additives, vitamin preparations, trace element solutions and lipid emulsions available on the market and to select a small range that in general will satisfy the requirements of the types of patients to be fed. Factors such as cost, ready availability and ease of manipulation also should be taken into consideration. When new products come on to the market these should be evaluated against the products currently in use
— evaluate equipment available for use in solution preparation and administration and select that which is most appropriate for the safe preparation and administration of nutrition solutions
— determine the method of solution preparation and testing procedures that are to be used by the pharmacist
— develop an accurate and quick method for formulating solution requirements
— develop a protocol for the preparation and use of parenteral nutrition solutions
— establish a data base of literature pertaining to parenteral nutrition and, in particular, stability and compatibility data.

Once the programme is established, the minimal ongoing responsibilities of the pharmacist include:

— receiving parenteral nutrition order

214

— checking order to make sure that:
  it is correctly written
  the amounts of additives prescribed are acceptable
  units are correctly specified
  rate of infusion is specified
— check order for physical and chemical incompatibilities
— derive formulation for preparing the solution
— check each solution container for cracks, punctures, precipitate and microbial growth
— prepare solution using proper aseptic technique in clean — laminar air flow cabinet — environment
— inspect the finished product for particulate contamination
— label the finished product correctly and completely as to contents, including electrolytes, vitamins and trace elements
— specify expiration date and time on label
— ensure solution is delivered to the correct patient and that it is properly administered
— if the solution is not administered immediately after preparation, the pharmacist must ensure correct storage of the solution
— assist the physician with any special formulation problems and answer any questions relating to the contents of the solution
— conduct routine checks on the sterility and contents of solutions selected on a random basis
— conduct routine tests on the integrity of equipment and cleanliness of the environment
— participate in in-service training programmes for pharmacy, medical, and nursing staff
— continue to update his knowledge of parenteral nutrition and pharmaceutical techniques.

The pharmacist should keep a record of the batch numbers of fluids and other pharmaceuticals used to compound parenteral nutrition solutions. The results of all qualitative and quantitative tests performed on these solutions should be filed with these records. Any anomalies in the results of the tests should be reported to the prescribing physician to facilitate the investigation of complications of therapy. In addition, steps should be taken by the pharmacist to avoid the anomaly from recurring.

The pharmacist should review other medications prescribed for patients receiving parenteral nutrition so that he can assist the physician to anticipate and avoid potential interactions between drugs and the nutritional support being provided. Some examples of clinical syndromes resulting from drug-nutrient interactions are listed in Table 26.1. An evaluation of drug therapy should be made with regard to the present nutritional support, laboratory parameters and the patient's clinical condition.

Table 26.1   Some clinical syndromes resulting from drug-nutrient interactions*

Drug	Nutrient	Syndrome
Alcohol	Thiamine (B_1)	Wernicke's encephalopathy
Antacids	Phosphate	Hypophosphataemia
aluminium-containing		
Anticonvulsants	Folate	Anaemia
phenobarbitone	Vitamin D	Childhood rickets
phenytoin		Adult osteomalacia
primidone	Vitamin K	Hypoprothrombinaemia
Antifolates	Folate	Stomatitis
methotrexate		
pyrimethamine		
trimethoprim		
Anti-infectives		
amphotericin	Magnesium	Hypomagnesaemia
	Potassium	Hypokalaemia
isoniazid	Pyridoxine (B6)	Peripheral neuropathy
	Niacin	Pellagra
tetracyclines	Calcium	Depress bone growth
	Magnesium	Disturbed mitochondrial enzyme functions
Beta-Blockers	Glycogen	Hypoglycaemia
Corticosteroids	Glucose	Hyperglycaemia and glycosuria
	Water	Fluid retention
	Sodium	Sodium retention
	Potassium	Hypokalaemia
	Calcium	Osteoporosis
Diuretics	Magnesium	Hypomagnesaemia
	Potassium	Hypokalaemia
Diuretics-thiazide	Glucose	Hyperglycaemia

* For a detailed review of drug-nutrient interactions, see Roe & Campbell, 1984.

Some areas of potential problems and/or concern that the pharmacist should address with the physician and other members of the nutrition team include:

1. *Chronic medication* — commonly used drugs such as steroids, antacids, diuretics, and anticonvulsants interfere with one or more nutritional substrates. Specific laboratory parameters may need to be checked to determine if a patient is at risk of developing a drug-induced deficiency.

2. *Chronic alcohol intake* — may cause various clinical syndromes including anaemia, due to reduced folic acid and B12 absorption, or Wernicke's encephalopathy due to reduced thiamine absorption.

3. *Fluid and electrolyte balance* — the aggressive use of insulin to treat hyperglycaemia or glycosuria may precipitate or worsen hypokalaemia, which, in patients receiving digoxin may precipitate digoxin toxicity. The total electrolyte content of drugs and other intravenous fluids should be considered. For example, a daily dose of 12–18 g of ticarcillin sodium will add an additional 62.5–93.5 mmol of sodium to the patient's daily intake.

Table 26.2 Compatibility of some commonly used liquid medicines with selected enteral products (Ensure, Ensure Plus, Osmolite, Vital). (Compiled from Altman & Cutie, 1984)

Product name (Brand)	pH of product	pH of mixture	Compatibility of mixture
Bactrim DS Suspension 10 ml (Roche)	5.6–5.7	6.0–6.2	C — Viscosity ↑ slightly, with small volumes of enteral product
Benadryl Elixir 10 ml (Parke Davis)	5.2	6.4–6.5	C — Viscosity ↑ slightly.
Dilantin Suspension 5 ml (Parke Davis)	4.9	5.5–6.0	C — Viscosity ↑ slightly, with small volumes of enteral product
Elixophyllin 15 ml (Berlex)	3.4	6.3–6.5	C — Add slowly, agitate well
Kayciel Elixir 15 ml (Berlex)	6.2	6.2–6.6	C — Mixes readily
Keflex Suspension 5 ml (Dista)	4.0–4.2	6.2–6.3	C — Add slowly, agitate well
Klorvess Syrup 15 ml (Dorsey)	2.4	3.4–4.3	I — Becomes viscous and gelatinous
Lanoxin Elixir 2 ml (Wellcome)	7.0	6.5–6.8	C — On mixing, compatible. On standing 24–48 hours, rubbery mass results
Lomotil Liquid 5 ml (Searle)	3.3–3.4	6.1–6.5	C — Add slowly, agitate well
Mandelamine Forte Suspension 10 ml (Parke Davis)	Oil Base	Oil Base	I — Tacky, gelatinous mixture results
Mandelamine Granules 1 pk. (Parke Davis)	Solid	6.4–6.6	C — Disperse and dissolve readily
MCT Oil 10 ml (Mead Johnson)	Oil	Oil	I — Immiscible
Melleril oral Solution 200 mg (Sandoz)	3.8	5.5–5.9	I — Causes granulation
Mylicon Drops 1.2 ml (Stuart)	4.5–4.6	6.2–6.4	C — Viscosity ↑ 20–30% when mixed with c. 15 ml enteral product
Pen VeeK 5 ml (Wyeth)	6.5	6.5–6.6	C — Identical pH favours chemical and physical stability
Phenergan Syrup 10 ml (Wyeth)	5.1–5.3	5.4–6.0	C — Viscosity ↑ slightly
Sudafed Syrup 10 ml (Wellcome)	2.5	4.5–4.8	I — Viscous, gelatinous mass forms instantly
Tylenol Elixir 10 ml (McNeil)	4.7	6.0–6.3	C — Compatible with products studied

C = Compatible
I = Incompatible
↑ = Increase

Malnourished and traumatised patients are at risk of developing sodium accumulation and oedema, hence the electrolyte input must be monitored closely. Aggressive diuretic therapy will increase potassium and chloride losses in addition to having the desired effects on sodium and water.

4. *Acid-base balance* — crystalline amino acid solutions have relatively high titratable acidities due to the buffering capacity of the amino acids. To avoid inducing metabolic acidosis, it is important to be aware of the titratable acidity of the solution used, and also the acid-base properties of the various amino acids present in this solution. Some amino acid solutions contain a high acetate load to compensate partially for the hydrogen load generated. If insufficient chloride is added to the solution, metabolic alkalosis may be induced or compounded in some patients.

5. *Enteral nutrition* — a common problem encountered in patients receiving enteral nutrition support involves crushing of sustained release or enteric coated tablets for administration as a slurry via the feeding tube. Prior to administration of any solid medications via the feeding tube, the possible effects of crushing the formulation must be considered. The bolus administration of concentrated electrolyte solutions such as 10% potassium chloride into the small bowel may result in cramps, diarrhoea and intestinal bleeding due to the high osmolarity (2600 mOsm/litre) of these solutions. The additive should be diluted in the tube feed, providing it is compatible, to avoid these complications (Table 26.2).

6. *Pharmacokinetics in malnutrition* — the available evidence suggests that the normal pharmacokinetic properties of a drug may be altered in malnourished patients (Table 26.3). Diarrhoea, malabsorption, reduced body cell mass, hypoalbuminaemia and impaired liver function are but a few of the factors that may affect a drug's pharmacokinetic properties. Close clinical monitoring of drug therapy is essential and serum drug concentrations should be obtained whenever possible in these patients.

Table 26.3 Some pharmacokinetic processes altered by malnutrition

Pharmacokinetic process	Alteration
Drug absorption	Rate and extent influenced
Protein binding	Hypoalbuminaemia, ↑ free fraction of normally highly bound drugs
Volume of distribution	Potentiation of pharmacologic effect if ↑ free fraction of drugs with small volume of distribution
Tissue uptake of drug	May vary qualitatively and quantitatively
Biotransformation, metabolism	May be altered: changes in drug metabolising enzymes; alteration in drug-binding by proteins; metabolic and hormonal influences
Excretion	Biliary excretion affected: changes in cardiac and renal function may indirectly influence excretion

For a summary of the effects of drugs on nutritional status, the reader is referred to the various pharmaceutical texts, and also to Grant's text (1979).

If the nutrition service extends to the provision of a home parenteral nutrition programme, then the pharmacist should assume the responsibilities of participating in the patients' education programme, development of a home parenteral nutrition training manual, coordination of the supply of solutions and ancillary equipment, and aspects discussed in Chapter 23 and summarised by Gaffron et al (1980).

Parenteral nutrition has been one of the most significant therapeutic advances in recent years, but it is not without serious complications. The pharmacist has a challenging and significant role to play in the formulation, preparation and delivery of solutions to ensure that the patient's nutritional requirements are met and that his safety is not jeopardised.

REFERENCES AND FURTHER READING

Altman E, Cutie A J Compatibility of enteral products with commonly employed drug additives. Nutr Supp Serv 1984; 4(12): 8–17
Bourbeau D, Vinay P, Lemieux G, Gougoux A, Duranceau A Acid-base balance during parenteral nutrition with Travasol*. In: Johnston IDA (ed) Advances in Parenteral Nutrition. MTP Press, Lancaster 1978; 391–401
(*Synthamin)
Gaffron R E, Fleming C R, Berkner S, McCallum D, Schwartau N, McGill D B Organization and operation of a home parenteral nutrition program with emphasis on the pharmacist's role. Mayo Clin Proc 1980; 55: 94–98
Gatlin L, Kulkarni P, Hussain A, DeLuca P P Determining osmolarities: a practical approach for multicomponent intravenous and parenteral nutrient solutions. Am J Hosp Pharm 1979; 36: 1357–1361
Grant A Section E: Drugs. Effects of drugs on nutritional status. In: Nutritional Assessment Guidelines (2nd edn). Seattle, 1979; 63–101
Ichikawa I, Purkerson M L, Klahr S, Troy J L, Martinez-Maldonado M, Brenner B M Mechanism of reduced glomerular filtration rate in chronic malnutrition. J Clin Invest 1980; 65: 982–988
Krishnaswamy K Drug metabolism and pharmacokinetics in malnutrition. Clin Pharmacokin 1978; 3: 216–240
Roe D A, Campbell T C (eds) Drug and nutrients: The interactive effects. Marcel Dekker, New York, 1984
Schiller W R, Long C L, Blakemore W S Creatinine and nitrogen excretion in seriously ill and injured patients. Surg Gynecol Obstet 1979; 149: 561–566
Sturgeon R J, Athanikar N K, Henry R S, Jurgens R W Jnr, Welco A D Titratable acidities of crystalline amino acid admixtures. Am J Hosp Pharm 1980; 37: 388–390
Vanderveen T W Drug-nutrition interrelationships — an expanded role for the nutritional support team pharmacist. ASPEN Update 1981; 3(2): 1–6

27

Enteral nutrition

Enteral tube feeding has a long history, early attempts being those of Capivacceus (1598), John Hunter (1790) and Baron Larrey (1812). Randall, in his Jonathan E Rhoads lecture, presented in 1984, gave a fascinating review of the development of enteral feeding. Included in this was a summary of John Hunter's ingenious approach to provision of nutrition for a 50 year old man who was unable to swallow. A tube made of whalebone and eelskin was attached to a bladder so that a mixture of eggs, milk, sugar and medicines could be squeezed into the stomach without interfering with lung function.

Many famous names are associated with the development of gastric tubes, including Astley Cooper, Kussmaul, Brown-Sequard, Boorhaave and Dupuytren. Although the danger of pulmonary aspiration was well recognised, prolonged nasogastric feeding was performed, with one such case of feeding for 21 years having been reported in the British Medical Journal, 1917.

Duodenal feeding was described by Eishorn in 1910, and he made reference to feed composition, temperature, volume and timing, matters which were subsequently ignored by many.

Surgical access to provide a route for enteral feeding also has a long history, most techniques having been described around the turn of the century by surgeons such as Witzel, Janeway, Stamm and Mayo.

Immediate jejunal feeding after gastroenterostomy was reported by Andresen in 1918. In a monograph on the subject by Pareira (1959) continuous drip feeding of a special-purpose liquid feed via a fine-bore polyvinyl chloride or polyethylene tube, and transanastomotic tube feeding were described.

Patients who cannot be fed orally, but whose gastrointestinal tract is accessible by nasogastric or nasoenteric tube, gastrostomy or enterostomy, should not be fed intravenously. Much of what has been said about parenteral nutrition is directly relevant to any discussion of enteral nutrition. Thus, attention to fluid balance, provision of known amounts of protein, carbohydrate, fat, electrolytes, trace elements and vitamins is essential. Monitoring, both clinical and biochemical, is also important. Home tube feeding, after adequate training, is entirely feasible, either via fine bore nasogastric tube, or an implanted jejunal catheter (see Ch 23).

INDICATIONS AND CONTRAINDICATIONS

Tube feeding is indicated in patients whose gastrointestinal tract is functional, and who cannot be fed orally (Table 27.1). It is contraindicated if the gastrointestinal tract is nonfunctional. Nasogastric or nasoduodenal feeding are the most common methods, but gastrostomy or enterostomy should not be forgotten. Page et al (1979) have reported a study of jejunostomy feeding of 199 patients for periods of up to 240 days post-operatively. Because small bowel motility is uninterrupted post-operatively, and absorption from the small bowel is unimpaired, even in the presence of gastric distension, enterostomy allows post-operative nutrition without the need for TPN. As with intravenous nutrition, major organ failure necessitates modification of the feed, but does not contraindicate it.

Table 27.1 Some indications for enteral nutrition

Neurological or psychiatric disorders
  Coma, severe depression, brainstem lesions
Oropharyngeal or oesophageal disorders
  Neoplasms, trauma, or fractures of the head and neck
Gastrointestinal disorders
  Gastrointestinal fistulae, short bowel syndrome, chronic pancreatic insufficiency
Post-trauma
  Head injuries, burns
Organ failure
  Renal or liver failure

NASOGASTRIC AND NASOINTESTINAL TUBES

There are now many types of tubes available. Selection should be based on the presence of features desired (see Appendix 2). In patients who are unconscious or who cannot protect their airway if they vomit, a tube large enough to allow aspiration of gastric contents is essential. In other patients, a fine bore tube is more comfortable and less likely to lead to oesophagitis. Commercially available tubes of this type are listed in Appendix 2. Tubes now used are modifications of those described by Fallis & Barron in 1952.

Dangers of tube insertion include stimulation of vomiting, and insertion into the trachea. Presence of the tube in the stomach, or duodenum, if this is required, should be confirmed (if necessary, radiographically) and the tube fixed to the nose by a method which is secure and yet does not produce pressure on the nostril. A piece of adhesive tape fixed to the bridge of the nose, with two tails wound in opposite spirals around the tube, is effective.

If the patient vomits after tube insertion, the tip of the tube may relocate itself in the oesophagus or pharynx.

Insertion of a nasogastric tube is most easily carried out by asking the patient to sit forward while the lubricated tube is gently advanced horizontally through the nostril. There is often slight resistance at the posterior nares, followed by a feeling that the tip is 'free' in the nasopharynx. As the tube is gently advanced, with the patient swallowing small sips of water, the tip is 'gripped' by the upper end of the oesophagus. From that point, the tube advances with the aid of oesophageal peristalsis until a sufficient length is in place. No attempt should be made to force fine bore tubes, nor should the stylet be reintroduced once withdrawn, since perforation of the oesophagus may occur.

In the unconscious patient the tube should be inserted with the patient lying slightly head down on his left side, so that regurgitation or vomiting of gastric contents does not result in pulmonary aspiration. If the patient does not have intact upper airway reflexes, endotracheal intubation may be required prior to passage of the gastric tube. If there is oesophageal obstruction, a tube may be placed with the aid of a gastroscope.

ENTERAL TUBES

Feeding by jejunostomy is a procedure with a long history. Its principal disadvantages are development of peritonitis from leakage at the jejunal opening, and production of intestinal obstruction. However, needle catheter jejunostomy, in which a needle is passed subserosally along the antimesenteric border of the jejunum, then into the lumen, and the catheter is inserted through the needle prior to its removal, appears not to have significant complications. A silk purse string closes the subserosal tunnel, and the catheter is sutured to peritoneum and to skin. Sriram has described an enterostomy tube which has a pair of silicone wings rather than a balloon. These wings facilitate construction of a Witzel tunnel and fixation to the abdominal wall. The tube also has a Dacron cuff similar to the Hickman catheter, which allows firm attachment to the subcutaneous exit tunnel. Feeding via this route is possible within 24 hours of operation, except in the presence of general peritonitis, bowel obstruction, or extensive retroperitoneal dissection. The technique is nutritionally efficient, compares favourably with TPN, and is applicable to children. Another approach to enteral feeding has been described by Moss (1981). A triple lumen nasogastric balloon tube, sited at laparotomy, allows aspiration of the oesophagus above a balloon at the gastrooesophageal junction, aspiration of the stomach and immediate post-operative duodenal feeding.

ADMINISTRATION SYSTEMS

Administration of the feed can be by bolus, intermittent gravity drip or continuous infusion. A variety of continuous administration systems has been devised. Most of these consist of a disposable reservoir of varying capacity, and an administration set without a filter, terminating in a tip which is incompatible with intravenous cannulae. Some suppliers provide a calibrated bottle, or a calibrated measuring chamber to allow accurate administration. In some patients, for example, those with short bowel syndrome, administration using a pump is preferable (see Appendix 3).

When intermittent feeding is used, an appropriate sized container attached to the end of the feeding tube is all that is required. Whichever system is used, attention must be paid to the risk of administering bacterially contaminated feed. Some of the available administration systems are listed in Appendix 2.

FEED COMPOSITION

The original approach to tube feeding was to use sloppy foods, or to blenderise a nutritious meal. The main problems with this approach are that the detailed composition of the feed is difficult to estimate, the fluid is thick, and the preparation is time-consuming. Early commercially available feeds were high in protein, and had a high osmolality. Diarrhoea was common, and uraemia was reported.

There are now many commercial tube feeds available. Chernoff has divided them into five groups (Chernoff, 1980):

1. *Intact nutrients containing milk* — 9 varieties, including Compleat B® (Doyle), Sustacal® and Sustagen® (Mead Johnson).
2. *Intact nutrients without milk* — 15 varieties, including Ensure® and Ensure Plus® (Ross), Isocal® (Mead Johnson), Osmolite® (Ross) and the Precision® range (Doyle).
3. *Predigested nutrients* (elemental) — 7 varieties, including Criticare HN (Mead Johnson), Vipep® (Cutter), Vivonex® and Vivonex HN® (Eaton).
4. *Special use nutrients* — 10 varieties, including Amin-Aid® (McGaw), and Sustacal-Pudding® (Mead Johnson).
5. *Single nutrients* — 12 varieties, including MCT Oil® (Mead Johnson), and Polycose® (Ross).

For practical purposes, a non-lactose containing isosmolar, non-elemental feed is generally tolerated well by most patients. As described by Randall (1984), 'comparisons of the efficacy of defined formula diets tube fed into a normal gastrointestinal tract with normal foods or their equivalents as partially solubilized polymeric feeds, has become an exercise in proving the obvious — that the human gastrointestinal tract is designed to maintain nutrition by the ingestion, digestion, and absorption of normal foods, and that such should be fed when possible'. The composition of some of these feeds is shown in Table 27.2.

Elemental diets are usually only indicated when there is a problem with

Table 27.2 Composition of some general purpose non-lactose tube feeds (per 2000 ml)

Content	Ensure (Ross)	Isocal (Mead Johnson)	Osmolite (Ross)	Survimed* (Fresenius)	Travasorb (Travenol)	Triosorbin L (Pfrimmer)
Protein (g)	74	68	74	81	70	80
Fat (g)	74	88	78	25	70	80
Carbohydrate (g)	290	266	290	441	274	236
Sodium (mmol)	74	45	48	140	61	84
Potassium (mmol)	80	65	54	72	61	84
Calcium (mmol)	26	32	26	33	25	26
Magnesium (mmol)	17.6	16	17.4	20	17	16
Chloride (mmol)	81	60	45	116	57	100
Phosphorus (mmol)	35	32	34	54	32	38
Zinc (μmol)	496	303	496	31	288	NS
Copper (μmol)	34	30	34	8	32	NS
Manganese (μmol)	76	89	76	14	73	NS
Iron (μmol)	342	321	342	356	321	468
Iodine (μmol)	1.25	1.2	1.25	0.4	1.2	NS
Vitamin B1 (mg)	3.2	4	3.2	2.3	3	2.0
Vitamin B2 (mg)	3.6	4.4	3.6	3.3	3.4	2.0
Vitamin B6 (mg)	4.2	5.2	4.2	2.6	4	2.4
Niacin/ Nicotinamide (mg)	42	52	42	22	40	21
Pantothenic acid (mg)	11	26	10.6	15	10	8.4
Vitamin B12 (μg)	12.8	15.8	12.6	6.6	12	5.6
Vitamin C (mg)	320	316	322	110	304	105
Vitamin A (U)	5274	4600	5286	4400	5000	5300
Vitamin D (U)	424	420	422	218	400	420
Vitamin E (U)	64	78	64	33	60	16
Vitamin K (μg)	76	260	76	230	1900	106
Folate (μg)	420	400	420	1100	400	420
Biotin (μg)	320	300	320	264	—	420
Choline (mg)	1120	520	1100	726	—	NS
mOsm/kg water	450	300	300	400	450	250
kJ/ml (kcal/ml)	4.4(1.05)	4.2(1)	4.4(1.05)	4.2(1)	4.4(1.05)	4.4(1.05)

NS = not stated.
* There is a low Na, low K formula of Survimed.

digestion or when a completely no-residue diet is required. Investigation of defined formula diets in patients with impairment of normal gastrointestinal function or metabolic errors of metabolism were sponsored by the National Aeronautics and Space Administration (NASA) to explore the possibility of using them for maintaining human nutrition during space exploration. Their complications have been listed by Russell (1975), and include unpalatability, diarrhoea and dehydration due to the high osmolality, hyperglycaemia, pancreatic acinar atrophy, alteration of gastrointestinal bacterial flora and reduced gastric emptying. The composition of some of these feeds is shown in Table 27.3. An erudite review of elemental diets has been provided by Russell (1981).

Table 27.3 Composition of some predigested (elemental) tube feeds (per 2000 ml)

Content	Criticare HN (Mead Johnson)	Travasorb STD (Travenol)	Vivonex (Norwich Eaton)
Protein (g)	76	60	44
Fat (g)	6	26.7	2.9
Carbohydrate (g)	444	380	460
Sodium (mmol)	54	80	40.8
Potassium (mmol)	68	59.5	60
Calcium (mmol)	26.5	25	28
Magnesium (mmol)	17	17	18
Chloride (mmol)	60	85.5	41
Phosphorus (mmol)	34	32	36
Zinc (μmol)	310	230	255
Copper (μmol)	40	32	34
Manganese (μmol)	100	46	57
Iron (μmol)	340	321	358
Iodine (μmol)	1.25	1.2	1.3
Vitamin B1 (mg)	4	1.5	1.6
Vitamin B2 (mg)	4.4	1.7	1.8
Vitamin B6 (mg)	5.2	2	2.2
Niacin (mg)	52	20	15
Pantothenic acid (mg)	26.4	10	11
Vitamin B12 (μg)	15.8	6	6.6
Vitamin C (mg)	318	90	66
Vitamin A (U)	5200	5000	5500
Vitamin D (U)	420	400	444
Vitamin E (U)	80	30	33
Vitamin K (μg)	264	1500	74
Folate (μg)	420	400	444
Biotin (μg)	318	—	333
choline (mg)	520	—	82
mOsm/kg water	650	400–450	500
kJ/ml (kcal/ml)	4.4(1.06)	4.2(1)	4.2(1)

If one examines the composition of some of the solutions that are currently in general use, the following observations can be made:

Ensure® (Ross): Protein derived from sodium and calcium caseinate and soy protein isolate. Lipid derived from corn oil. Carbohydrate derived from corn syrup solids and sucrose. Ensure Plus® is also available. It contains 6.3 kJ/ml (1.5 kcal/ml), and has increased amounts of protein, lipid and carbohydrate. The osmolality of 600 mOsm/kg water renders it more likely to cause diarrhoea than Ensure®, in some patients.

Flexical® (Mead Johnson): Protein source is casein hydrolysate, plus methionine, tyrosine and tryptophan. Fat is in the form of medium chain triglycerides and soy oil. Carbohydrate consists of sucrose and glucose oligosaccharides. Flexical® has one of the lowest sodium contents of all the feeds.

Isocal® (Mead Johnson): Protein source is sodium caseinate and soy protein isolate. Fat consists of medium chain triglycerides and soy oil. Carbohydrate is derived from corn syrup solids. Sodium content is one of the lowest of all the feeds. Isocal HCN® contains 8.4 kJ/ml (2 kcal/ml), has an osmolality of 690 mOsm/kg water, and increased nitrogen fat and carbohydrate content.

Osmolite® (Ross): Protein source is sodium and calcium caseinate, soy protein isolate. Fat source is medium chain triglycerides, corn and soy oil. Carbohydrate source is polycose, a glucose polymer. Sodium and potassium contents are both low. Osmolite HN® is also available. It has a higher nitrogen content, but remains at 4.2 kJ/ml (1 kcal/ml).

Travasorb® (Travenol): Protein source is caseinates. Fat source is corn and soy oil. Carbohydrate source is oligosaccharides, corn syrup solids and sucrose. The Travasorb range now includes Travasorb HN®, Travasorb MCT®, Travasorb Renal and Travasorb Hepatic.

Travasorb STD® (Travenol): Protein source is lactalbumin and peptides. Fat source is medium chain triglycerides. Carbohydrate source is oligosaccharides, corn syrup solids. Fat content is low.

Triosorbin L® (Pfrimmer): Protein source is lactoproteins. Fat source is soy bean oil. Carbohydrate consists of mono, oligo, and polysaccharides.

Vivonex® (Norwich-Eaton): Protein source is amino acids. Fat source is safflower oil. Carbohydrate source is glucose. Vivonex HN® contains twice the amount of nitrogen, with a lower content of fat and carbohydrate. The fat content of Vivonex® is extremely low.

Flexical®, Isocal® and Osmolite® have the lowest sodium content; Vipep® and Osmolite® the lowest potassium content. Other special formulae now available include Criticare HN® (Mead-Johnson), an elemental diet, and TraumaCal® (Mead Johnson). The proper place and value of many of the special purpose preparations is not established, while their increased cost is. The essential differences in protein, fat, carbohydrate and energy content of some of the special formulae, compared with 'standard' formulae, are shown in Table 27.4. Detailed composition of three special formulae is given in Table 27.5.

Table 27.4   Some differences between standard and special formulae (per 1000 ml)

	Protein (g)	Fat (g)	Carbohydrate (g)	kJ/ml (kcal/ml)	mOsm/kg
Ensure[1]	37	37	145	4.4(1.05)	450
Ensure plus[1]	55	53	200	6.3(1.5)	600
Isocal[2]	34	44	133	4.2(1)	300
Isocal HCN[2]	75	91	225	8.4(2)	690
Osmolite[1]	37	39	145	4.4(1.05)	300
Osmolite HN[1]	44	37	141	4.2(1)	310
Sustagen[2]	61	9	169	4.2(1)	740
Traumacal[2]	83	68	143	6.3(1.5)	550
Vivonex[3]	22	1.5	230	4.2(1)	500
Vivonex HN[3]	44	0.9	211	4.2(1)	810
Criticare HN[2]	38	3	222	4.4(1.06)	650

1. Ross Laboratories
2. Mead Johnson & Co
3. Norwich-Eaton

Table 27.5   Composition of some special purpose tube feeds (per 2000 ml)

Content	Enrich* (Ross)	Traumacal[†] (Mead Johnson)	Ensure plus (Ross)
Protein (g)	79.4	166	110
Fat (g)	73.9	136	107
Carbohydrate (g)	323.2	286	400
Sodium (mmol)	73.4	104	100
Potassium (mmol)	80	72	120
Calcium (mmol)	35	37.5	32
Magnesium (mmol)	24	16.7	26
Chloride (mmol)	81	90	112
Phosphorus (mmol)	46	48	41
Zinc (μmol)	496	460	744
Copper (μmol)	46	50	50
Manganese (μmol)	116	100	77
Iron (μmol)	472	330	154
Iodine (μmol)	1.9	1.2	1.7
Vitamin B1 (mg)	3.2	3.8	5.4
Vitamin B2 (mg)	3.6	4	5.5
Vitamin B6 (mg)	4.2	5	6.3
Niacin (mg)	42	50	63
Pantothenic acid (mg)	21	25	17
Vitamin B12 (μg)	12.6	15	19
Vitamin C (mg)	254	300	320
Vitamin A (U)	7172	5000	7510
Vitamin D (U)	574	400	590
Vitamin E (U)	63	75	90
Vitamin K (μg)	102	250	111
Folate (μg)	844	400	634
Biotin (μg)	320	300	640
Choline (mg)	1120	500	1060
mOsm/kg	480	550	600
kJ/ml (kcal/ml)	4.6(1.1)	6.3(1.5)	6.3(1.5)

* Enrich contains 42 g soy polysaccharide as fibre source.
† Traumacal contains a high content of branched chain amino acids.

There are small groups of patients in whom discrete nutritional requirements cannot be easily met. Smith & Heymsfield (1983) have described a system of formula preparation from modular ingredients which results in a variety of diets to meet almost any need. They describe seven protein modules from different sources with different amino acid compositions, three lipid modules based on MCT or LCT oil, and seven carbohydrate modules of different carbohydrate source and osmolality. Examples of this approach are shown in Table 27.6.

As these authors point out, digestion and absorption of nutrients depends on many factors, including the amino acid composition, the carbohydrate source, fat source and pH of solution. Stability of the modular formulae is influenced by nutrient composition, moisture content, mixing procedures, and temperature. Longer stability is a feature of low fat content, presence of emulsifiers, use of whole or hydrolysed proteins and complex carbohydrates and blenderisation at room temperature. Powders store better than liquids.

DRUG: NUTRIENT INTERACTIONS

A topic often not considered by those who order enteral nutrition is that of drug:nutrient interactions. Many drugs interfere with absorption of one or more components of enteral feeding mixtures. Most of these are not of great importance in most patients, but because of potentially serious effects in the occasional patient, a check list has been provided in Table 27.7.

REGIMENS

Our practice is to commence with 30 ml of water or diluted feed per hour, and increase to a volume and strength, which will provide the daily fluid and energy requirements in 2 hourly boluses. Initially, the tube is aspirated prior to each feed to ensure that the previous one has been tolerated. Feeding is then continued as second hourly boluses, or changed to continuous gravity feeding via a fine tube. Intolerance may become evident by increasing residual volumes, nausea, vomiting, diarrhoea, tachycardia, abdominal discomfort or sweating.

The volume of residual contents which is acceptable varies from patient to patient. It has been our practice to accept a residual volume of 200 ml and continue feeding, but to have the patient reviewed if the residual is greater than this.

Hiebert et al (1981) in a comparison of continuous versus intermittent tube feedings, using Isocal®, found that continuous feeding produced less diarrhoea and a better nutritional response than intermittent feeding. Campbell et al (1983) on the other hand, reported lower resting oxygen consumption and better cumulative nitrogen balance with intermittent bolus, rather than continuous nasogastric feeding with Clinifeed®.

Table 27.6 Examples of modular formulae (per 2000 kcal). (Modified from Smith & Heymsfield, 1983)

Component	ml	kJ	Protein source (g)	Carbohydrate source (g)	Lipid source (g)	Maximum refrigeration storage (hour)	Comments
1. Vital (Ross)	1500	6280	Whey Meat Soy (63)	Corn Syrup Sucrose (283)	Safflower MCT (16)	<12	Protein and fat malabsorption
MCT Oil	64	2090			MCT (60)		
2. Osmolite (Ross)	1000	4435	Casein Soy (37)	Glucose Polymers (145)	MCT (50%) Corn Soy (39)		
Polycose (Ross)	300	2510		Glucose polymers (150)		<72	Renal failure
Microlipid (Organon)	76	1420			Safflower Oil (38)		
3. Casec (Mead Johnson)	45	700	Calcium Caseinate (40)				
Moducal (Mead Johnson)	346	5510		Maltodextrin (329)		<72	Hepatic encephalopathy
Microlipid (Organon)	115	2150			Safflower Oil (115)		

Table 27.7 Drug-nutrient interactions (Enteral nutrition)

Drugs	May cause decreased absorption or loss of:
Biguanides Chloramphenicol Chlorpromazine Kanamycin Neomycin Tetracycline	*Amino acids and protein*
Biguanides Irritant laxatives Neomycin	*Carbohydrate*
Colchicine Cholestyramine Neomycin Para-Amino Salicylic Acid	*Lipid*
	Minerals
Aluminium antacids	Phosphate
Aspirin Cholestyramine Non-steroidal anti-inflammatory drugs	Iron
Irritant laxatives	Calcium and potassium
	Vitamins
Anticonvulsants Cholestyramine	Folic acid
Cholestyramine Neomycin Potassium chloride	Cyanocobalamin
Cholestyramine Mineral oil Neomycin	A
Cholestyramine Irritant laxatives Mineral oils	D
Antibiotics (broad spectrum) Cholestyramine Mineral oils	K

COMPLICATIONS

Reported complications of nasogastic tube feeding include vomiting or regurgitation, and aspiration of gastric contents, trauma to the nose, rhinitis, sinusitis and oesophagitis. Metabolic complications have included uraemia, due to inadequate water and excess protein, hyperosmolar coma and electrolyte imbalance. Diarrhoea, the bugbear of the older feeds, is uncommon with the newer ones. It has been attributed to large volumes, cold fluid, high osmolality, infection, and lactose intolerance.

There has been an increasing number of reports recently regarding misplacement of fine bore nasogastric tubes, including insertion into the tracheobronchial tree, and into the pleural space. Theodore et al (1984) has recently listed complications of placement of nasoenteric tubes as including intracranial penetration of the cribiform plate, nasopharyngeal perforation, tracheobronchial intubation, pneumothorax, oesophageal perforation and pneumomediastinum. He has identified as risk factors, malnourishment, age, altered mental status, chronic illness, nasal trauma or surgery, and recommends seven procedures for safe tube placement:

— gauge the length of tube required, and check stylet position
— insert the tube gently, and let the patient swallow it
— suspect misplacement if there is resistance, or difficulty removing stylet
— aspirate fluid and check pH
— check for air movement in the tube
— use endoscopic guidance if tube passage is difficult
— confirm position radiologically.

Insufflation of air with auscultation over the stomach for bubbling is an inadequate test for proper position of the tube.

The apparent paucity of complications of enteral feeding in most hospitals is probably because they are not sought. A prospective study of 253 patients over a 12 month period in one hospital revealed an overall incidence of complications of 11.7%. The most frequent complications were diarrhoea, inadequate gastric emptying, tube obstruction and vomiting. Pulmonary aspiration occurred in 0.8% of patients.

A potential problem with continuous tube feeding is the inadvertent connection of the drip set to an intravenous cannula, which is avoidable if distinctive administration equipment is used.

VALUE OF TUBE FEEDING

There are many studies of the value of enteral feeding. Allardyce & Groves (1974) compared elemental diet enteral feeding with TPN in 20 patients with intraperitoneal abscesses or fistulas. They found that jejunal feeding was the most effective way of providing nutrition for an extended period.

In a study of 12 cachectic patients fed nasogastrically with Isocal® or Vivonex®, (Bethel et al, 1979) there was an increase in weight, serum albumin, urine creatinine and triceps skinfold thickness.

Heymsfield et al (1979) have reviewed both enteral nutrition as an alternative to parenteral nutrition with reference to selection of patients, route of nutrition, composition of solutions, use of tubes and monitoring. They pointed out that enteral nutrition maintains structural and functional integrity of the small intestine, that it provides a more complete diet, and that it is both cheaper and safer than TPN.

A recent study (Lim et al, 1981) in which gastrostomy feeding and TPN were used to prepare patients for operation for carcinoma of the oesophagus showed that TPN resulted in better nitrogen balance and weight gain, with a lower morbidity and mortality.

In a series of infants weighing less than 1500 g, fed either parenterally or transpylorically, it was concluded that TPN did not confer any appreciable benefit, and should be reserved for infants in whom enteral nutrition is impossible.

Deitel (1983) has made the following points regarding choice of mode of nutrition for management of patients with enterocutaneous gastrointestinal fistulae:

1. Full diet stimulates gastric pancreatobiliary and duodenal secretion, which digests and enlarges the fistula and maximally stimulates gut activity.
2. Elemental diets do not stimulate pancreatic and gastrointestinal secretions, but with high small bowel fistulae there is substantial volume and nutritional loss through the fistula. There is some increase in gut activity.
3. TPN maximally suppresses gastric, pancreatic and duodenal digestive enzyme secretions, and maximally reduces gut activity.
4. Elemental diets may be used effectively if delivered distal to proximal gut fistulae, or proximal to low fistulae.
5. TPN is the nutrition method of choice in most gastroduodenal and upper small bowel fistulae, fistulae associated with prolonged adynamic ileus, and those in which insertion of a jejunostomy tube is inadvisable.

It is fair to say that the availability of new tubes, new techniques and new formulations has made safe cheap enteral nutrition available to many patients previously thought manageable only with TPN. A good review is that of Rombeau & Barot (1981). It should be remembered that the ratio of cost of hospital prepared tube feeds: intact nutrient packaged feeds: elemental feeds: TPN, is of the order of 1:3:7:30, excluding staff preparation time.

HOME ENTERAL NUTRITION

Home enteral nutrition is simpler and easier to manage than home parenteral nutrition. It requires a patient, with family support, who is capable of learning and carrying out the nutritional plan. The patient needs to learn how to prepare and store feeds, how to administer them, and how to look after equipment. Help must be available if required, from a resource team.

Instruction and planning should be begun early, and tailored to the patient's ability to learn and perform. A simple instruction booklet providing information on preparation of feeds, storage, equipment use, complications, etc, is of great value. Apparently minor details should not be overlooked, including storage details and the need to bring feeds to room temperature before administration.

Patients develop preferences for many aspects of home enteral nutrition. Some prefer bolus administration, and others continuous infusion or intermittent gravity drip. Some become adept at intermittent tube insertion. Patients on home enteral nutrition via an ostomy, may benefit from advice from a stoma nurse regarding care of the tube entry site.

REFERENCES AND FURTHER READING

Allardyce D B, Groves A C A comparison of nutritional gains resulting from intravenous and enteral feeding. Surg Gynecol Obstet 1974; 139: 179–184

Andrassy R J, Mahour G H, Harrison M R, Muenchow S K, Mishalany H G, Woolley M M The role and safety of early postoperative feeding in the pediatric surgical patient. J Pediatr Surg 1979; 14: 381–385

Andresen A F R Immediate jejunal feeding after gastro-enterostomy. Ann Surg 1918; 67: 565–566

Bayer L M, Scholl D E, Ford E G Tube feeding at home. Am J Nurs 1983; 83: 1321–1325

Bethel R A, Jansen R D, Heymsfield S B, Ansley J D, Hersh T, Rudman D Nasogastric hyperalimentation through a polyethylene catheter: an alternative to central venous hyperalimentation. Am J Clin Nutr 1979; 32: 1112–1120

Campbell I T, Morton R P, Cole J A, Raine C H, Shapiro L M, Stell P M A comparison of the effects of intermittent and continuous nasogastric feeding on the oxygen consumption and nitrogen balance of patients after major head and neck surgery. Am J Clin Nutr 1983; 38: 870–878

Cataldi-Betcher E L, Seltzer M H, Slocum B A, Jones K W Complications occurring during enteral nutrition support: a prospective study. JPEN 1983; 7: 546–552

Chernoff R Enteral feedings. Am J Hosp Pharm 1980; 37: 65–74

Deitel M Elemental diet and enterocutaneous fistula. World J Surg 1983; 7: 451–454

Delany H M, Carnevale N J, Garvey J W Jejunostomy by a needle catheter technique. Surgery 1973; 73: 786–790

Dunn E L, Moore E E, Bohus R W Immediate postoperative feeding following massive abdominal trauma — the catheter jejunostomy. JPEN 1980; 4: 393–395

Enteral Nutrition Group of the Royal Adelaide Hospital. Fine bore enteral feeding: a simple alternative to intravenous feeding. Med J Aust 1980; 2: 363–368, 397

Fairfull-Smith R, Abunassar R, Freeman J B, Maroun J A Rational use of elemental and nonelemental diets in hospitalized patients. Ann Surg 1980; 192: 600–603

Fallis L S, Barron J Gastric and jejunal alimentation with fine polyethylene tubes. Arch Surg 1952; 65: 373–381

Gault M H, Dixon M E, Doyle M, Cohen W M Hypernatremia, azotemia, and dehydration due to high-protein tube feeding. Ann Int Med 1968; 68: 778–791

Glass E J, Hume R, Lang M A, Forfar J O Parenteral nutrition compared with transpyloric feeding. Arch Dis Child 1984; 59: 131–135

Heimburger D C, Weinsier R L Guidelines for evaluating and categorizing enteral feeding formulas according to therapeutic equivalence. JPEN 1985; 9: 61–67

Heymsfield S B, Bethel R A, Ansley J D, Nixon D W, Rudman D Enteral hyperalimentation: an alternative to central venous hyperalimentation. Ann Int Med 1979; 90: 63–71

Hiebert J M, Brown A, Anderson R G, Halfacre S, Rodeheaver G T, Edlich R F Comparison of continuous vs intermittent tube feedings in adult burn patients. JPEN 1981; 5: 73–75

Hoover H C Jnr, Ryan J A, Anderson E J, Fischer J E Nutritional benefits of immediate postoperative jejunal feeding of an elemental diet. Am J Surg 1980; 139: 153–159

Howman-Giles R H, Roy L P Extreme hypernatraemia in a child receiving gastrostomy feeding. Aust Paediatr J 1976; 12: 167–170

Hulten L, Andersson H, Bosaeus I, Fasth S, Hellberg R, Isaksson B et al Enteral alimentation in the early postoperative course. JPEN 1980; 4: 455–459

Kaminski M V, Freed B A Enteral hyperalimentation: prevention and treatment of complications. Nutr Supp Serv 1981; 1(4): 29–40

Lim S T K, Choa R G, Lam K H, Wong J, Ong G B Total parenteral nutrition versus gastrostomy in the preoperative preparation of patients with carcinoma of the oesophagus. Br J Surg 1981; 68: 69–72

Moss G Maintenance of gastrointestinal function after bowel surgery and immediate enteral full nutrition. II: Clinical experience, with objective demonstration of intestinal absorption and motility. JPEN 1981; 5: 215–220

Muggia-Sullam M, Bower R H, Murphy R F, Joffe S N, Fischer J E Postoperative enteral versus parenteral nutritional support in gastrointestinal surgery. A matched prospective study. Am J Surg 1985; 149: 106–112

Olivares L, Segovia A, Revuelta R Tube feeding and lethal aspiration in neurological patients: a review of 720 autopsy cases. Stroke 1974; 5: 654–657

Page C P, Carlton P K, Andrassy R J, Feldtman R W, Shield C F III Safe, cost-effective postoperative nutrition. Defined formula diet via needle-catheter jejunostomy. Am J Surg 1979; 138: 939–945

Pareira M D Therapeutic nutrition with tube feeding. Charles C Thomas, Springfield, Illinois, 1959

Randall H T Enteral nutrition: tube feeding in acute and chronic illness. Sixth Annual Jonathan E Rhoads Lecture. JPEN 1984; 8: 113–136

Rombeau J L, Barot L R Enteral nutritional therapy. Surg Clin N Am 1981; 61: 605–620

Russell R I Progress report — elemental diets. Gut 1975; 16: 68–79

Russell R I (ed) Elemental diets. CRC Press, Boca Raton, 1981

Smith J L, Heymsfield S B Enteral nutrition support: formula preparation from modular ingredients. JPEN 1983; 7: 280–288

Sriram K, Gray D S Home enteral hyperalimentation catheter: surgical technique and problem-solving. Nutr Supp Serv 1984; 4(3): 32–36

Theodore A C, Frank J A, Ende J, Snider G L, Beer D J Errant placement of nasoenteric tubes. Chest 1984; 86: 931–933

Welch R G Feeding jejunostomy. Aust N Z J Surg 1971; 41: 35–39

Worthen D B, Lorimer J R A key to the literature of total enteral nutrition. Drug Intell Clin Pharm 1984; 18: 794–803

28

State of the art

The material covered in this book has been aimed at providing up-to-date, practical and relevant information on parenteral and enteral nutrition, with the intent of contributing to better, safer and more widespread patient nutrition. For this to be achieved, the concept of a team approach to nutrition must be stressed. With enteral feeding, the nutritionist and dietitian may be heavily involved, as well as the nurse, pharmacist and physician. In parenteral nutrition, while the nutritionist and dietitian may be involved, the pharmacist often plays a key role, the nurse is vital, but the physician bears the responsibility for prescribing, and establishing a system of patient care.

Advances in both enteral and parenteral nutrition over the last 15 years, with increased knowledge, better formulations and improved equipment, have made it possible for many patients in both hospital and home settings, to be offered parenteral or enteral nutrition relatively easily. It should no longer be a one man or one woman entrepreneurial activity to provide this care, but a readily available extension of routine medical care. In difficult situations, where the patient has complex medical problems, referral to a major centre will remain appropriate.

Those interested in pursuing the subject further are advised to read the state of the art reviews listed below, which have appeared over the years. Advances in parenteral and enteral nutrition over the next few years, on an individual patient basis, will depend on the wide, careful application of existing knowledge and techniques rather than on newer solutions and technological advances.

REFERENCES AND FURTHER READING

Apelgren K N, Wilmore D W Nutritional care of the critically ill patient. Surg Clin N Am 1983; 63: 497–507
Brennan M F, Horowitz G Total parenteral nutrition in surgical patients. Adv Surg 1984; 17: 1–36
Chernoff R Enteral feedings. Am J Hosp 1980; 37: 65–74
Cuthbertson D P The metabolic response to injury and its nutritional implications:

retrospect and prospect. Second Annual Jonathan E. Rhoads Lecture. JPEN 1979; 3: 108–129

Dudrick S J Current status of total parenteral nutrition. The Arvid Wretlind lecture. Acta Chir Scand 1980; Suppl 498: 12–19

Easton L B, Halata M S, Dweck H S Parenteral nutrition in the newborn: a practical guide. Ped Clin N Am 1982; 29: 1171–1190

Heird W C, Winters R W Total parenteral nutrition. The state of the art. J Pediatr 1975; 86: 2–16

Hill G L, Church J Energy and protein requirements of general surgical patients requiring intravenous nutrition. Br J Surg 1984; 71: 1–9

Johnston I D A The role of parenteral nutrition in surgical care. Ann Roy Coll Surg Engl 1972; 50: 196–206

Kaminski M V Jnr Humanism in hyperalimentation. JPEN 1981; 5: 1–6

Moore F D Energy and the maintenance of the body cell mass. Third Annual Jonathan E Rhoads Lecture. JPEN 1980; 4: 228–260

Ota D M, Imbembo A L, Zuidema G D Total parenteral nutrition. Surgery 1978; 83: 503–520

Randall H T Enteral nutrition: tube feeding in acute and chronic illness. Sixth Annual Jonathan E Rhoads Lecture. JPEN 1984; 8: 113–136

Rombeau J L, Barot L R Enteral nutritional therapy. Surg Clin N Am 1981; 61: 605–620

Wretlind A Parenteral nutrition. Nutr Rev 1981; 39: 257–265

Appendix 1

Central venous catheters

The procedure described in Chapter 4 (Venous access) is based on the use of the Arrow subclavian catheter, which is one of many central venous catheter sets available. Choice of unit is influenced by the following features:

— ease of insertion and experience of operator
— flexibility, stiffness, and need for stylet
— catheter length, internal and external diameters, and tip characteristics
— catheter material (Table A1.1), surface smoothness, method of manufacture, chemical inertness and thrombogenicity
— hub/catheter junction stability
— wings or groove for suture safety
— needle length, bevel and removability
— sterility
— radiopacity
— cost.

There are arguments which may be advanced for the relative importance of each of these points. Complications of central venous catheters are discussed in Chapter 4. The following list of catheters is only a partial one, and the only general comment which can be made is that use of a fine bore needle-guidewire-catheter is a far superior technique when compared with the use of a catheter through wide bore needle, with its attendant hazards. Polyvinyl chloride catheters have been superceded by newer materials. Of these, polyurethane seems to be superior to other materials at present.

Table A1.1 Catheter material

Polyvinyl chloride (PVC)
Polytetrafluoroethylene (Teflon)
Polyethylene
Polyurethane
Silicone rubber (Silastic)

Abbott Laboratories, North Chicago, Illinois 60064, USA	Drum cartridge catheter
Arrow International Inc, Reading, Pennsylvania 19610, USA	Central vein catheterization set
C R Bard Inc, Murray Hill, New Jersey 07974, USA	Bard advanset
C R Bard International Ltd, Sunderland, UK	Bard-I-Cath
B Braun, Melsungen AG, Germany	Cavafix MT
Burron Medical Inc, 824 Twelfth Avenue, Bethlehem, Pennsylvania 18018, USA	Accuguide
CardioSearch PO Box 24126, Tampa, Florida 33623, USA	Erythrocath
W A Cook Australia Pty. Ltd, 22A Stirling Crescent, Surrey Hills, Australia 3127	Subclavian catheter
Cormed Inc, 591 Mahan Street, Medina, New York 14103, USA	Corcath
Cormed Inc, 591 Mahan Street, Medina, New York 14103, USA	Mediport
The Deseret Company, Sandy, Utah 84070, USA	EZ Cath
The Deseret Company, Sandy, Utah 84070, USA	Intracath
The Deseret Company, Sandy, Utah 84070, USA	Subclavian jugular catheter set

Evermed, PO Box A, Kirkland, Washington 96033, USA	Broviac
Evermed, PO Box A, Kirkland, Washington 96033, USA	Hickman
Extracorporeal Medical Specialties Inc, King of Prussia, Pennsylvania 19406, USA	Parenteral alimentation catheter
Health Care Group Laboratories Inc, 1117 S Milwaukee Avenue, Suite 1, Forum 11, Libertyville, Illinois 60048, USA	Hirsch
Quinton Instrument Co, 2121 Terry Avenue, Seattle, Washington 98121, USA	RAAF Cath
Sherwood Medical Industries, St. Louis, Missouri 63103, USA	Intramedicut (Argyle)
Sorenson Research Company, Salt Lake City, Utah, USA	Intrafusor
Travenol Laboratories Inc, Vicra Division, Dallas, Texas 75220, USA	Centrasil
Universal Medical Instrument Cor, Box 100, Ballston 5PA, New York 12020, USA	CVP Monitoring set
Vygon Pharmaceutical Laboratories, Ecouen, France	Intravenous catheter
HG Wallace Ltd., Colchester, Essex, UK	Wallace central venous catheter

REFERENCES AND FURTHER READING

American Society for Parenteral and Enteral Nutrition. Product Resource Manual. 2nd ed revised American Society for Parenteral and Enteral Nutrition, Washington DC, 1982

Burri C, Ahnefeld F W The caval catheter. Springer Verlag, Berlin, 1978; 32–38

Hecker J F, Fisk G C, Farrell P C Measurement of thrombus formation on intravascular catheters. Anaesth Intens Care 1976; 4: 225–231

Lindner L E, Curelaru I, Gustavvsun B, Hansson H A, Stenquist O, Wojciechowski J Material thrombogenicity in central venous catheterization: a comparison between soft, antebrachial catheters of silicone elastomer and polyurethane. JPEN 1984; 8: 399–406

Prian G W, Way C W Van III The long arm silastic catheter: a critical look at complications. JPEN 1978; 2: 124–128

Rosen M, Latto I P, Ng W S Handbook of percutaneous central venous catheterisation. W B Saunders, London, 1981; 7–18

Appendix 2

Enteral feeding equipment

The tube we currently use is one of many gastrointestinal feeding tubes available. Choice of tube is influenced by the following:

— ease of insertion and experience of operator
— flexibility, stiffness, and need for stylet
— tube length, internal and external diameters, and tip characteristics
— tube material, surface smoothness, method of manufacture, chemical inertness
— radiopacity
— cost
— need to aspirate gastric contents
— hub incompatibility with intravenous infusion sets.

In a similar way, choice of an enteral feed delivery system is influenced by the following:

— container should be of adequate size, non-leak, easy to fill, and with reliable hanger. It should be distinguishable from IV containers
— measuring chamber should be of adequate size with readable markings
— tubing should be of adequate length and have an end connection which is incompatible with IV cannulae. The drip controller should be reliable
— the set should accommodate a variety of formulae.

There are arguments which may be advanced for each of these points. The following list is only a partial one, and includes tubes, administration sets and reservoir bags:

AHS/Australia Pty. Ltd,   AHS Enteral feeding bags, sets,
25–27 Paul Street,   tubes
North Ryde, NSW 2113, Australia

American McGaw,   EFS Enteral feeding system
PO Box 11887,
Santa Ana,
California 92711, USA

J

Biosearch Medical Products Inc,
  PO Box 1700,
  Somerville,
  New Jersey 08876, USA

Biosearch
  Enteral feeding bag
  Tube feeding/jejunostomy kit
Top-fill enteral feeding bag
Dobbhoff enteral feeding bag
Dobbhoff enteral feeding tube
K-tube enterostomy tube
Entriflex enteral feeding tube
Entri-pak delivery system

Chesebrough-Pond's Inc,
  33 Benedict Place,
  Greenwich,
  Connecticut 06836, USA

Kangaroo bag pump set

Corpak Company,
  140 W Hintz Road,
  Wheeling,
  Illinois 60090, USA

Polyurethane feeding tube
Feeding bag and set

Gil-Med Industries Inc,
  PO Box 748,
  Skokie,
  Illinois 60076, USA

ETO Enteral nutrition system

The Health Care Group
Laboratories Inc,
  1117 S Milwaukee Avenue,
  Suite 1, Forum 11,
  Libertyville,
  Illinois 60048, USA

Vitafeed gavage feeding container

Ethox Corporation,
  251 Seneca Street,
  Buffalo,
  New York 14204, USA

Rella-flo enteral feeding system

IVAC Corporation,
  10300 Campus Point Drive,
  San Diego,
  California 92121, USA

Keofeed enteral feeding bag
Keofeed enteral feeding tube
Rombeau gastrostomy-jejunal tube
Surgifeed needle catheter
jejunostomy kit

Norwich Eaton Pharmaceuticals
Inc,
  17 Eaton Avenue,
  Norwich,
  New York 13815, USA.

Vivonex jejunostomy kit
Vivonex Moss tube
Vivonex tungsten tip tube

J Pfrimmer & Co,
  Erlangen, West Germany

Enteral feeding tube
Nutriset bag

Quest Medical Inc,
  3312 Wiley Post Road,
  Carroliton,
  Texas 75006, USA

Duo-tube nasogastric catheter

Ross Laboratories,
  625 Cleveland Avenue,
  Columbus,
  Ohio 43216, USA

Flexitainer feeding container
Flexiflo gavage set
Flexiflo enteral feeding tube

Roussel Laboratories Ltd,
  Wembley Park,
  UK

Clinifeeding system 1 nasogastric
tube, bag and administration set

Superior Plastic Products Corp,
  Cumberland,
  Rhode Island 02804, USA

Superior enteral feeding tube

Travenol Laboratories Inc,
  Deerfield,
  Illinois 60075, USA

Travasorb enteral feeding kits

Tuta Laboratories,
  Lane Cove,
  New South Wales 2066, Australia

Tuta enteral feeding bag and set

Vygon Pharmaceutical Laboratories,
  Ecouen, France

Vygon nasogastric tube

REFERENCES AND FURTHER READING

Anon. Nutritional Support Services Companies. Nutr Supp Serv 1984; 4 (5): 24–26
Anon. Nutritional Support Services Brand Name Index. Nutr Supp Serv 1984; 4 (5): 10–24
Anon. Nutritional Support Services Buyers Guide — company section. Nutr Supp Serv 1984;
  4(11): 6–24
Anon. Nutritional Support Services Buyers Guide — product section. Nutr Supp Serv 1984;
  4(11): 25–29

Appendix 3

Pumps

There are a number of risk factors associated with the use of gravity-clamp controlled systems for the infusion of parenteral nutrition solutions. These include physicochemical factors such as the volume of solution in the container, viscosity of the solution and drop size, effect of a final filter on flow rate, distortion of the plastic tubing by the clamp resulting in 'cold flow' and slipping of the clamp. In addition, patient factors such as variations in blood pressure, position and movements, and clot formation may influence the flow rate. Wide variations have been reported in blood insulin and glucose concentrations when hypertonic solutions of glucose were infused by gravity. During constant infusion using a peristaltic pump, the blood insulin and glucose concentrations remained relatively constant and the risk of inducing either hyperglycaemia or hypoglycaemia was minimised.

In recent years the infusion control device market has grown rapidly. There is a multitude of electronic devices available on the market to facilitate the infusion of parenteral solutions, and now a number of pumps have been designed specifically for the infusion of enteral feeds. These infusion devices may be classified according to their pumping mechanism.

CONTROLLER

The controller works on the concept of gravity and exerts no pressure on the infused fluid. Thus, some of the problems associated with the gravity-clamp controlled system are inherent in the controller. The controller either counts drops electronically or extrudes volumes of fluid mechanically and electronically at a rate which may range from 1–99 drops per minute. It has no moving parts, is less complex than the pump and presents fewer maintenance problems. Accuracy of the volume infused may vary from as much as −10% to +10%, depending on the viscosity of the fluid. Most controllers can be operated by battery in the event of power failure and feature a small range of audiovisual alarms. Some require a specific administration set, others can be operated using a standard intravenous administration set.

244

Examples of *controllers* include:

FLO-GARD 3000 Controller (accepts standard IV sets)
  Travenol Laboratories,
  Deerfield, Illinois 60015, USA
IMED 350 and IMED 380 Piggyback Controllers (require Accudot sets)
  IMED Corporation,
  San Diego, California 92131, USA
Infutrol 2000 Volumetric Controller
  ValleyLab Incorporated,
  Boulder, Colorado 80301, USA
IVAC 230 and IVAC 260 Volumetric Controllers (accept standard IV sets)
  IVAC Corporation,
  San Diego, California 92121, USA
Rateminder II Volumetric Controller (requires Rateminder set)
  Kendall-Anatross Corporation,
  San Jose, California 95131, USA

SYRINGE PUMP

The syringe pump was one of the earliest infusion pumps to be marketed. A synchronous motor drives the syringe plunger, discharging the fluid at a pre-set rate which may range from 0.01 to 299 ml/hour, depending on the model and syringe size. The accuracy with which the fluid is delivered is in the range of -2% to $+2\%$, and is influenced by the type and size of syringe used. Syringe pumps are used by some centres for the delivery of nutrition solutions to neonates.

Examples of *syringe pumps* include:

Autosyringe AS5B (operates on AC battery)
  Auto-Syringe Inc,
  Hooksett, New Hampshire 03104, USA
Harvard Syringe Infusion 2620 and Harvard Syringe Infusion 2681
  Harvard Apparatus Co. Inc,
  Millis, Massachusetts 02054, USA
Injectomat 50 and Injectomat 30
  Fresenius Medizintèchnik KG,
  Bad Homburg, v.d.H.1, West Germany
Perfusor ED and Perfusor VI
  B Braun,
  Melsungen A G, West Germany
Sage Infusion 242
  Sage Instruments,
  Division of Orion Research,
  Cambridge, Massachusetts 02139, USA

PERISTALTIC PUMP

The peristaltic pump may be either of the linear or rotary type. The action of the pump consists of the movement of the pumping chamber wall as a result of an externally applied force. The application and relaxation of pressure on the tubing propels the fluid towards the patient. The linear peristaltic pump flow rate is regulated by drop counting and thus accuracy is subject to the viscosity of the fluid. The flow rate range is from 1 to 999 ml/hour. A number of linear peristaltic pumps may be operated using a standard intravenous administration set. These pumps can be operated on AC current and battery, and feature a range of audiovisual alarms.

Examples of *linear peristaltic pumps* include:

American McGaw AccuPro Pump
  American McGaw,
  Division of American Hospital Supply Corporation,
  Santa Ana, California 92711, USA
IVAC 560 Infusion Pump
  IVAC Corporation,
  San Diego, California 92121, USA

The rotary peristaltic pumps generally require special sets incorporating a segment of silicone tubing. These silicone chambers are manufactured to very exact specifications with a precise internal diameter and deliver a predictable volume of fluid. Variations in drop size due to the vicosity of the fluid do not affect the accuracy of delivery, which is in the range of -5% to $+5\%$. The volume of fluid delivered ranges from 1 to 999 ml/hour. Most rotary peristaltic pumps operate on AC current and battery, and feature a range of audiovisual alarms.

Examples of *volumetric rotary peristaltic pumps* include:

AS70 Volumetric Pump (requires specific set)
  Air-Shields,
  Hatboro, Pennsylvania 19040, USA
Cormed Ambulatory Infusion Pump ML 6–8 (battery operation only) (requires Cormed set)
  Cormed Inc,
  Medina, New York 14103, USA
Critikon Simplicity 2100A Pump (requires Critikon set)
  Critikon Incorporated,
  Tampa, Florida 33607, USA
Extracorporeal 2100 Infusion Pump (requires Extracorporeal pump set)
  Extracorporeal Medical Specialties Inc,
  King of Prussia, Pennsylvania 19406, USA
FLO-GARD 6100 (accepts Travenol solution administration and standard sets)
  Travenol Laboratories,

Deerfield, Illinois 60015, USA

Holter 900 Series and 920 Series Infusion (require Extracorporeal-Holter sets)
  Extracorporeal Medical Specialties Inc,
  King of Prussia, Pennsylvania 19406, USA

Infusomat II (requires Infusomat set)
  B Braun,
  Melsungen A G, West Germany

Secura IV Volumetric Infusion Pump
  Diatek Incorporated,
  San Diego, California 92121, USA

Examples of *enteral rotary peristaltic pumps* include:

Biosearch Enteral Feeding Pump (No. 14–7005)(requires Biosearch pump set)
  Biosearch Medical Products Incorporated,
  Somerville, New Jersey 08876, USA

Corpak VTR 300 Enteral Pump (requires Corpak set)
  Corpak Company,
  Wheeling, Illinois 60090, USA

Ethox/Barron 2000 Enteral Feeding and Ethox Relia-Flo 4000 Pumps (require Ethox pump sets)
  Ethox Corporation,
  Buffalo, New York 14210, USA

Flexiflo Enteral Nutrition Pumps as Flexiflo II, Flexiflo III (require Flexiflo enteral pump set)
  Ross Laboratories,
  Columbus, Ohio 43216, USA

Frenta System for continuous tube feeding (requires Fresenius transfer set)
  Fresenius,
  Bad Homburg, v.d. H.1, West Germany

Flo-Gard 2000 Pump
  Travenol Laboratories,
  Deerfield, Illinois 60015, USA

IMED 430 Enteral Pump
  IMED Corporation,
  San Diego, California 92131, USA

IVAC Keofeed Enteric Feeding Pump 3000
  IVAC Corporation,
  San Diego, California 92121, USA

Kangaroo 220 Feeding Pump and Kangaroo 330 Feeding Pump (require Kangaroo or Universal feeding pump sets)
  Chesebrough-Pond's Inc, Hospital Products Div.
  Greenwich, Connecticut 06830, USA

Vygon Enteral Feeding Pump (requires Vygon Enteral Administration set)

Vygon Pharmaceutical Laboratories,
Ecouen, France
(Exco-Vygon, Wall, New Jersey 07719, USA)

PISTON VOLUMETRIC PUMP

This type of volumetric pump has a metered chamber, or cassette, which is operated by the pump as an integral part of the fluid pathway, to measure and pump the fluid towards the patient. In contrast to the peristaltic volumetric pumps, fluid flow is not continuous as the piston (cassette) mechanism has two cycles — a filling cycle and a delivery cycle. These devices operate with a high degree of accuracy, generally in the range of −2% to +2%, and their mechanism of operation is independent of drop size and fluid viscosity. Fluid is delivered within a range of 1–999 ml/hour. These pumps operate on both AC current and battery, and include a range of audiovisual features, and require special administration/pump sets.

Examples of *piston volumetric pumps* include:

IMED Volumetric Infusion Pumps, Models 922, 927, 960 (require Accuset cassette set; also accept Travenol volumetric pump cassette set)
   IMED Corporation,
   San Diego, California 92131, USA
IMED 965 Micro Volumetric Pump (requires IMED microset)
   IMED Corporation,
   San Diego, California 92131, USA
IVAC 630 Volumetric Infusion and IVAC 1500 Infu-Chek Pumps (require volumetric cassette sets)
   IVAC Corporation,
   San Diego, California 92121, USA

CHAMBER VOLUMETRIC PUMP

The chamber volumetric pump operates on Archimedes' fluid principle — as fluid enters the filled chamber, fluid is displaced out the other side, thus providing continuous delivery of fluid to the patient. The mechanism of operation is independent of drop size and fluid viscosity. The range of flow rate is from 1 to 999 ml/hour. These pumps offer similar features to the piston volumetric pumps.

Examples of *chamber volumetric pumps* include:

Dependaflo Volumetric Infusion Pump (requires Dependaflo set)
   Cutter Medical Laboratories Inc.
   Berkeley, California 94710, USA.
FLO-GARD 8000 Volumetric Infusion Pump (requires Travenol chamber cassette set)

Travenol Laboratories,
Deerfield, Illinois 60015, USA
LifeCare Model 3 Pump (requires LifeCare pump set)
Abbott Laboratories,
North Chicago, Illinois 60064, USA
ValleyLab Infutrol Pumps, Models 7000, 6000b, 6006b (require ValleyLab
pump sets)
ValleyLab Incorporated,
Boulder, Colorado 80301, USA

Example of *dual chamber volumetric pump*:

AVI Guardian 100 and Micro 110 (require specific AVI pump set)
AVI Incorporated,
St. Paul, Minnesota 55112, USA

AVI Incorporated has introduced the dual chamber rolling diaphragm, which is a dual chamber mechanism intended to provide a constant flow by filling one chamber while the other one is pumping fluid to the patient. Both pumps use the same set.

The pumps most suited to the infusion of parenteral nutrition solutions are the peristaltic (volumetric) pumps, the piston volumetric pumps and the chamber volumetric pumps. In selecting one of these pumps, consideration should be given to a number of criteria, including ease of setting the flow rate, flow rate range per hour, flow rate accuracy, ability to operate on both AC current and battery, and portability. The pump should feature a range of audiovisual alarms to indicate empty container or air embolism, infiltration, occlusion, rate variation, volume delivery variation, infusion complete, low battery and electrical malfunction. The unit should meet electrical safety standards for current leakage, grounding resistance and use of a safety plug. The pump should be reasonably priced, reliable and require minimum maintenance or repairs. If special sets are required, these should be reasonably priced and readily available.

REFERENCES AND FURTHER READING

Anon. Evaluation. Infusion pumps. Health Devices 1983; 13: 31–62
Anon. Evaluation. Enteral feeding pumps. Health Devices 1984; 14: 9–30
Finkelstein J W, Boley S J, Kream J, Cohen M I Profile of 24-hour plasma glucose and insulin concentrations. Their variation with two methods of total parenteral nutrition administration. Arch Surg 1979; 114: 1433–1437
Pipp T L Intravenous infusion pumps justification and selection and utilization. Infusion 1978; 2: 45–58
Runciman W B, Ilsley A H, Baker D, Shepherd T M An evaluation of intravenous infusion devices. Anaesth Intens Care (in press) 1986

Appendix 4

Pharmaceutical data

This Appendix contains relevant pharmaceutical data in table form:

Table A4.1 Trace elements (Micrograms, micromoles per micrograms of salts)

Element — μg per 1 μmol	Salts of element — molecular weight	% Element content	μg Salt containing 1 μg element	μg Salt containing 1 μmol element
Chromium 51.996	Chromic chloride, hexahydrate $CrCl_3.6H_2O$ 266.48	19.51	5.125	266.48
Copper 63.54	Cupric chloride, dihydrate $CuCl_2.2H_2O$ 170.48	37.27	2.68	170.48
	Cupric sulphate, pentahydrate $CuSO_4.5H_2O$ 249.69	25.45	3.93	249.69
Fluorine 18.998	Sodium fluoride NaF 42.00	45.23	2.21	42.0
Iodine 126.904	Sodium iodide NaI 149.92	84.65	1.18	149.92
	Potassium iodide KI 166.02	76.44	1.31	166.02
Iron 55.847	Ferric citrate $FeC_6H_5O_7. \times H_2O$ 244.95 (anhydrous)	22.80 (anhydrous)	4.39 (anhydrous)	244.95 (anhydrous)
Manganese 54.94	Manganese chloride $MnCl_2.4H_2O$ 197.91	27.76	3.60	197.91

Element — µg per 1 µmol	Salts of element — molecular weight	% Element content	µg Salt containing 1 µg element	µg Salt containing 1 µmol element
	Manganese sulphate MnSO$_4$.H$_2$0 169.01	32.51	3.08	169.01
Molybdenum 95.94	Ammonium molybdate H$_{24}$Mo$_7$N$_6$O$_{24}$ 1163.89	57.70	1.73	166.27
Selenium 78.96	Selenious acid H$_2$O$_3$Se 128.98	82.30	1.63	95.94
	Selenomethionine C$_5$H$_{11}$NO$_2$Se 196.11	40.26	2.48	196.13
	Sodium selenite Na$_2$O$_3$Se 172.95	45.65	2.19	172.97
Zinc 65.37	Zinc chloride ZnCl$_2$ 136.29	47.96	2.08	136.29
	Zinc sulphate, heptahydrate ZnSO$_4$.7H$_2$O 287.55	22.73	4.40	287.55

Table A4.2   Amino acids — molecular weights, nitrogen content

Amino acid	Formula	Molecular weight	% Nitrogen content	g AA containing 1 g N
Isoleucine	C$_6$H$_{13}$NO$_2$	131.17	10.68	9.36
Leucine	C$_6$H$_{13}$NO$_2$	131.17	10.68	9.36
Lysine	C$_6$H$_{14}$N$_2$O$_2$	146.19	19.16	5.22
Methionine	C$_5$H$_{11}$NO$_2$S	149.21	9.39	10.65
Phenylalanine	C$_9$H$_{11}$NO$_2$	165.19	8.48	11.79
Threonine	C$_4$H$_9$NO$_3$	119.12	11.76	8.50
Tryptophan	C$_{11}$H$_{12}$N$_2$O$_2$	204.22	13.72	7.29
Valine	C$_5$H$_{11}$NO$_2$	117.15	11.96	8.36
Alanine	C$_3$H$_7$NO$_2$	89.09	15.72	6.36
Arginine	C$_6$H$_{14}$N$_4$O$_2$	174.20	32.16	3.11
Aspartic acid	C$_4$H$_7$NO$_4$	133.10	10.52	9.50
Cysteine	C$_3$H$_7$NO$_2$S	121.16	11.56	8.65
Glutamic acid	C$_5$H$_9$NO$_4$	147.13	9.52	10.50
Glycine	C$_2$H$_5$NO$_2$	75.07	18.66	5.36
Histidine	C$_6$H$_9$N$_3$O$_2$	155.16	27.08	3.69
Ornithine	C$_5$H$_{12}$N$_2$O$_2$	132.16	21.20	4.72
Proline	C$_5$H$_9$NO$_2$	115.13	12.17	8.22
Serine	C$_3$H$_7$NO$_3$	105.09	13.33	7.50
Taurine	C$_2$H$_7$NO$_3$S	125.14	11.19	8.94
Tyrosine	C$_9$H$_{11}$NO$_3$	181.19	7.73	12.93
n-Acetyl-L-Cysteine	C$_5$H$_9$NO$_3$S	163.20	8.58	11.66
n-Acetyl-L-Tyrosine	C$_{11}$H$_{13}$NO$_4$	223.24	6.27	15.95

Table A4.3   Electrolytes (Millimoles, milliequivalents per milligrams of commonly used salts)

Ion	mg per 1 mmol	Commonly used salts	Molecular weight of salts	mg salt containing 1 mmol Ion	mg salt containing 1 mEq Ion
Sodium Na^+	22.99	Sodium chloride NaCl	58.45	58.45	58.45
		Sodium acetate anhydrous CH_3COONa	82.04	82.04	82.04
		Sodium phosphate dibasic $Na_2HPO_4.12H_2O$	358.17	179.09	179.09
		Sodium acid phosphate $NaH_2PO_4.2H_2O$	156.03	156.03	156.03
Potassium K^+	39.102	Potassium chloride KCl	74.55	74.55	74.55
		Potassium acetate CH_3COOK	98.14	98.14	98.14
		Potassium phosphate dibasic K_2HPO_4	174.18	87.09	87.09
		Potassium acid phosphate KH_2PO_4	136.09	136.09	136.09
Magnesium Mg^{++}	24.312	Magnesium chloride $MgCl_2.6H_2O$	203.33	203.33	101.67
		Magnesium sulphate $MgSO_4.7H_2O$	246.49	246.49	123.25
Calcium Ca^{++}	40.08	Calcium chloride dihydrate $CaCl_2.2H_2O$	147.02	147.02	73.51
		Calcium gluconate $C_{12}H_{22}CaO_{14}.H_2O$	448.40	448.40	224.20
Chloride Cl^-	35.45	Sodium chloride NaCl	58.45	58.45	58.45
		Potassium chloride KCl	74.55	74.55	74.55
		Magnesium chloride $MgCl_2.6H_2O$	203.33	101.67	101.67
		Calcium chloride dihydrate $CaCl_2.2H_2O$	147.02	73.51	73.51
Acetate CH_3COO^-	59.05	Sodium acetate CH_3COONa	82.04	82.04	82.04
		Potassium acetate CH_3COOK	98.14	98.14	98.14
Phosphate PO_4^{3-}	94.97	Sodium phosphate dibasic $Na_2HPO_4.12H_2O$	358.17	358.17	★
		Sodium acid phosphate $NaH_2PO_4.2H_2O$	156.03	156.03	★
(Phosphorus P 30.97)		Potassium phosphate dibasic K_2HPO_4	174.18	174.18	★
		Potassium acid phosphate KH_2PO_4	136.09	136.09	★

★ Determination of phosphate species:
Phosphate, unlike other electrolytes, exists in aqueous solution as the following species: H_3PO_4, $H_2PO_4^-$, $HPO_4^=$, PO_4^{3-}. Within the range pH 4 through 10, the principal phosphate species are $H_2PO_4^-$ and $HPO_4^=$, with H_3PO_4 and PO_4^{3-} being present in negligible amounts. At pH 7.4, the ratio of $HPO_4^=$:$H_2PO_4^-$ is approximate 4:1 and the average valence is 1.8. At pH 5.4, the ratio of $HPO_4^=$:$H_2PO_4^-$ is approximately 4:100 and the average valence is 1.04.

Because the average valence of phosphate changes as the pH changes, it is necessary to define the pH before the valence can be determined in order to calculate and express phosphate in milliequivalents. Thus, to avoid any confusion or ambiguity, the desired phosphate or phosphorus content should be expressed in millimoles.

Table A4.4   Some conversion factors used in text

Component	'Old' unit	'New' (SI) unit
Energy		
quantity of heat	1 kcal	4.184 kJ
dextrose anhydrous, 1 g	3.76 kcal	15.73 kJ
alcohol, 1g	7 kcal	29.29 kJ
fat, 1 g	9 kcal	37.66 kJ
glycerol, 1 g	4.32 kcal	18.0 kJ
Vitamins		
A, all-trans vitamin A acetate	1 IU	0.344 μg
A, all-trans retinol	1 IU	0.3 μg
D, cholecalciferol or ergocalciferol	1 IU	0.025 μg
E, dl-alpha-tocopheryl acetate	1 IU	1 mg

Table A4.5   Calculation of water of metabolism. (Adapted from Consolazio et al, 1963)

Nutrients (1 g)	Water of metabolism	Nutrients (representative 24 h input)	Water of metabolism
Protein	0.41 ml	50 g Amino Acid	26
Amino Acid	0.52 ml★	200 g Carbohydrate	120
Carbohydrate	0.60 ml	100 g Fat	107
Fat	1.07 ml		
		Water of metabolism (ml)	253

★ Factor derived from Shenkin & Wretlind (1978).

REFERENCES AND FURTHER READING

Consolazio C F, Johnson R E, Pecora L J Physiological measurements of metabolic functions in man. McGraw-Hill Book Company, New York 1963; 314
Shenkin A, Wretlind A Parenteral nutrition. Wld Rev Nutr Diet 1978; 28: 1–111

Appendix 5

A regimen, *or* putting it all together — practically

In this section an attempt will be made to paint a picture around a patient needing parenteral nutrition, incorporating the principles outlined in the book.

The patient is a 54 year old man admitted 7 days previously with bowel obstruction due to carcinoma of the descending colon. At laparotomy, left hemicolectomy and primary anastomosis were performed. Five days later he was taken back to the operating theatre because of a burst anastomosis. Colostomy was performed and a paralytic ileus developed. The patient was previously in good health and on no medications. The participants in the scenario are Mr Jones (the patient), Nurse Smith (the Ward Nurse), Dr Brown (the patient's Surgeon), Dr Phillips (from the TPN Team), and Miss Odgers (the Pharmacist). Dr. Phillips arrives in the ward to see the patient with a view to commencing TPN at the request of the Surgeon.

'Good morning Nurse, Dr Brown has asked me to see Mr Jones with a view to commencing him on TPN'. 'Good morning Doctor. Yes, I was expecting you, and Dr Brown has spoken to Mr Jones about the TPN. Here is his medical record. When you're ready I'll take you to the patient'.

The medical record indicated that Mr Jones had been kept in good fluid, electrolyte and acid-base balance, had a normal haemoglobin and white cell count, and no coagulation defect. He was receiving opioids and antibiotics, but was not on corticosteroids, insulin or anticoagulants. His pulse, blood pressure, respiratory rate and temperature were within normal limits, and he had not had glycosuria. His weight was 50 kg, having been 55 kg on admission. Intravenous fluids since operation had included plasma, blood, isotonic glucose and electrolyte solutions. The previous day's laboratory results are shown in Table A5.1.

'Thank you Nurse. I'll see Mr Jones now'. 'Yes, Doctor. Come this way'. 'Mr Jones, Dr Phillips is here'. 'Hello, Mr Jones. Dr Brown has asked me to see you about starting some intravenous feeding'. 'Yes, Doctor, Dr Brown explained everything to me. When will you start?' 'I'll just get some details from you and examine you while Nurse is getting the equipment ready'.

Table A5.1 Laboratory results

JONES, John UR No. 999999	7/2/1986	Normal values mmol/l
Na	140	132–144
K	4	3.1–4.8
Cl	101	93–108
HCO_3	27	21–32
Urea	6	3–8
Creatinine	0.08	0.06–0.12
Glucose	4	3–5.5
Total protein	75	60–85
Albumin	38	30–50
Bilirubin	15	<20
Prothrombin ratio	1.0	1.0
Ca	2.1	2.05–2.55
PO_4	1.0	0.6–1.25
Mg	1.0	0.75–1
Hb	13.6	
WCC	7000	
Platelets	200 000	

A full history and physical examination are essential prior to commencing TPN to determine the presence of any heart, lung, liver or renal disease, and to assess nutritional and fluid status. In the case of this patient, the indication for TPN was clear, there were no contraindications, and no reason why an uncomplicated regimen should not be followed.

'As soon as Nurse is ready, Mr Jones, we'll move you into the Procedure Room, take off your jacket, and lie you flat on the bed, which we'll tip head-down to make it easier to insert the feeding tube. I will clean the skin of your chest with antiseptic, inject some local anaesthetic, then insert a plastic tube through a needle into a vein near your collar bone. The procedure won't take long, and will be only slightly uncomfortable. After it's finished you can sit up again, and the running of the drip won't worry you or immobilise you at all'. 'OK, Doc'. 'All ready, Doctor. I've opened a sterile tray and set up a drip set with glucose 10%'. 'Thank you, Nurse. We'll get on with insertion of the catheter, then'.

After insertion of the catheter a chest X-ray was ordered to confirm the presence of the tip of the catheter in the superior vena cava and exclude a pneumothorax. Glucose 10% was ordered at a rate of 2 litres in 24 hours, and the peripheral IV infusion was discontinued.

'Dr Brown's resident would like to discuss the TPN orders and monitoring routine with you, Dr Phillips'. 'Yes, Nurse. Ah, here he is now. Let's run through that together. First, the ordering. I'll order a mixture of 500 ml glucose 40% and 500 ml of 10% amino acid solution, with 40 mmol Na, 40 mmol K, 2 mmol Ca, 2.5 mmol Mg and 15 mmol PO_4 per litre of the mixture. 2 litres of the mixture will provide approximately his daily requirements'. 'What about chloride?' 'The pharmacist uses appropriate salts to produce a balance of chloride and acetate, to prevent development of hyper- or hypochloraemia and associated metabolic acid-base problems'. 'Vitamins and trace elements?' 'Yes, I add 1 ampoule of vitamin B with C per litre of solution, and 2 mg of zinc chloride. In addition, I give vitamin K_1 10 mg, vitamin B_{12} 100 mcg, and folic acid 15 mg intramuscularly once a week. If his TPN has to be continued for more than 2 or 3 weeks, I will change to MVI-12®, which contains fat soluble vitamins in addition to most of the water soluble vitamins, and a trace element mixture, which includes zinc, chromium, iodine, copper and manganese'. 'You mentioned monitoring'. 'Yes, the most important form of monitoring is, of course, clinical observation and careful fluid balance, supplemented by weighing, and by 4th hourly urinalysis to detect glycosuria, or ward glucose estimations. Routine investigations should include daily blood urea, creatinine, electrolytes and sugar, as well as twice weekly liver function tests, serum calcium, magnesium and phosphate, prothrombin, haemoglobin, white cell and platelet counts'.

Two days later a number of problems had developed. The dressing on the catheter entry site had lifted, the infusion had stopped, the patient had developed profuse colostomy fluid loss, become oliguric, and developed a fever.

'Mr Jones is not well today, Doctor Phillips'. 'The Resident is on his way, so we'll review the situation systematically. Are there any worries from the nursing point of view?' 'Mr Jones has a pulse of 110 per minute, BP 140/70 mmHg, respiratory rate 24 per minute, and a temperature of 39°C. He has an irritating cough'. 'I'll examine him then. Let's see. He is certainly febrile, tachypnoiec and has a tachycardia. He has signs of consolidation at his left base and looks somewhat dehydrated, but otherwise there is no change in findings from 2 days ago'. 'The Resident is here, Doctor'. 'Good, now, let's look at the laboratory data (Table A5.2). Low sodium and magnesium would fit with excess colostomy fluid loss. Low potassium also, although that is probably contributed to by inadequate potassium intake in a patient who was potassium deficient. Administration of hypertonic glucose often results in hypokalaemia as well. Hypophosphataemia is common also when TPN is commenced. The elevated urea, creatinine and haemoglobin confirm dehydration, and the increased white cell count suggests infection'. 'What's the best way to correct the fluid and electrolyte problems, Sir?' 'Well, clearly the patient needs more water, sodium, potassium, chloride, magnesium and phosphate. As well as the colostomy losses, he has increased insensible water loss because of his fever and tachypnoea. In view of the fact that his blood sugar is elevated, perhaps due to the infection, I don't think we should increase the volume of TPN.

Let's leave the infusion rate the same, but increase the sodium, potassium and magnesium concentrations by 50%, and the phosphate concentration to 20 mmol per litre and review the laboratory results tomorrow'. 'I'll correct the fluid deficit via a peripheral intravenous infusion of elec-

Table A5.2   Laboratory results

JONES, John UR No. 999999	7/2/86	9/2/86	Normal values mmol/l
Na	140	132	132–144
K	4	2.8	3.1–4.8
Cl	101	93	93–108
CO_2	27	22	21–32
Urea	6	12	3–8
Creatinine	0.08	0.14	0.06–0.12
Glucose	4	14	3–5.5
Total protein	75	70	60–85
Albumin	38	30	30–50
Bilirubin	15	15	<20
Prothrombin ratio	1.0	1.0	1.0
Ca	2.1	2.0	2.05–2.55
PO_4	1.0	0.5	0.6–1.25
Mg Hb	1.0	0.6	0.75–1
Hb	13.6	15	
WCC	7000	13 000	
Platelets	200 000	220 000	

trolyte replacement solution then?' 'Yes, that's reasonable at present. The colostomy fluid is likely to contain about 70 mmol per litre sodium and 15 mmol per litre potassium, but that can be checked in the laboratory. With normally functioning kidneys some extra sodium won't be a problem'. 'What about the pyrexia and raised white cell count?' 'There is reasonable evidence of a chest infection. Let's do a chest X-ray, obtain sputum for culture and commence an appropriate antibiotic. The physiotherapist should review his therapy with you. There's no indication that the central line is a problem'. 'Can I flush the catheter, Doctor?' 'Yes, Nurse. Provided an aseptic technique is used I think that is reasonable. The dressing needs replacing also, and would you make sure the night staff are aware of the importance of keeping the drip running?'

Two days later Dr Phillips, Dr Brown, Miss Odgers and the Ward Nurse met to review the patient.

'How do you feel the patient is progressing, Nurse?' 'His fever is down and his breathing more comfortable, but his colostomy loss remains about 2 litres a day. His urine output has improved'. 'How is he from the surgical point of view, John?' 'His ileus persists, but there is no evidence of further intraabdominal complications. I would like to continue the TPN for at least another 10 days'. 'I notice from the lab results (Table A5.3) that we have corrected the low sodium, potassium and magnesium, and his hydration is improved. However, he still requires increased phosphate and also more calcium. Is that a problem, Chris?' 'Based on some preliminary studies we have undertaken with this particular amino acid-glucose-electrolyte combination I could increase the concentrations of both electrolytes to, say, 22.5 mmol per litre of phosphate and 4 mmol per litre of calcium. But, it is important that no other drugs are added to

Table A5.3 Laboratory results

JONES, John UR No. 999999	7/2/86	9/2/86	11/2/86	Normal values mmol/l
Na	140	132	136	132–144
K	4	2.8	3.8	3.1–4.8
Cl	101	93	97	93–108
CO_2	27	22	25	21–32
Urea	6	12	8	3–8
Creatinine	0.08	0.14	0.12	0.06–0.12
Glucose	4	14	6	3–5.5
Total protein	75	70	65	60–85
Albumin	38	30	28	30–50
Bilirubin	15	15	17	<20
Prothrombin ratio	1.0	1.0	1.1	1.0
Ca	2.1	2.0	1.8	2.05–2.55
PO_4	1.0	0.5	0.6	0.6–1.25
Mg	1.0	0.6	0.8	0.75–1
Hb	13.6	15	14	
WCC	7000	13 000	11 000	
Platelets	200 000	220 000	210 000	

the TPN solution as only a slight increase in the solution pH may result in calcium phosphate precipitation'. 'Good, then I'll increase the phosphate to 22.5 mmol per litre and the calcium to 4 mmol per litre. I think we could stop the peripheral drip, which would please Mr Jones, and increase the TPN to 3 litres per day. He should tolerate an increased glucose load. We will need to increase the sodium content to cope with the colostomy loss, but decrease the potassium content per litre so the daily intake remains the same. I will summarise the changes in TPN orders in the notes' (Table A5.4). 'What about fat?' 'A good point. Let's see. He will be receiving 2256 kcal from glucose, plus 120 grams protein (20.25 g N) per day, with a calorie: nitrogen ratio of 110:1. 500 ml 20% lipid emulsion would provide a further 900 kcal per day, which would be quite reasonable, as he appears to be entering the recovery phase of his illness from the metabolic point of view. If the extra glucose results in glucose intolerance, we could reduce the glucose concentration'. 'Why not add insulin if he becomes glucose intolerant?' 'No, recent evidence indicates that there is no benefit to be gained from doing that unless, of course, the patient is diabetic'. 'But isn't administration of lipid a problem technically?' 'No, it is true the emulsion can crack if it is allowed to mix with other solutions under certain circumstances, but it can be run through the central venous catheter with the TPN mixture via a sidearm close to the patient, with no problems'. 'Well then, I'll explain the situation to Mr Jones, John, and provided we continue our surveillance we shouldn't run into any major problems between now and when he is to commence oral intake'.

A week later the patient was tolerating oral fluids, TPN had been reduced

Table A5.4 TPN orders

	7/2/86	9/2/86	11/2/86
Content per litre:			
Volume (ml)	1000	1000	1000
Glucose (g)	200	200	200
Protein (g)	40	40	40
Na (mmol)	40	60	85
K (mmol)	40	60	50
Ca (mmol)	2	2	4
Mg (mmol)	2.5	3.75	3.75
PO_4 (mmol)	15	20	22.5
Cl (mmol)	46	71.2	76.5
Acetate (mmol)	65	71.2	76.5
Gluconate (mmol)	4	4	8
Content per day:			
Volume (ml)	2000	2000	3000
Glucose (g)	400	400	600
Protein (g)	80	80	120
Na (mmol)	80	120	255
K (mmol)	80	120	150
Ca (mmol)	4	4	12
Mg (mmol)	5	7.5	11.25
PO_4 (mmol)	30	40	67.5
Cl (mmol)	92	142.4	229.5
Acetate (mmol)	130	142.4	229.5
Gluconate (mmol)	8	8	24

+ Vitamins and trace elements: Vitamin B group with C 2 ml & Zn 2 mg/litre

to 1 litre a day, and the glucose concentration had been reduced to 10% in preparation for cessation, when a new problem arose.

'Good morning, Nurse. I've come to stop Mr Jones' TPN'. 'Good morning, Doctor. I'm afraid there's been a setback. Mr Jones appears to have had a stroke during the night. He is conscious, but can't swallow. No doubt you will want to continue the TPN'. 'No, his bowel is functioning and he has been tolerating a light diet. The best method of nutrition now is nasogastric feeding via a fine bore tube. I'll put one down while I'm here, and you can commence one of the isotonic, predigested diets. It may be best to start with intermittent bolus feeding, and then change to a continuous infusion later once we are sure there is no risk of vomiting or regurgitation'. 'You mean an elemental diet, Doctor?' 'No, Nurse. They are not indicated in Mr Jones because he has normal digestive and absorptive capacity. Also, they provide a higher osmotic load than the predigested diets and are more likely to cause diarrhoea'. 'What about the TPN?' 'Stop that, remove the catheter and send the tip for culture'. 'What about monitoring?' '2 litres of tube feed will provide a balanced diet. Clinical assessment and weekly laboratory tests should be quite adequate. I will ask the dietitian to come up and discuss dietary management with you from now on'. 'Thank you, Doctor'.

This case report was very straightforward, but some are extremely complex — for example, a patient with pancreatic sepsis, cardiac, respiratory, renal and hepatic failure, with multiple electrolyte abnormalities, and difficult venous access can be extremely difficult to feed parenterally or enterally.

Index